# Medical Terminology and Clinical Procedures
## 3rd Edition (Revised)

**Mary Bird** SRN RN FAMS

Chief Examiner Medical Terminology for AMSPAR
(The Association of Medical Secretaries, Practice
Managers, Administrators and Receptionists)

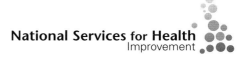

National Services for Health
Improvement

**Medical Terminology and Clinical Procedures. 3rd Edition (Revised)**
**Copyright © Mary Bird 2010**

The rights of Mary Bird to be identified as the author of this work
has been asserted by her in accordance with the Copyright , Designs
and Patent Act 1988.

**ISBN 978-0-9554803-6-2**

Published in the UK by:
National Services for Health Improvement
Nucleus@The Bridge, London Science and Business Park
Brunel Way, Darford, Kent DA1 5GA

www.nshi.co.uk

Printed in the UK by Nuffield Press Ltd, Abingdon.

# Medical Terminology
# Clinical Procedures
## 3rd Edition (Revised)

# Contents

# Contents

# Contents

# Contents

As President of The Association of Medical Secretaries, Practice Managers, Administrators and Receptionists (AMSPAR) I am delighted to have this opportunity to write the foreword to this essential publication.

In the ever changing health environment it is all too easy to underestimate the huge contribution made by non-clinical staff to the smooth running of both Primary and Secondary Care for the benefit and general well-being of patients.

Primary Care has seen the arrival of Practice Based Commissioning and the Quality and Outcomes Framework. This has placed greater demands on managers and all staff, and as a consequence there has been an influx of staff from outside the health sector whose knowledge of the terminology and 'jargon' is often limited. New members of staff have to learn about their new field and gain a basic grasp of the terminology used in their new environment quickly. This book will enable them to do just that.

Secondary Care has seen a move to outsourcing some clerical work and the re-emergence of 'typing pools' with a reliance on computer software. This often proves to be false economy – there can be no substitute for genuine knowledge.

AMSPAR continues to promote training and continuing professional development to its members and others. Our Medical Terminology qualifications, now run in conjunction with City and Guilds, continue to prove increasingly popular. This new edition of Mary Bird's book is an invaluable tool for those embarking on the courses, for reference purposes, or for having immediately to hand at your work station for use on a day-to-day basis.

*Elaine Guy*
President, AMSPAR

Mary Bird was born in Dorset, attended the local grammar school in the immediate post war period and began registered nursing training locally, upon leaving school. She gained wide experience in all branches of nursing, (including medical, surgical, orthopaedic, paediatrics, ophthalmology, neurology, ENT and theatre) during this period and had the benefit of the influence of a charismatic matron, with extremely high standards. Awarded numerous prizes for differing specialities, she gained the equivalent hospital 'Gold Medal' award, (the Sanderson Wells Award), as the best student nurse of her year.

Qualifying as an SRN in 1957 and marrying in the same year, she moved to Devon. Mary gained further experience in the casualty department and medical wards prior to the birth of her first child in 1960. Her second child was born in 1962. A period of time out from nursing between 1960 and 1964, enabled Mary to spend important time with her family prior to returning in a part time capacity as a District Nursing Sister and later in Intensive Care.

In 1971, Mary together with her family, moved to Essex where she continued nursing, including a period as an Industrial Nursing Sister and also as a School Nurse at a busy comprehensive school. She also gained invaluable experience as a Practice Nurse for a busy general practice.

In 1976, Mary commenced lecturing in medical terminology, anatomy and physiology at a College of Further Education. Among her students were pre-nursing cadets, community care students and AMSPAR medical secretaries and receptionists.

Eventually she became the Course Director for AMSPAR students, including those students who were studying for the Diploma for Practice Managers. Mary was appointed by AMSPAR, first as an Examiner and then, in 1989, as Chief Examiner for the Medical Aspects section. Involvement in NVQ training and assessing led to her appointment as an OCR/AMSPAR External Verifier. Retiring from college teaching in 1994, Mary continued with providing independent training for various Health Authorities and hospitals, under the name of Medicus Enterprises. She continues this at the present time as well as her role of Chief Examiner for the AMSPAR Medical Terminology Certificate, of which she is author. She was awarded an AMSPAR Fellowship in 1997, in recognition of her contribution to AMSPAR.

Involvement in teaching and examining for the Voluntary Aid Societies, St John Ambulance and the British Red Cross, are also important aspects of her life and in 1965 she was presented with the Royal Humane Society Award for the resuscitation of a youth from drowning.

Both of her children have chosen medical subjects for their careers; her daughter is a well-known psychologist and her son is a Professor of Molecular Endocrinology, in the USA. She and her husband, a retired solicitor, enjoy their grandchildren and hobbies of gardening, swimming and reading – now that there is time to do so!

This book is intended to provide an insight into medical terminology and the common clinical procedures met in the everyday work of health workers, including secretaries, receptionists, administrators and managers, as well as students in many other disciplines.

The breakdown of medical words into the basic prefixes, roots and suffixes, aims to help unravel the mystery of medical language and enable the reader to build a vast vocabulary in a surprisingly short time. Basic anatomy and physiology of the body have been included in order to provide further explanation and interest for the reader. Medical terms and abbreviations are grouped together with the appropriate body system, wherever possible, eg: 'Angina pectoris' and 'Blood pressure' are explained in Chapter 5: The Cardiovascular System.

At the end of each chapter you will find lists of abbreviations, terminology, diseases and disorders, as well as procedures and equipment related to that body system. The index at the end of the book contains all the full terms mentioned in the text. The appendices provide further lists of prefixes roots suffixes, abbreviations and eponyms.

Chapters on drugs and preventive medicine, including immunisation schedules and notifiable diseases are included. Areas concerning the work of the pathology and imaging/X-ray departments are intended to provide more knowledge of the principles of common tests performed on patients.

In this new edition, numerous procedures have been added to the text in an attempt to keep up with the ever growing changes in medical procedures and investigations.

At the outset of my career, I was encouraged always to remember that the welfare of the patient was the priority. I express the hope that this book, by giving a better understanding, will enable all those involved in patient care to deal more effectively with that most important person – the patient!

*Mary Bird*
July 2010

# Acknowledgements

This book is dedicated with grateful thanks to:

*All my AMSPAR students*, *past and present,*
*from whom I have learnt so much.*

*Olga de Souza*, *my predecessor as*
*AMSPAR Chief Examiner, for her very high standards,*
*which I have tried my best to maintain.*

*Michael*, *Susan*, *Ian*, *Beth* and *Iain*,
*for all their support and encouragement,*
*without which this book would never have been written!*

*And with love to my grandchildren*
*James*, *Sarah*, *Jennifer* and *Christopher*.

*Mary Bird*

# Chapter 1

# Understanding terminology

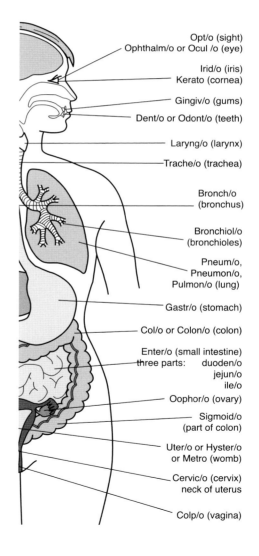

Opt/o (sight)
Ophthalm/o or Ocul /o (eye)

Irid/o (iris)
Kerato (cornea)

Gingiv/o (gums)

Dent/o or Odont/o (teeth)

Laryng/o (larynx)

Trache/o (trachea)

Bronch/o
(bronchus)

Bronchiol/o
(bronchioles)

Pneum/o,
Pneumon/o,
Pulmon/o (lung)

Gastr/o (stomach)

Col/o or Colon/o (colon)

Enter/o (small intestine)
three parts:     duoden/o
jejun/o
ile/o

Oophor/o (ovary)

Sigmoid/o
(part of colon)

Uter/o or Hyster/o
or Metro (womb)

Cervic/o (cervix)
neck of uterus

Colp/o (vagina)

# The origin and construction of medical terms

To the uninitiated, medical terms can seem frightening and unintelligible. As with any specialty, a language has developed which separates those 'within' from outsiders, conveying a mystique which appears hard to penetrate. However, it is necessary to have a precise language to describe a medical condition or procedure, in order that other members of the medical profession may accurately interpret diagnoses etc. Most medical words are derived from Greek and Latin sources – international languages until the eighteenth century. Some Arabic, Anglo-Saxon and German origins are also involved. Understanding and following some basic rules can reveal the mystery of medical terminology.

## Basic construction of medical terms

Medical terms consist of the following parts:

- a **prefix**
- a **root** or **stem**
- a **suffix**
- a **combining vowel**.

## Prefix

This part of the word is found before the stem and qualifies, (i.e. tells us more about), the stem.

e.g. **poly** – meaning 'many'.

Not all words have a prefix.

## Root or stem

This is the main part of the word, which gives the information about that which is being described.

e.g. **neur** – meaning 'nerve'.

## Suffix

This part of the word is found following the stem and gives further information about the stem.

e.g. **-itis** – meaning 'inflammation of'.

All medical terms have a suffix.

e.g. **polyneuritis**

| Prefix | | Root/stem | | Suffix |
|--------|---|-----------|---|--------|
| **poly** | / | **neur** | / | **itis** |

## Combining vowel

This is a vowel which is added to the stem, when necessary, to allow easy pronunciation; it is usually an **o**.

If the suffix begins with a vowel then it is not required.

e.g. **poly/neur/itis** meaning 'inflammation of many nerves' where the suffix **-itis** begins with a vowel and so does not require a 'combining vowel'

### Some further examples

**En/cephal/o/gram**

means 'a recording of brain waves'.

As there is no vowel in the suffix, **o** is inserted between the stem and suffix.

- **en-** is a prefix meaning 'within'.
- **-cephal-** is a stem meaning 'head', i.e. the brain.
- **-gram** is a suffix meaning 'a tracing or writing'.

**Peri/card/itis**

meaning 'inflammation of the pericardium' (the layer of tissue around the heart).

- **peri-** is a prefix meaning 'around'.
- **-cardi-** is a stem meaning 'heart'.
- **-itis** is a suffix meaning 'inflammation'.

However, there is a vowel at the end of the stem **cardi** as well as a vowel **i** at the beginning of **itis**. One of the **i**s is dropped to form the word 'pericarditis'. No added **o** is necessary.

The letter **h** is also treated as a vowel sound and is dropped when combining with another vowel, or where the pronunciation would be clumsy:

**An/aem/ia**

literally means 'lack of blood', but in medical terms it is the reduction of red cells or haemoglobin content in the blood.

- **an-** is a prefix meaning 'absence of'.
- **-haem-** is a stem meaning 'blood'.
- **-ia** is a suffix meaning 'condition of'.

The **h** of the stem is dropped as 'anhaemia' is difficult to pronounce.

**Leuc/o/rrhoea**

meaning 'white discharge'.

**leuc-** is a stem meaning 'white'.

**-o-** is a combining vowel added to the stem.

**-rrhoea** is a suffix meaning 'running or discharge'.

By following the rules illustrated above, many terms can be understood or constructed. Some examples are given below:

## Examples of common prefixes

| | |
|---|---|
| **a- or an-** | meaning absence of |
| **anti-** | meaning against |
| **ante-** | meaning before |
| **dys-** | meaning difficult/ abnormal/painful |
| **endo-** | meaning inside |
| **haemo-** | meaning blood |
| **hypo-** | meaning under/low |
| **hyper-** | meaning above/high |

## Examples of common suffixes

*Surgical procedures*

| | |
|---|---|
| **-otomy** | meaning cutting into or dividing, e.g. **osteotomy** meaning cutting into bone |
| **-ostomy** | meaning making an artificial opening, e.g. **tracheostomy** meaning making an artificial opening into the trachea |

N.B. Note the difference between tracheotomy and tracheostomy. In a tracheostomy the hole is left open, whereas a tracheotomy is a simple cutting into and then closing.

| | |
|---|---|
| **-orrhaphy** | means a sewing or repair, e.g. **herniorrhaphy** meaning repair of a hernia |
| **-ectomy** | means surgical removal, e.g. **appendicectomy** meaning surgical removal of the appendix |
| **-pexy** | meaning fixation, e.g. **orchiopexy** meaning fixation of an undescended testicle |

*Other surgical and procedure suffixes*

| | |
|---|---|
| **-oscopy** | meaning examination with a lighted instrument |
| **-plasty** | meaning reshape or form |
| **-tripsy** | meaning crushing |
| **-centesis** | meaning puncturing and drawing off (tapping) |
| **-gram** | meaning record/picture |
| **-graph** | meaning instrument that records |
| **-graphy** | meaning procedure of recording |
| **-opsy** | meaning looking at |
| **-stasis** | meaning stopping |
| **-clasis** | meaning breaking |

*Examples of other important suffixes*

| | |
|---|---|
| **-ia, -iasis** | |
| **-osis, -ism** | all meaning condition of |
| **-itis** | meaning inflammation of |
| **-pathy** | meaning disease of |
| **-genic** | meaning produced from or originating from |
| **-al, -ic, -iac** | meaning pertaining to |
| **-oid** | meaning shape or form |
| **-ology** | meaning scientific study of |
| **-cyte** | meaning cell |

## Common roots or stems

The following is a list of common roots or stems together with combining vowel. Some have two different stems, one from the Greek and one from the Latin, e.g. **phleb/o** (Greek) and **ven/o** (Latin) both meaning 'vein'.

| Stem | Meaning |
|---|---|
| **abdomin/o, lapar/o** | abdomen/abdominal wall |
| **aden/o** | gland |
| **adipo** | fat |
| **amyl** | starch |
| **an/o** | anus |
| **andr/o** | man |

3

# Roots for body parts and organs

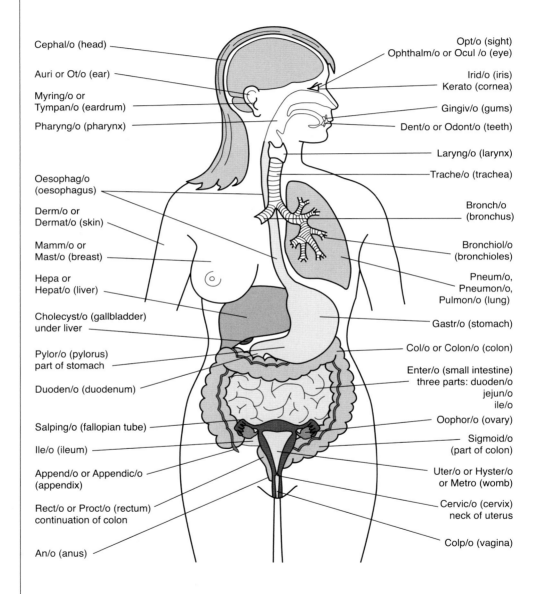

Cephal/o (head)

Auri or Ot/o (ear)

Myring/o or
Tympan/o (eardrum)

Pharyng/o (pharynx)

Oesophag/o
(oesophagus)

Derm/o or
Dermat/o (skin)

Mamm/o or
Mast/o (breast)

Hepa or
Hepat/o (liver)

Cholecyst/o (gallbladder)
under liver

Pylor/o (pylorus)
part of stomach

Duoden/o (duodenum)

Salping/o (fallopian tube)

Ile/o (ileum)

Append/o or Appendic/o
(appendix)

Rect/o or Proct/o (rectum)
continuation of colon

An/o (anus)

Opt/o (sight)
Ophthalm/o or Ocul /o (eye)

Irid/o (iris)
Kerato (cornea)

Gingiv/o (gums)

Dent/o or Odont/o (teeth)

Laryng/o (larynx)

Trache/o (trachea)

Bronch/o
(bronchus)

Bronchiol/o
(bronchioles)

Pneum/o,
Pneumon/o,
Pulmon/o (lung)

Gastr/o (stomach)

Col/o or Colon/o (colon)

Enter/o (small intestine)
three parts: duoden/o
jejun/o
ile/o

Oophor/o (ovary)

Sigmoid/o
(part of colon)

Uter/o or Hyster/o
or Metro (womb)

Cervic/o (cervix)
neck of uterus

Colp/o (vagina)

**Figure 1:** Gyne (woman). Anterior view showing intestinal tract, female reproductive organs,
lung and airway *Redrawn after Prendergast A: Medical Terminology, 2nd edition, Addison-Wesley, 1983.*

| Stem | Meaning |
|---|---|
| angi/o, vas/o | vessel |
| appendic/o | appendix |
| arteri/o | artery |
| arthr/o | joint |
| aur/i, ot/o | ear |
| bili | bile |
| bronch/o | bronchus |
| bronchiol/o | bronchiole (small termination of bronchial tubes) |
| cardi/o | heart |
| carpo | wrist |
| cephal/o | head |
| cerebr/o | cerebrum (part of brain) |
| cheil/o | lip |
| cheir/o | hand/surgery |
| chole | bile |
| cholecyst/o | gallbladder |
| choledoch/o | common bile duct |
| chondr/o | cartilage |
| col/o | colon (large intestine) |
| cost/o | rib |
| crani/o | cranium (skull containing brain) |
| cyst/o | bladder |
| cyto | cell |
| dacryo | tear |
| dactyl | finger |
| dent/o, odont/o | tooth |
| derm/o, dermat/o | skin |
| duoden/o | duodenum (part of small intestine) |
| encephal/o | brain |
| gastr/o | stomach |
| gingiv/o | gums |
| gloss/o, lingu/o | tongue |
| glyco | sugar |
| gynaec/o | woman |

| Stem | Meaning |
|---|---|
| hep/o, hepat/o | liver |
| histo | tissue |
| hydro | water, fluid |
| hyster/o, metr/o, uter/o | womb/uterus |
| iatro | physician |
| ile/o | ileum (part of small intestine) |
| ili/o | ilium (bone of pelvis) |
| irid/o | iris (of eye) |
| karyo | nucleus |
| kerat/o | cornea of eye |
| lacrim/o | tear |
| lacto | milk |
| lamina | part of vertebra |
| lip/o | fat |
| lob/o | lobe (e.g. of lung) |
| lympho | lymphatic |
| mast/o, mamm/o | breast |
| metro | measure, uterus |
| my/o, myos | muscle |
| myco, myceto | fungus |
| myel/o | bone marrow/spinal cord |
| myring/o, tympan/o | eardrum |
| nas/o, rhin/o | nose |
| nephr/o, ren/o | kidney |
| neur/o | nerve |
| oesophag/o | oesophagus |
| onycho | nail |
| oo | egg/ovum |
| oophor/o | ovary |
| ophthalm/o | eye |
| orchi/o, orchid/o | testicle/testis |
| oro | mouth |
| oste/o | bone |
| paedo | child |
| pancreat/o | pancreas |
| patho | disease |
| pharmaco | drugs/chemist |

## Roots for body parts and organs

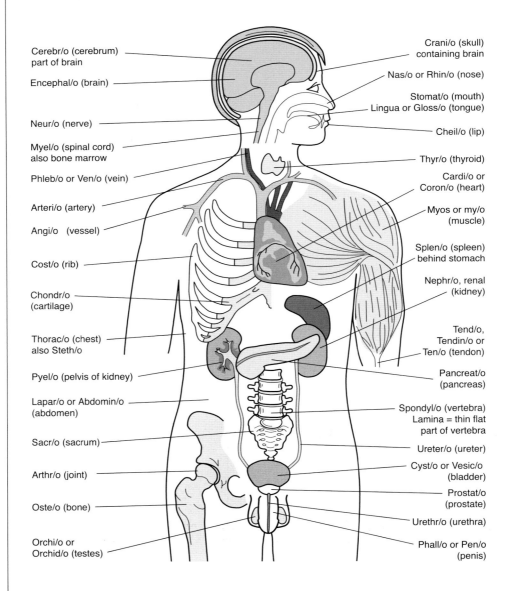

Cerebr/o (cerebrum) part of brain

Encephal/o (brain)

Neur/o (nerve)

Myel/o (spinal cord) also bone marrow

Phleb/o or Ven/o (vein)

Arteri/o (artery)

Angi/o (vessel)

Cost/o (rib)

Chondr/o (cartilage)

Thorac/o (chest) also Steth/o

Pyel/o (pelvis of kidney)

Lapar/o or Abdomin/o (abdomen)

Sacr/o (sacrum)

Arthr/o (joint)

Oste/o (bone)

Orchi/o or Orchid/o (testes)

Crani/o (skull) containing brain

Nas/o or Rhin/o (nose)

Stomat/o (mouth)
Lingua or Gloss/o (tongue)

Cheil/o (lip)

Thyr/o (thyroid)

Cardi/o or Coron/o (heart)

Myos or my/o (muscle)

Splen/o (spleen) behind stomach

Nephr/o, renal (kidney)

Tend/o, Tendin/o or Ten/o (tendon)

Pancreat/o (pancreas)

Spondyl/o (vertebra)
Lamina = thin flat part of vertebra

Ureter/o (ureter)

Cyst/o or Vesic/o (bladder)

Prostat/o (prostate)

Urethr/o (urethra)

Phall/o or Pen/o (penis)

**Figure 2:** Andro (man). Anterior view showing male reproductive organs, urinary tract, heart, spleen, pancreas, hip joint and some shoulder muscles
*Redrawn after Prendergast A: Medical Terminology, 2nd edition, Addison-Wesley, 1983.*

| Stem | Meaning |
|------|---------|
| **pharyng/o** | pharynx |
| **phleb/o, ven/o** | vein |
| **phren/o** | diaphragm |
| **pleuro** | pleura/rib/side |
| **pneumo** | air |
| **pneumon/o,** | |
| **pneum/o** | lungs |
| **podo** | foot |
| **proct/o** | rectum/anus |
| **prostat/o** | prostate gland |
| **psycho** | mind |
| **pyel/o** | pelvis of kidney |
| **pylor/o** | part of stomach |
| **pyo** | pus |
| **pyro** | fire, heat |
| **radio** | radiation |
| **rect/o** | rectum |
| **sacr/o** | sacrum (part of vertebrae) |
| **salping/o** | fallopian tube |
| **sial/o** | salivary gland |
| **splen/o** | spleen |
| **spondyl/o,** | |
| **vertebr/o** | vertebra |
| **steato** | fat |
| **stomat/o** | mouth |
| **tarso** | foot, eyelid |
| **ten/o, tendin/o** | tendon |
| **thermo** | heat |
| **thorac/o,** | |
| **steth/o** | thorax (chest) |
| **thrombo** | blood clot |
| **thyr/o** | thyroid gland |
| **tox, toxico** | poison |
| **trache/o** | trachea (windpipe) |
| **trich/o** | hair |
| **ureter/o** | ureter (urinary system) |
| **urethr/o** | urethra |
| **uro** | urine |
| **vaso** | vessel |

## Common prefixes

The following is a list of common prefixes for combining with stems and suffixes.

| Prefix | Meaning |
|--------|---------|
| **a-** or **an-** | absence of, without |
| **ab-** | away from |
| **acro-** | extremity |
| **ad-** | towards |
| **ambi-** | both |
| **ana-** | up, excessive |
| **aniso-** | unequal |
| **ante-** | before |
| **anti-** | against |
| **auto-** | self |
| **bi-** | two |
| **bio-** | life |
| **brady-** | slow |
| **centi-** | hundred |
| **chrom-** | colour |
| **circum-** | around |
| **co-/con-** | together with |
| **contra-** | against |
| **cryo-** | cold |
| **crypto-** | hidden |
| **cyano-** | blue |
| **de-** | away from/reversing |
| **demi-** | half |
| **dextro-** | to the right |
| **di-** | two |
| **dia-** | through |
| **dys-** | difficult, painful |
| **ecto-** | without, outside |
| **endo-** | within, inside |
| **epi-** | upon |
| **ery-/erythro-** | red |
| **eu-** | good, normal |
| **ex-** | out |
| **extra-** | outside |
| **flavo-** | yellow |

| Prefix | Meaning |
|---|---|
| gen- | referring to birth or producing |
| haemo- | blood |
| hemi- | half |
| hetero- | different, other |
| homeo- | like |
| homo- | same |
| hyper- | above, in excess of normal |
| hypo- | below, under, less than normal |
| idio- | peculiar to the individual |
| in- | in |
| infra- | below |
| inter- | between |
| intra- | within |
| iso- | equal, same |
| kypho- | humped, rounded |
| leuco- | white |
| macro- | large |
| mal- | bad, abnormal |
| mega- | big, enlarged |
| melano- | black, dark, pigment |
| meta- | beyond |
| micro- | small |
| multi- | many |
| narco- | stupor |
| neo- | new |
| nocto-/nycto- | night |
| oligo- | scanty |
| ortho- | straight |
| os- | opening, bone |
| pachy- | thick |
| pan- | all |
| para- | alongside, close to |
| ped- | foot, child |
| penta- | five |
| per- | through |
| peri- | around |
| polio- | grey |
| poly- | many |
| post- | after |

| Prefix | Meaning |
|---|---|
| pre-/pro- | before |
| proto- | first |
| pseudo- | false |
| quadri- | four |
| retro- | behind |
| sub- | below |
| supra- | above |
| syn- | with, union |
| tachy- | fast, rapid |
| tetra- | four |
| tri- | three |
| ultra- | beyond |
| uni- | one |
| xantho- | yellow |
| xer/o- | dry |

## Roots used as prefixes and suffixes

Some root word parts may also be used as prefixes if they are used at the beginning of a word to qualify or describe a following root word part.

e.g. **haem/o/thor/ax**
blood in the thoracic (chest) cavity

**haem** meaning blood, used here as a prefix referring to **thor**, the root for chest cavity

**o** combining vowel

**thor** root for chest cavity

**ax** suffix for the singular ending of the noun.

e.g. **hist/o/path/ology**
study of the disease of tissues

**hist** meaning tissue, used here as a prefix, referring to **path** the root for disease

**o** combining vowel

**path** root for disease

**ology** suffix for the 'study of'

## Common suffixes

| Suffix | Meaning |
|---|---|
| -aemia | blood |
| -aesthesia | sensibility |
| -al | pertaining to |
| -algia | pain |
| -an | pertaining to |
| -blast | immature cell |
| -cele | swelling/protrusion/herniation |
| -centesis | puncture, drawing off |
| -cide | killing, destroying |
| -cision | cutting |
| -clasis | breaking |
| -coccus | round cell, type of bacteria |
| -cyte | cell |
| -derm | skin |
| -desis | binding together |
| -dynia | pain |
| -ectasis | dilatation |
| -ectomy | removal of |
| -form | having the formation or shape of |
| -genesis | forming or origin |
| -genic | producing or forming |
| -gram | a picture |
| -graph | a machine which records |
| -graphy | the procedure of recording |
| -iasis | condition of/state of |
| -iatric | pertaining to medicine/physician |
| -ism | condition of |
| -itis | inflammation of |
| -kinesis | movement, activity |
| -lith | stone |
| -lithiasis | condition of stones |
| -lysis | breaking down (keep splitting) |
| -malacia | softening |
| -megaly | enlargement |

| Suffix | Meaning |
|---|---|
| -meter | measure |
| -oid | likeness, resemblance |
| -ology | scientific study of |
| -oma | tumour |
| -opia | condition of the eye |
| -ose | sugar |
| -osis | condition of |
| -ostomy | making an opening (to remain) |
| -otomy | to cut into, divide |
| -ous | like, similar to |
| -paresis | weakness |
| -pathy | disease |
| -penia | lack of, decreased |
| -pexy | fixation of |
| -phage | eating, ingesting |
| -phagia | swallowing |
| -phasia | speech |
| -philia | loving, affinity for |
| -phobia | irrational fear of |
| -phylaxis | protection, prevention |
| -plasia | formation |
| -plasty | form, mould, reconstruct |
| -plegia | paralysis |
| -pnoea | breathing |
| -poiesis | making |
| -rhythmia | rhythm |
| -rrhage | to burst forth (heavy bleeding) |
| -rrhaphy | sewing, repair |
| -rrhexis | rupture of |
| -rrhoea | flowing, discharge |
| -sclerosis | hardening |
| -scope | lighted instrument used for examination |
| -scopy | examination with lighted instrument |
| -somatic | pertaining to the body |
| -stasis | cessation of movement/flow |

| Suffix | Meaning |
|---|---|
| **-staxis** | dripping (blood) |
| **-stenosis** | narrowing |
| **-sthenia** | strength |
| **-taxia** | co-ordination, order |
| **-tome** | cutting instrument |
| **-tripsy** | crushing of stones |
| **-trophy** | nourishment |
| **-uria** | condition of urine |

## Common plural forms

The following rules apply when forming plural words:

| Singular | Plural |
|---|---|
| **-us** | **-i** |

e.g. staphylococcus / staphylococci

| | |
|---|---|
| **-a** | **-ae** |

e.g. vertebra / vertebrae

| | |
|---|---|
| **-um** | **-a** |

e.g. atrium / atria

| | |
|---|---|
| **-is** | **-es** |

e.g. diagnosis / diagnoses

| | |
|---|---|
| **-oma** | **-omata** |

e.g. stoma / stomata

| | |
|---|---|
| **-ix** | **-ices** |

e.g. cervix / cervices

| | |
|---|---|
| **-ax** | **-aces** |

e.g. thorax / thoraces

| | |
|---|---|
| **-on** | **-a** |

e.g. ganglion / ganglia

## Americanisms

In American versions of medical terms, spellings are altered in the following ways. It is common to drop the silent double vowels (diphthong) as used in English spellings, e.g. **ae** becomes **e.**

The English stem **haem**, in American spelling is **hem** (meaning blood).

Other examples include:

| English | American |
|---|---|
| **anaemia** | **anemia** |
| **anaesthesia** | **anesthesia** |
| **oedema** | **edema** |
| **dyspnoea** | **dyspnea** |
| **leucocyte** | **leukocyte** |
| **paediatric** | **pediatric** |

With the advent of word checks on computers, American style spellings of medical words is increasing in use. However, the English interpretation is used throughout this book.

# Chapter 2

# The structure and function of the human body

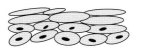

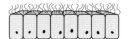

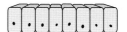

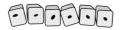

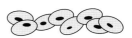

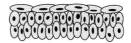

## Anatomy and physiology

**Anatomy**      is the study of
                 the structure of the body.

**Physiology**   is the study of
                 the function of the body.

## The basic elements

The human body is an incredibly complex creation, much of which is still not fully understood. In order to appreciate its complexity, the basic elements must be examined. The following are the main structures of which it is composed:

**cells, tissues, organs** and **systems**

### Cells

The human body is composed of billions of tiny living materials known as cells. Cells vary in form and size, each type being adapted in structure to the function it performs.

The cell is composed of **protoplasm** containing numerous inclusions. It is surrounded by a selective semi-permeable membrane; i.e. it will allow some substances in and out through the membrane, but not others.

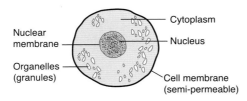

Nuclear membrane — Cytoplasm — Nucleus — Organelles (granules) — Cell membrane (semi-permeable)

**Figure 3:** The human cell

At some stage in every cell's life, there is a **nucleus** surrounded by a similar membrane known as the nuclear membrane *(see Figure 3)*. It is here within the nucleus that the chromosomes are found, consisting of **DNA** (deoxyribonucleic acid). Each human cell normally contains 23 pairs of **chromosomes**, and it is upon these structures that the genetic blueprint is found, known as **genes**. These determine the individual characteristics of each cell.

The sex cells (**gametes**) of the ovum from the female and the spermatazoon from the male contain only 23 single chromosomes, which upon fusion at fertilisation enables the mixing of the genetic materials to form a new unique human being.

### Tissues

Similar types of cells are grouped together to form tissues *(see Figure 4)*. Each type of tissue has a particular function.

*Abbreviations*

**Ca**     carcinoma

**SA**     sarcoma

**TNM**    tumour nodes metastases

**T**      tumour

*Types of tissues*

There are four main types of tissue in the human body:

**1. Epithelial**
covering and lining of organs and cavities, (known as endothelium when lining internal organs).

**2. Connective**
supporting tissue, includes fibrous and elastic fibres, ligaments, cartilage and bone-blood.

**3. Muscle**
voluntary muscle (skeletal) attached to the skeleton; involuntary muscle (smooth) forming many internal organs, e.g. the stomach; **cardiac muscle** is a specialised muscle found only in the heart.

**4. Nerve**
a highly specialised tissue containing neurones forming the central, autonomic and peripheral nervous systems as well as special sensory organs, e.g. retina of eye (see Chapter 13).

### Organs

Differing types of tissues are grouped together to form organs which perform special functions.

### Systems

Organs working together to perform particular functions are known as systems. In health, each system normally works in harmony with others to maintain the body in its correct state (homeostasis).

# Tissue cells

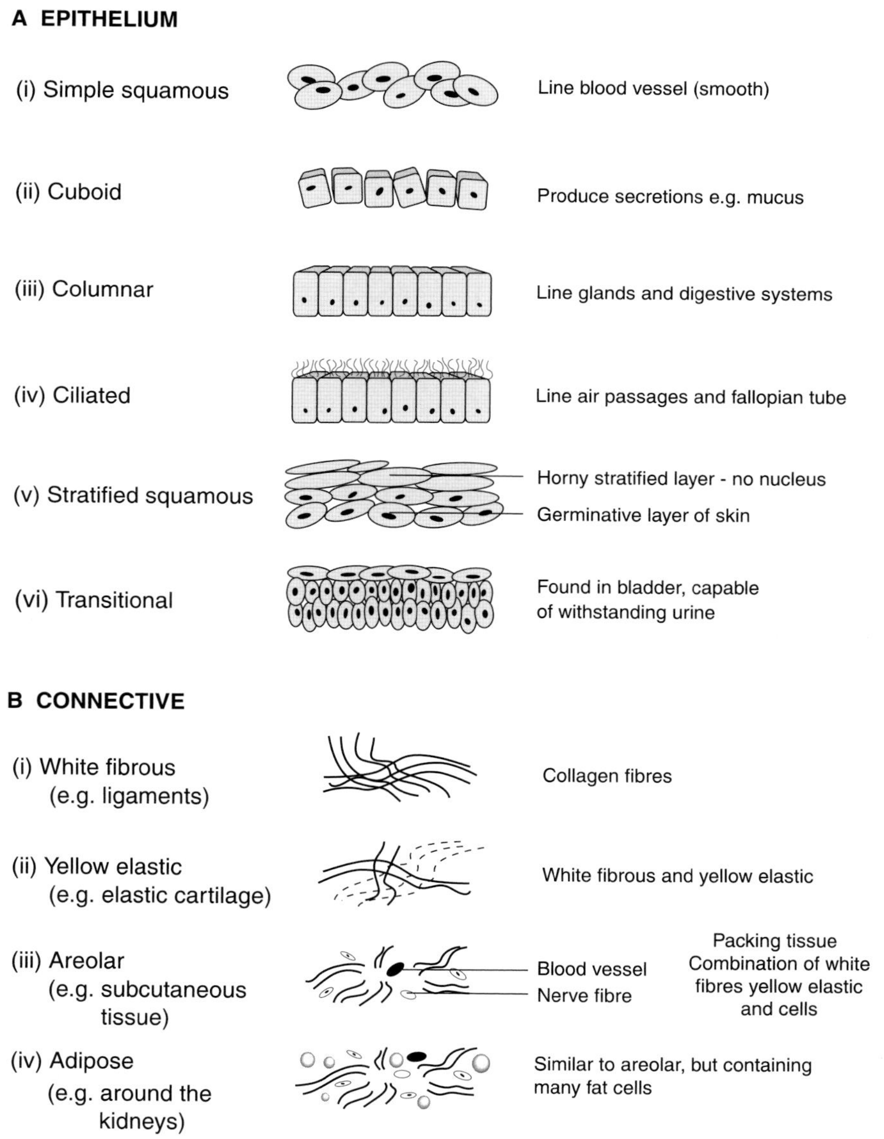

## A EPITHELIUM

(i) Simple squamous          Line blood vessel (smooth)

(ii) Cuboid          Produce secretions e.g. mucus

(iii) Columnar          Line glands and digestive systems

(iv) Ciliated          Line air passages and fallopian tube

(v) Stratified squamous          Horny stratified layer - no nucleus

Germinative layer of skin

(vi) Transitional          Found in bladder, capable of withstanding urine

## B CONNECTIVE

(i) White fibrous
    (e.g. ligaments)          Collagen fibres

(ii) Yellow elastic
    (e.g. elastic cartilage)          White fibrous and yellow elastic

(iii) Areolar
    (e.g. subcutaneous
        tissue)          Blood vessel          Packing tissue
                         Nerve fibre          Combination of white
                                              fibres yellow elastic
                                              and cells

(iv) Adipose
    (e.g. around the
        kidneys)          Similar to areolar, but containing many fat cells

**Figure 4:** Tissue Cells

## Properties of living organisms

All living organisms, as opposed to non-living matter, have the following qualities:

**Respiration**
the process of producing energy in order to carry out all the metabolic processes required. In humans, this involves the absorption of oxygen for use in the cells together with glucose, and the production of waste products for excretion of carbon dioxide and water.

**Nutrition**
the process by which food is obtained for use as energy for growth or repair of the body.

**Excretion**
the process by which the body eliminates the waste products of metabolism.

**Growth and repair**
the ability to increase in size and repair damage to cells as well as producing new, similar cells (by **mitosis** division).

**Reproduction**
the process by which new individuals are produced (by **meiosis** division).

**Sensitivity**
the ability to detect changes in the environment.

**Movement**
capability of some movement.

## Non-living materials

The following materials are also present in the body and are essential to life:

**Water**
- $H_2O$ forming the largest component of all.

**Mineral salts** including
- Sodium      Na
- Potassium      K
- Calcium      Ca
- Magnesium      Mg
- Iron      Fe
- Phosphates, carbonates, chlorides and other trace elements.

The balance of salts in the body is vital to life, and the electrolytes or electrolytic balance (balance of ions or mineral salts) are often measured in blood tests.

## Metabolism

Metabolism is the basic working of the body cells. It concerns the continuous chemical changes that occur to sustain life. Energy is produced as a by-product of the reactions.

## Osmosis

This is the passage of fluid across a semi-permeable membrane, which allows equalisation of the concentration of solutions either side of the membrane. Tissue fluid is drawn back into the venous capillaries of the body by the presence of large plasma proteins, after it has given up its nutrients etc. to the tissue cells.

## Glands

These are structures which produce and secrete their own substance. There are two types:

**1. Exocrine glands (with ducts)**
These pour their secretions through ducts to another organ, or directly upon the surface of a membrane, e.g. mucus secretions from epithelial tissue, or **bile** from the liver to the bile-duct.

**2. Endocrine glands (ductless)**
These produce secretions known as **hormones**, which are secreted directly into the blood supply for stimulation of another target organ (see Chapter 15, Endocrine system).

## Membranes

These are special tissues covering and lining areas of the body. There are three types:

**1. Mucous membranes**
tissue containing mucus-secreting cells which moisten and lubricate surfaces.

**2. Serous membranes**
a double-layered tissue composed of smooth, simple squamous epithelial cells which secrete

a thin fluid between the two layers known as serous fluid, e.g. **pleura** covering the lungs and **peritoneum** covering abdominal organs.

**3. Synovial membranes**
a single membrane which produces a thick glairy fluid known as synovial fluid, found at freely moveable joints preventing friction and wear.

## Anatomical position and planes

The body is described facing forwards, feet apart, arms at sides and palms facing forward, as illustrated in Figure 5.

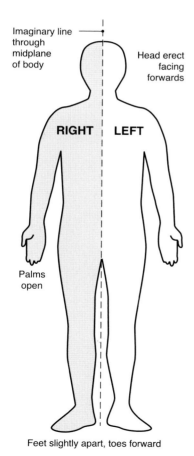

Imaginary line through midplane of body

Head erect facing forwards

RIGHT | LEFT

Palms open

Feet slightly apart, toes forward

**Figure 5:** Anatomical position

The following terms are used to describe anatomical positions:

| | |
|---|---|
| **Superior** | above |
| **Inferior** | below |
| **Anterior** | front or in front |
| **Posterior** | back or back of |
| **Medial** | midline towards centre |
| **Lateral** | side or away from midline |
| **Proximal** | nearest to a point of origin |
| **Distal** | furthest from a point of origin |
| **Superficial** | nearest body surface |
| **Deep** | away from surface |
| **Ventral** | front |
| **Dorsal** | back |
| **Cortex** | outer region, e.g. of kidney |
| **Medulla** | inner region, e.g. of kidney |
| **Peripheral** | relating to the outer surface or circumference |
| **Plantar** | referring to sole of foot |
| **Palmar** | referring to palm of hand |

The following terms are used to describe anatomical planes (*see Figure 6*):

| | |
|---|---|
| **Sagittal** | lengthwise (vertically) from front to back |
| **Frontal or coronal** | lengthwise (vertically) from side to side dividing body into ventral and dorsal sections |
| **Horizontal or transverse** | divides body across into upper and lower parts |
| **Cranial** | head or upper section |
| **Caudal** | tail or lower section |

## Cavities of the body

The main cavities of the body are the:

- **thoracic cavity**

- **abdominal cavity**

- **pelvic cavity**

## Regions of the abdomen

The abdominal and pelvic areas of the trunk are divided into **quadrants**, as shown in Figure 7.

The abdomen is also divided into the **regions** shown in Figure 8.

## Terminology

| | |
|---|---|
| **Anaplasia** | abnormal cells without a regular nucleus (malignant) |
| **Atrophy** | wastage of an organ |
| **Cortex** | outer portion of an organ |
| **Cytology** | study of cells |
| **Dysplasia** | formation of abnormal cells |
| **Fundus** | the area of a hollow organ, which is opposite the main opening, e.g. of the uterus |
| **Genome** | a map of the genetic material of the species |
| **Hilum** | a depression on the surface of an organ where blood and other vessels, and ducts enter and leave |
| **Histology** | study of tissues |
| **Hypertrophy** | enlargement of an organ with its own tissue |
| **Infarct** | a wedge-shaped area of tissue deprived of its blood supply |
| **Interstitial** | type of supporting tissue |
| **Ischaemia** | lack of blood to a part |
| **Medulla** | inner portion of an organ |
| **Metaplasia** | type of cell growing beyond where usually found |
| **Oncology** | study of tumours |
| **Viscus** | organ |

## Anatomical planes

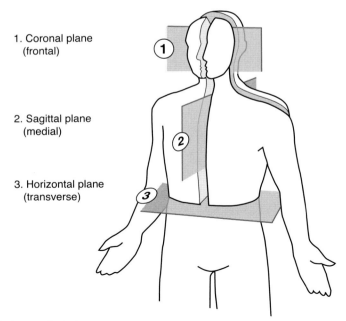

1. Coronal plane (frontal)

2. Sagittal plane (medial)

3. Horizontal plane (transverse)

**Figure 6:** Anatomical planes

## Diseases and disorders

**Adenoma**     tumour of a gland

**Benign**     favourable for recovery, opposite of malignant

**Carcinoma**     cancerous, abnormal malignant cells growing in the body

**Chondroma**     benign tumour of cartilage

**Chondrosarcoma**     malignant tumour of cartilage and bone

**Contusion**     bleeding beneath the skin (bruise)

**Embolism**     obstruction of a blood vessel by a detached, travelling particle of blood, fat or air

**Embolus**     blood clot, fat or air detached from another place and travelling in the blood stream

## Quadrants of the abdominopelvic regions and regions of the abdominal cavity

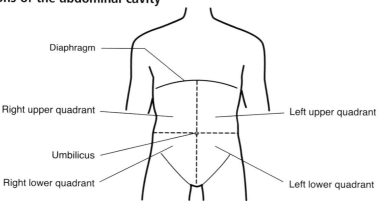

**Figure 7:** Quadrants of the abdominopelvic regions of the body

1. Right hypochondriac region
2. Epigastric region
3. Left hypochondriac region
4. Right lumbar region
5. Umbilical region
6. Left lumbar region
7. Right iliac fossa
8. Hypogastric region
9. Left iliac fossa

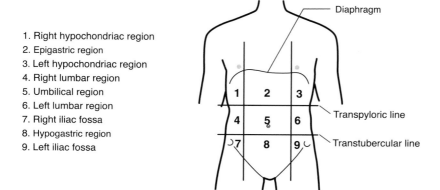

**Figure 8:** Regions of the abdominal cavity

| | |
|---|---|
| **Epithelioma** | tumour of epithelial tissue (lining and covering organs), e.g. of the epidermis |
| **Fibroma** | tumour of fibrous tissue |
| **Fibrosis** | formation of scar tissue |
| **Haematoma** | swelling containing blood |
| **Ischaemia** | deficiency of blood supply to a part |
| **Keloid scar** | abnormal overgrowth of fibrous tissue in the healing of a wound |
| **Lesion** | morbid (abnormal) change in tissue |
| **Lipoma** | tumour composed of fat |
| **Malignant** | virulent/dangerous, likely to have a fatal outcome (disease or tumour) |
| **Myalgia** | painful muscles |
| **Myasthenia gravis** | disease causing abnormal fatigue and weakness in voluntary muscles |
| **Myoma** | tumour composed of muscle |
| **NG** | new growth |
| **Necrosis** | death of tissue |
| **Necrotising fasciitis** | destruction of soft tissue by overwhelming infection, usually post-operatively, by haemolytic streptococcus bacteria (Group A) |
| **Neoplasm** | new growth or tumour |
| **Oedema** | free fluid in the tissues |
| **Papilloma** | wart-type benign tumour |
| **Peritonitis** | inflammation of the peritoneum (the lining of the abdomen and pelvic cavities) |
| **Pleurisy** | inflammation of the pleura (the covering of the lungs) |
| **Sarcoma** | cancer arising in the connective tissue, e.g. bone, blood |
| **Sebaceous cyst** | swelling caused by blockage of sebaceous gland duct in the skin |

## Procedures and equipment

| | |
|---|---|
| **Biopsy** | removal of a portion of living tissue for microscopic investigation |

## Classification of diseases

| | |
|---|---|
| **Acquired** | acquired after birth |
| **Acute** | rapid onset and progress |
| **Allergic** | hypersensitivity to foreign proteins |
| **Chronic** | slow onset and progress |
| **Congenital** | present at birth |
| **Cryptogenic** | of doubtful or hidden origin |
| **Endocrine** | associated with hormone dysfunction |
| **Familial** | occurs in families |
| **Functional** | no anatomical abnormality demonstrated but associated with dysfunction |
| **Iatrogenic** | a disease produced by the treatment given for a primary illness |
| **Idiopathic** | peculiar to the individual |
| **Infectious** | caused by micro-organisms readily passed on to other people |
| **Local** | involving an area or one part of the body only |
| **Metabolic** | disorder of basic working (physiology) of the body |
| **Neoplastic** | associated with development of new growths (e.g. malignant or benign tumours) |
| **Nosocomial** | infection acquired from hospital, e.g. MRSA |
| **Organic** | structural abnormality demonstrated |
| **Silent** | no symptoms apparent or obvious signs |
| **Systemic** | involving the entire body |
| **Traumatic** | involving injury |

# Chapter **3** | The locomotor system

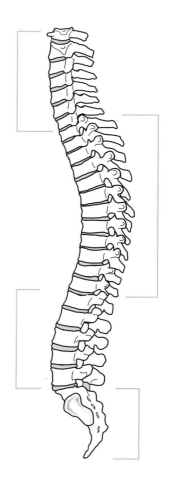

# The locomotor system

The locomotor system consists of the bones, muscles, ligaments, cartilage and tendons. It is mainly concerned with movement.

## Bone

There are two different types of bone structure known as:

- **Compact** (hard)
- **Cancellous** (spongy)

Cancellous bone tissue forms the red bone marrow. All bones are covered in a membrane known as the **periosteum**, which provides nourishment.

**Hyaline cartilage tissue** is found at the ends of long bones where joints are formed, preventing wear. In fetal life, bone is generally developed from cartilage tissue by the laying down of calcium salts by specialised bone cells. This continues after birth and is known as **ossification.**

**Vitamin D** and **calcium** are essential for healthy bone formation. There are 206 bones in the adult human body.

### Descriptive terms of bones

| | |
|---|---|
| **Articulation** | a joint between two bones |
| **Border** | edge separating two surfaces of bone |
| **Condyle** | rounded enlargement at the ends of bone |
| **Crest** | elevated ridge on a bone |
| **Facet** | a small articulating surface |
| **Foramen** (pl: -mina) | hole or opening in a bone |
| **Fossa** | depression or hollowed out area on the surface of a bone |
| **Lamina** | thin plate or layer (usually of bone) |
| **Process** | projection from a bone |
| **Trochanter** | large, rough eminence on a bone |
| **Tuberosity** | large protuberance on a bone |
| **Tubercle** | small rounded prominence |

# The skeleton

This is made up of five classifications of bones:

**1. long bones**
forming limbs and having a cavity

**2. short bones**
having no cavity, found in the hands and feet

**3. flat bones**
forming the cranium and scapula

**4. irregular bones**
face bones and vertebrae

**5. sesamoid bones**
formed in a tendon, e.g. patella and hyoid bones

The bony framework of the body (see Figure 9) has the following functions:

| | |
|---|---|
| **Support** | provides a framework for the body and gives shape |
| **Leverage** | provides levers for muscle attachment allowing movement and articulation |
| **Protection** | protects organs, e.g. brain within the cranium |
| **Storage** | stores calcium salts |
| **Production** | manufactures blood cells in the bone marrow |

There are two parts to the skeleton:

**1. The axial skeleton**
formed from the skull, vertebrae, rib cage and breast bone - made up of 80 bones

**2. The appendicular skeleton**
consisting of 126 bones forming the limb bones and their girdles.

### Some unusual adjectives of bones

| | |
|---|---|
| **Clavicular** | relating to the clavicles |
| **Coccygeal** | relating to the coccyx |
| **Femoral** | relating to the femur |
| **Fibular** | relating to the fibula |
| **Humeral** | relating to the humerus |
| **Phalangeal** | relating to the phalanges |
| **Scapular** | relating to the scapula |
| **Ulnar** | relating to the ulna |

# The skeleton

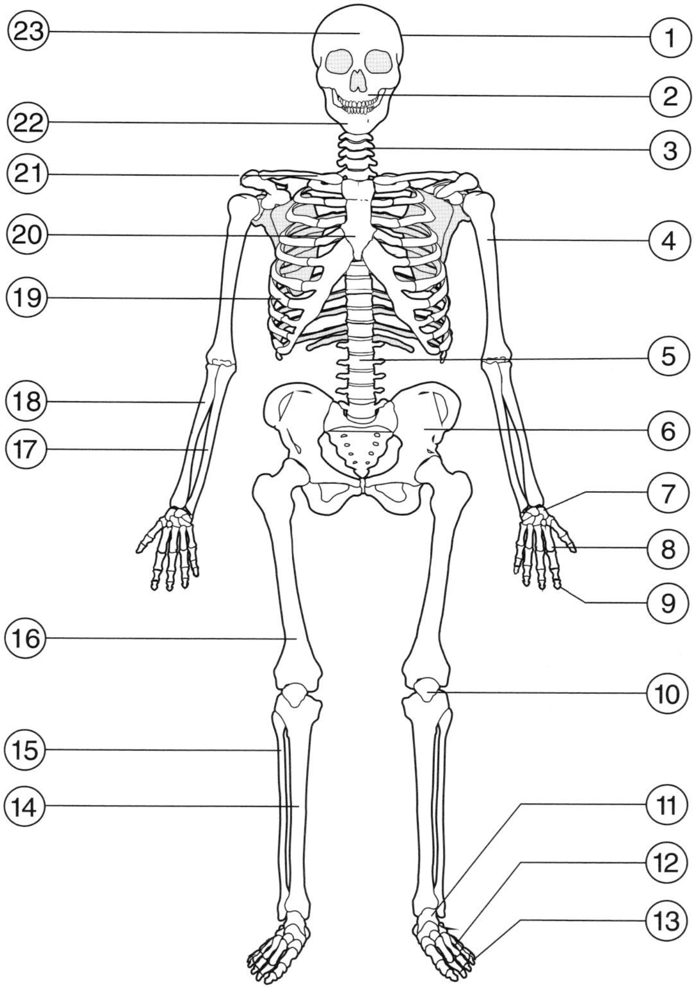

1. Skull
2. Maxilla
3. Cervical vertebrae
4. Humerus
5. Lumbar vertebrae
6. Pelvis
7. Carpals
8. Metacarpals

9. Phalanges
10. Patella
11. Tarsals
12. Metatarsals
13. Phalanges
14. Tibia
15. Fibula
16. Femur

17. Ulna
18. Radius
19. Ribs
20. Sternum
21. Clavicle
22. Mandible
23. Frontal bone

**Figure 9:** The skeleton

## The skull

This includes the bones of the face and the bones which form the **cranium** containing the brain and beginning of the spinal cord (*see Figure 10*). The lobes of the **cerebrum** (part of brain) are named by the bones under which they lie.

### Bones of the cranium

These consist of the following individual bones:

- One **occipital**
- Two **parietal**
- Two **temporal**
- One **frontal**
- One **sphenoid**
- One **ethmoid**

### Fontanelles

The uniting of the cranial bones by **sutures** (fibrous immovable joints) occurs after birth. Because the bones are not united in the fetus, moulding of the skull to aid delivery is able to occur during childbirth.

The anterior fontanelle is a 'soft spot' which can be felt until its closure at approximately 18 months. The 'soft spot' allows the skull bones to continue to grow to accommodate the increasing size of the brain.

The posterior fontanelle closes at approximately three months (*see Figure 11*).

### Bones of the face

These consist of the following individual bones:

- One **mandible**   lower jaw
- Two **maxilla**    upper jaw
- Two **malar** or **zygomatic**   cheek bones
- One **nasal**      part of nose
- One **vomer**      part of nasal septum
- Two **lacrimal (lacrymal)**   bony orbit
- Two **palatine**   hard palate in mouth
- Two **turbinate**  inside nose

## Bones of the skull

1. Parietal*
2. Sphenoid*
3. Temporal*
4. Occipital*
5. Mastoid portion of temporal lobe
6. Mandible
7. Malar or zygomatic
8. Maxilla
9. Ethmoid*
10. Nasal
11. Lacrimal
12. Frontal*

   * form the cranium

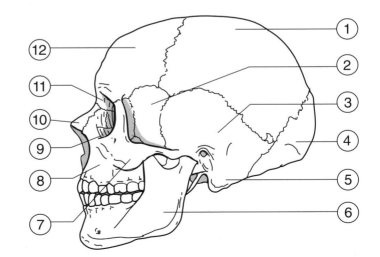

**Figure 10:** Bones of the skull

## Fontanelles of the skull

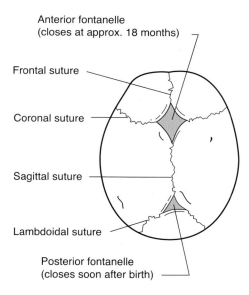

Anterior fontanelle
(closes at approx. 18 months)

Frontal suture

Coronal suture

Sagittal suture

Lambdoidal suture

Posterior fontanelle
(closes soon after birth)

**Figure 11:** Fontanelles of the skull

### Air sinuses of the skull

These are cavities containing air within the bone tissues which lighten the skull. They are lined with mucous membrane which may become infected. They are found in the following bones:

- **Frontal**

- **Maxillary**

- **Ethmoid**

- **Sphenoid**

### Hyoid bone

The **hyoid** bone is a small bone to which the tongue is attached. It is often found to be fractured in cases of strangulation.

## Vertebrae

There are 33 irregular bones in the vertebral column or **spine**, stacked one upon the other and bound together by strong ligaments. The spine combines great strength with mobility. Its function is to:

- Provide a framework for attachment of other structures

- Protect the spinal cord and nerves

- Provide locomotion

- Absorb shock

- Form strong joints

Vertebrae are in groups and are named after the region in which they are situated. They become larger and heavier in size as they descend, although the neural or vertebral **foramen** (hole through which the spinal cord travels) becomes smaller.

The vertebrae are described as **typical** (having similar features) or **atypical** (not having the typical features).

### Typical vertebrae

A typical vertebra *(see Figure 12)* contains the following features:

- A **body**

- Four **articulating processes** (surfaces) – forming joints with the vertebrae above and below

- Two **pedicles**

- Two **transverse processes**

- Two **lamina**

- A **spinous process** – formed from the uniting of the lamina

- Two **intervertebral notches** – through which spinal nerves travel from each side of the spinal cord

- A **vertebral (neural) foramen** – through which the spinal cord travels

## Vertebrae

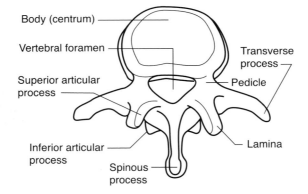

Body (centrum)

Vertebral foramen

Superior articular process

Transverse process

Pedicle

Inferior articular process

Lamina

Spinous process

**Figure 12:** A typical vertebra

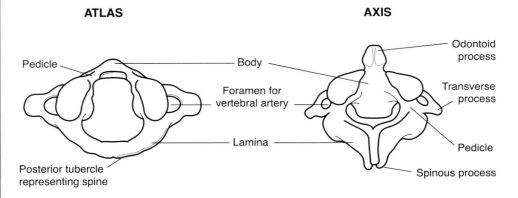

**ATLAS**

Pedicle

Body

Foramen for vertebral artery

Lamina

Posterior tubercle representing spine

**AXIS**

Odontoid process

Transverse process

Pedicle

Spinous process

**ATLAS AND AXIS IN POSITION**

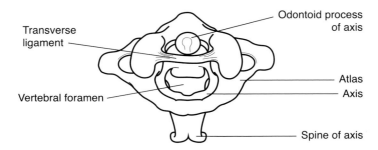

Transverse ligament

Odontoid process of axis

Atlas

Axis

Vertebral foramen

Spine of axis

**Figure 13:** The atlas and axis (anterior view)

## Atypical vertebrae

These consist of the **atlas** and **axis** (the first and second cervical vertebrae), and the **sacrum** and **coccyx** which are formed of fused vertebrae. They do *not* possess the typical features described above.

The atlas forms a joint (**articulates**) with the occipital bone of the skull above, and allows the movement of nodding the head. The atlas and axis form a pivot joint which allows movement of the head from side to side *(see Figure 13)*.

## Intervertebral discs

Between the bodies of each vertebra are the intervertebral discs, pads of cartilage filled with a fluid. These act as shock absorbers, preventing damage to the structure.

## Regions of the vertebral column

- **cervical**      seven bones
- **thoracic**     12 bones
- **lumbar**       five bones
- **sacral**       five fused bones
- **coccyx**       four fused bones

## Curvatures

The curvatures of the vertebral column are initially formed in fetal development, while the developing fetus is curled up in the mother's uterus. These are the **thoracic** and **sacral** curvatures *(see Figure 14)*.

After birth, the **cervical curvature** is formed when the baby is able to support its own head, from approximately three months. The lumbar curvature forms when the child stands and supports his/her body at 12-18 months.

## Rib cage (thoracic)

This is made up of the following structures *(see Figure 15)*:

- One **sternum**   (breast bone)
- 12 pairs of **ribs**
- 12 **thoracic vertebrae**

## Sternum

This flat bone forms the front (**anterior**) part of the rib cage, and it is to this that the ribs and collar bone (**clavicle**) are attached. It is composed of three parts known as the **manubrium**, **body** and **xiphoid** portions. Beneath this bone lies the heart, and it is this bone which is depressed in the rendering of **cardiopulmonary resuscitation** (**CPR**).

The ribs form the bony lateral walls of the chest cavity and form joints (**articulate**) with

## Vertebral column and curvatures

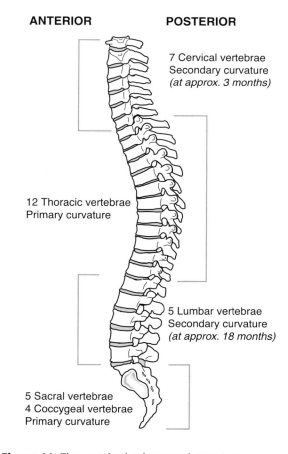

**ANTERIOR**          **POSTERIOR**

7 Cervical vertebrae
Secondary curvature
*(at approx. 3 months)*

12 Thoracic vertebrae
Primary curvature

5 Lumbar vertebrae
Secondary curvature
*(at approx. 18 months)*

5 Sacral vertebrae
4 Coccygeal vertebrae
Primary curvature

**Figure 14:** The vertebral column and curvatures

the **thoracic vertebrae** at the rear (**posteriorly**). The first 10 pairs of ribs are attached to the sternum **anteriorly** by the attachment of **costal cartilages**, the first seven directly and the lower three indirectly as shown in Figure 15. The last two pairs of ribs are known as **floating ribs** as they remain unattached to the sternum.

The rib cage protects the organs lying within it: heart, lungs, oesophagus, major blood vessels etc.

**Intercostal muscles** are attached to the ribs between the rib spaces and are involved in the process of **inspiration** and **expiration**. The rib cage swings outwards and upwards on inspiration, which increases the capacity of the thoracic cavity, allowing expansion of the lung tissue (see Chapter 7).

## Pelvis

This structure is composed of the following bones:

- Two **innominate bones**
- **Sacrum** (part of the vertebrae)

These structures are bound together by ligaments to form the pelvic basin (*see Figure 16*). The innominate bone is composed of three separate bones which are fused together:

- **Ilium**
- **Ischium**
- **Pubis**

The area within the pelvis is known as the

## The rib cage

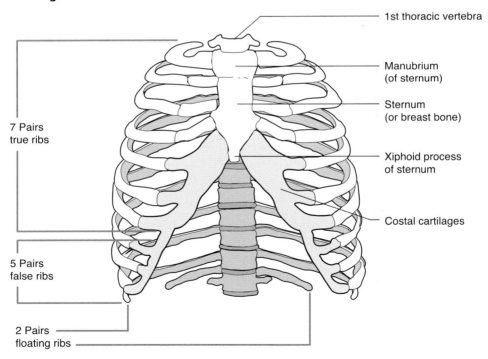

1st thoracic vertebra

Manubrium
(of sternum)

Sternum
(or breast bone)

Xiphoid process
of sternum

Costal cartilages

7 Pairs
true ribs

5 Pairs
false ribs

2 Pairs
floating ribs

**Figure 15:** The rib cage

## The pelvis

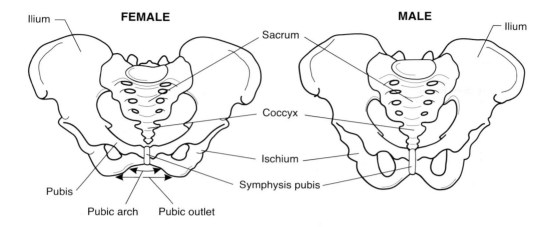

**Figure 16:** The pelvis

**pelvic cavity** and contains important structures, such as the intestine, rectum and anus, bladder, ureters, urethra, prostate gland, some organs of the male reproductive system, female reproductive organs, blood vessels, nerves etc., which are protected by the bony frame.

### The hand

The hand comprises a number of small bones (shown in Figure 17).

### The foot

The foot comprises a number of small bones (shown in Figure 18).

### Joints

Joints are formed wherever two or more bony surfaces are attached to each other.

### Types of joint

**Fixed joints**
formed of fibrous tissue where no movement is possible, e.g. sutures of cranium

**Slightly moveable**
cartilaginous joints which allow only slight movement, e.g. intervertebral joints between the bodies of vertebrae

**Freely moveable synovial joints**
which allow free movement according to the shape of the joint. *(see Figures 19 and 20)*

Synovial joints are lined with a synovial membrane which produces synovial fluid, a thick glairy fluid which acts as a lubricant preventing friction and wear. The ends of the bones which form these joints are covered in **hyaline cartilage** *(see Figure 20).*

# Bones of the hand and foot

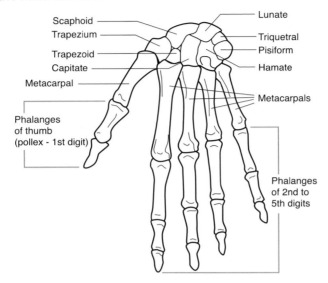

Scaphoid
Trapezium
Trapezoid
Capitate
Metacarpal

Lunate
Triquetral
Pisiform
Hamate

Metacarpals

Phalanges
of thumb
(pollex - 1st digit)

Phalanges
of 2nd to
5th digits

**Figure 17:** The hand

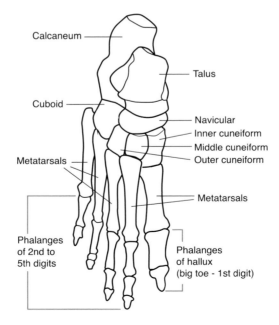

Calcaneum

Talus

Cuboid

Navicular
Inner cuneiform
Middle cuneiform
Outer cuneiform

Metatarsals

Metatarsals

Phalanges
of 2nd to
5th digits

Phalanges
of hallux
(big toe - 1st digit)

**Figure 18:** The foot

## Body movements and positions

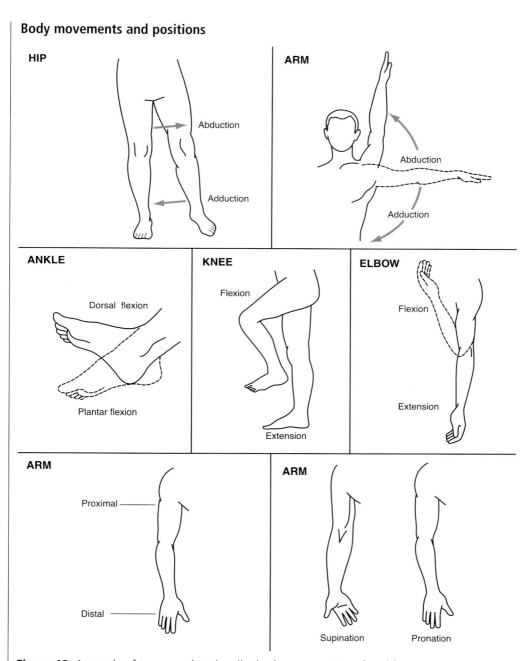

**HIP**

Abduction

Adduction

**ARM**

Abduction

Adduction

**ANKLE**

Dorsal flexion

Plantar flexion

**KNEE**

Flexion

Extension

**ELBOW**

Flexion

Extension

**ARM**

Proximal

Distal

**ARM**

Supination

Pronation

**Figure 19:** A sample of terms used to describe body movements and positions

*Redrawn after Prendergast A: Medical Terminology, 2nd edition, Addison-Wesley, 1983*

## A synovial joint

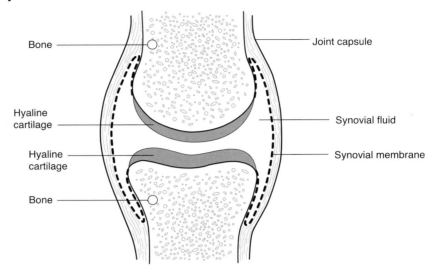

Bone

Joint capsule

Hyaline cartilage

Synovial fluid

Hyaline cartilage

Synovial membrane

Bone

**Figure 20:** A synovial joint

### Bursa

This is a sac lined with synovial membrane containing synovial fluid, usually found between a tendon and a bone near the surface of the body in order to prevent friction on movement. Inflammation of these is common in conditions such as **housemaid's knee**.

### Ligaments

These are composed of tough fibrous tissue and bind bone to bone.

### Muscles

These are strong elastic tissue, well supplied with blood (vascular), capable of contraction and relaxation. In life, muscles are always partially contracted, and this is known as muscle tone.

### Types of muscle

There are three types of muscle in the body:

1. **Voluntary (striated)**
   attached to the skeleton and under control of the will

2. **Involuntary (unstriated)**
   smooth and controlled automatically by the autonomic nervous system; these form the walls of major organs, e.g. stomach

3. **Cardiac (myogenic)**
   special muscle exclusive to the heart, forming its walls; controlled by the autonomic nervous system. It's capable of independent contraction causing quivering of the heart if the nerve supply within is interrupted.

Skeletal or striated muscle is often named from its shape, e.g. **deltoid** (triangular), or the number of heads it has, e.g. **triceps**. Muscles usually work in groups and in co-ordination.

## Diaphragm

This is an important muscle which divides the **thoracic** (chest) cavity from the abdominal cavity. It is essential for the act of **respiration** (breathing). Also involved are the **intercostal muscles** which move the rib cage (see Chapter 7).

## Tendons

These are specialised fibrous bands found at the ends of muscles which attach muscle to bone, or muscle to muscle.

## Energy

Muscles require a good blood supply to provide oxygen and nutrients. Glucose is converted and stored in muscle tissue ready for its release when required. Cramp occurs when there is insufficient oxygen available for the chemical reaction to occur and **lactic acid** is produced. The remedy for cramp is to extend the muscle.

## Hernia

This condition arises from a weakness in the muscle which allows part of an organ to **prolapse** through the space created by the weakness.

### Types of hernia
#### Inguinal hernia
This is common in men. It arises in an area known as the **inguinal canal**, which is a tunnel in the abdominal muscles where the spermatic cord and testis travel to descend into the scrotum in fetal life. Protrusion of the intestine through this area can occur and may lead to strangulation, i.e. the blood supply to this intestinal area becomes deprived.

#### Femoral hernia
This is a condition where the weakness is in the groin where the **femoral artery** travels to the leg. Hernias in this area are more common among women.

#### Hiatus hernia
This is a condition where the weakness is in the diaphragm. Part of the **oesophagus** (gullet) and/or the stomach travels through the space created by the weakness causing symptoms of 'heart burn' due to gastric juices affecting the oesophagus.

#### Umbilical hernia
In this condition, the weakness is in the area of muscle through which the umbilical cord travelled in the fetus and may give rise to an intestinal protrusion.

## Abbreviations

| | |
|---|---|
| **BI** | bone injury |
| **C1, C2 etc** | cervical vertebrae |
| **CDH** | congenital dislocation of the hip |
| **CPT** | carpal tunnel syndrome |
| **L1, L2 etc** | lumbar vertebrae |
| **NBI** | no bone injury |
| **OA** | osteoarthritis |
| **PID** | prolapsed intervertebral disc (can also mean pelvic inflammatory disease) |
| **RA** | rheumatoid arthritis |
| **RTA** | road traffic accident |
| **T1, T2 etc** | thoracic vertebrae |
| **THR** | total hip replacement |
| **TKR** | total knee replacement |

## Terminology and roots/stems

| | |
|---|---|
| **acetabul/o** | acetabulum, area where femur/thigh bone, forms joint with innominate bone |
| **arthr/o** | joint |
| **articul/o** | joint |
| **carp/o** | carpals, hand bones, wrist |
| **chondr/o** | cartilage |
| **clavicul/o** | clavicle, collar bone |
| **cost/o** | rib |

| | |
|---|---|
| **coccyg/o** | coccyx, part of spine/ rudimentary tail |
| **crani/o** | cranium (skull containing brain) |
| **disc/o** | disc between vertebrae |
| **ethmoid/o** | part of cranium |
| **femor/o** | femur, thigh bone |
| **fibul/o** | fibula, lower leg bone |
| **front/o** | frontal bone part of cranium |
| **humer/o** | humerus, upper arm |
| **ischi/o** | ischium, part of innominate bone |
| **ili/o** | ilium (bone of pelvis), part of innominate bone |
| **intra-articular** | directly into a joint, e.g. injected |
| **lacrim/o** | lacrimal bone of eye orbit/socket |
| **lamin/o** | lamina, arch of vertebra, thin sheet of bone |
| **mal/o** | malar, cheek bone |
| **mandibul/o** | mandible, lower jaw |
| **maxill/o** | maxilla, upper jaw |
| **menisc/o** | meniscus, cartilage of knee |
| **metacarp/o** | metacarpals, hand bones |
| **metatars/o** | metatarsals, foot bones |
| **my/o (myos)** | muscle |
| **myel/o** | bone marrow (also spinal cord) |
| **nas/o** | nasal bone, part of skull |
| **occipit/o** | occipital, part of cranium |
| **olecran/o** | part of elbow joint |
| **orbit/o** | orbital, part of eye socket |
| **oste/o** | bone |
| **palat/o** | palatine bones (in roof of mouth) |
| **pariet/o** | parietal, part of cranium |
| **patell/o** | patella, knee cap |
| **phalange/o** | phalanges, fingers/toes |
| **pub/o** | pubis, part of innominate bone |
| **radi/o** | radius, main lower arm bone |
| **sacr/o** | sacrum, part of spine |

| | |
|---|---|
| **scapul/o** | scapula, shoulder blade |
| **sphenoid/o** | sphenoid, part of cranium |
| **spondyl/o (vertebr/o)** | vertebra/spine |
| **stern/o** | sternum, the breast bone |
| **synov/o** | synovial |
| **tars/o** | tarsals, foot bones |
| **tempor/o** | temporal bone, part of cranium |
| **ten/o, tendin/o** | tendon |
| **tibi/o** | tibia, lower leg bone |
| **turbin/o** | turbinate bones in the nose |
| **uln/o** | ulna, lower arm bone adjective: ulnar |
| **vertebr/o** | vertebra |
| **zyg/o, zygomat/o** | cheek bone |

## Diseases and disorders

| | |
|---|---|
| **Ankylosing spondylitis** | fixation of the vertebrae with fibrous tissue causing loss of movement |
| **Ankylosis** | immobilisation and solidification of a joint |
| **Arthritis** | inflammation of a joint |
| **Arthrodynia** | pain in a joint |
| **Bursitis** | inflammation of the pad of synovial membrane protecting a bone near the surface of the body, e.g. the elbow or knee |
| **Callus** | an outgrowth of partly bony tissue produced in the body's process of the mending of bones |
| **Exostosis** | an overgrowth of bone |
| **Genu valgum** | knock knee |
| **Genu varum** | bow legged |
| **Hallux valgus** | bunion/deviation of the large toe joint |
| **Kyphosis** | hunchback/excessive curvature of the thoracic vertebrae |

| | |
|---|---|
| **Lordosis** | 'sway back'/excessive inward curvature of the lumbar spine |
| **Luxation** | complete dislocation of a joint |
| **Osteoarthritis** | degenerative disease of ageing – large joints of knee, hip etc. |
| **Osteoma** | tumour of bone |
| **Osteomalacia** | rickets – softening of bone due to lack of vitamin D and deposit of calcium salts |
| **Osteomyelitis** | inflammation of the bone marrow |
| **Osteoporosis** | brittle bones due to ageing and lack of oestrogen hormone which affects the ability to deposit calcium in the matrix of bone |
| **Polyarthritis** | arthritis involving many joints |
| **Rheumatoid arthritis** | disease causing inflammation of small joints, usually hands and feet |
| **Scoliosis** | a lateral S-shaped deformity of the vertebrae |
| **Spina bifida** | failure of the spinous processes to unite in fetal development, causing various degrees of deformity, with or without the meninges (covering of spinal cord) and/or spinal cord protruding through to the surface of the body |
| **Spondylitis** | inflammation of one or more vertebrae |
| **Spondylosis** | degenerative disease of the spine, crumbling occurs |
| **Still's disease** | a form of rheumatoid polyarthritis in children |
| **Subluxation** | partial dislocation of a joint |
| **Synovitis** | inflammation of a synovial (moveable) joint |
| **Talipes** | club foot deformity |
| **Valgus** | deviation outwards |
| **Varus** | deviation inwards |

## Procedures and equipment

| | |
|---|---|
| **Arthroclasia** | surgical breaking of a joint to provide movement |
| **Arthrocentesis** | puncture of a joint cavity to remove fluid |
| **Arthrodesis** | surgical stiffening of a joint |
| **Arthroplasty** | reshaping or moulding of a joint |
| **Arthroscopy** | examination of a joint with a lighted instrument |
| **Bursectomy** | removal (excision) of bursa |
| **Laminectomy** | surgical removal of the lamina of a vertebra to relieve pressure in 'slipped disc' |
| **Meniscectomy** | surgical removal of the semi-lunar cartilage of the knee joint |
| **Open reduction** | using surgery to reduce a dislocation of a joint or fracture as opposed to a closed reduction where manipulation alone is used |
| **Osteotomy** | cutting or dividing of bone |
| **Prosthesis** | artificial part or replacement, e.g. hip, leg or breast |
| **Synovectomy** | surgical removal of synovial (lining) membrane |
| **Tenotomy** | surgical dividing or cutting of a tendon |

## Fractures

| | |
|---|---|
| **Fracture** | a break in the continuity of the bone – includes cracks as well as complete breaks (*See Figure 21 for types of fracture*) |
| **Avulsion** | fragmented bone at the site of a ligament or tendon attachment |
| **Colles'** | fracture of the wrist, both the radius and ulna are fractured and cause the typical dinner fork deformity |

| | | | |
|---|---|---|---|
| **Comminuted** | a fracture where there are several breaks in the bone | | is not as ossified (hardened with mineral salts), but is rather like a green branch of a tree in its splitting – heals quickly |
| **Complicated** | fracture in which there is associated damage to vital neighbouring structures | | |
| **Compound/open** | a break in a bone where there is communication with the outside air through the skin – danger of infection | **Impacted** | a fracture where the ends of the bone are forced into one another |
| | | **Oblique** | fracture that is not directly across the axis of the bone |
| **Depressed** | fracture of the skull with depressed segments | **Pott's** | fracture of the ankle involving both the tibia and fibula |
| **Greenstick** | type of fracture in children where the bone does not completely break as it | **Transverse** | fracture at right angles to the axis of the bone |

## Types of fracture

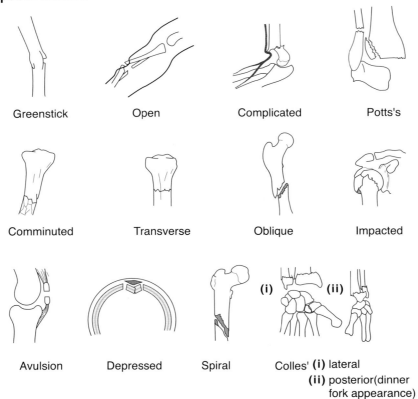

Greenstick    Open    Complicated    Potts's

Comminuted    Transverse    Oblique    Impacted

Avulsion    Depressed    Spiral    Colles' **(i)** lateral
**(ii)** posterior(dinner fork appearance)

(i)    (ii)

**Figure 21:** Types of fracture

Chapter **4** | # The blood

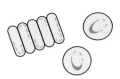

## Function

The function of blood can be summarised as both the transportation of substances throughout the body and also a defence system.

## Structure

Blood consists of a slightly alkaline (*pH* 7.35) straw-coloured fluid known as plasma that contains blood cells suspended within it. It is the main transport system of the body, travelling within a closed system of blood vessels.

An adult has five to six litres (eight to10 pints) of blood.

## Plasma

The fluid which forms 55% of the blood and contains numerous substances, including:

- **Water** (91%)
- **Mineral salts**
  including sodium chloride,
  the largest component at 0.9%
- **Food materials**:
  - amino acids (proteins)
  - glucose
  - fats known as lipids
- **Plasma proteins**
  albumin, globulin and the clotting factors fibrinogen and prothrombin
- **Waste materials**
  carbon dioxide in solution, urea and uric acid
- **Antibodies** and **antitoxins**
- **Vitamins**
- **Hormones**
- **Enzymes**
- **Oxygen** – in solution.

## Serum

When the clotting factor fibrinogen has been removed from plasma, it is known as serum.

## Cells

These consist of three main groups (*see Figure 22*):

- **Red cells** known as **erythrocytes** (around 5 million per cubic millimetre – *see Tables 1 and 2*)
- **White cells** known as **leucocytes** (around 8,000 per cubic millimetre)
- **Platelets** known as **thrombocytes** (around 350,000 per cubic millimetre).

### Erythrocytes

These are smaller than the white cells and have no nuclei. This gives them a biconcave shape and enables them to carry more **haemoglobin** (an orange-coloured substance containing iron, which combines with oxygen in the blood contained in the capillary network of the lungs). This is then carried in the blood stream, ready to supply the tissues where oxygen is released. Their function is to carry oxygen, and they are small enough to travel within the capillaries.

Haemoglobin combines with oxygen to form **oxyhaemoglobin:**

$$\text{Haemoglobin} + O_2 \longleftrightarrow \text{oxyhaemoglobin}$$
$$\text{(reversible)}$$

Erythrocytes are manufactured in the bone marrow, live for approximately 3 months and are destroyed by the spleen and liver. The part containing iron is stored by the liver and the residue is excreted as bile pigments (bilirubin) in the faeces, and it is this pigment which gives the faeces their colour.

## Anaemia

Anaemia may be defined as a condition in which there is an insufficient amount of oxygen-carrying capacity in the blood. It may be caused by too few normal erythrocytes or by red blood cells not being mature and fully

**Table 1:** Meaning of pathology values for red blood cells

| Term | Meaning of term |
|---|---|
| Erythrocyte count | Number of red blood cells per litre or per cubic millimetre of blood |
| Haemoglobin | Weight of haemoglobin in whole blood expressed as grams per decilitre |
| Mean cell volume | Average volume of cells expressed in femtolitres |
| Mean corpuscular (cell) haemoglobin | Average amount of haemoglobin in each cell expressed in femtolitres |
| Mean corpuscular (cell) haemoglobin concentration | Amount of haemoglobin in 100 ml (1 decilitre) of blood |
| Packed cell volume or haematocrit | Volume of red cells in 1 litre (100 millilitres) of whole blood |

charged with haemoglobin. Varying conditions of anaemia may give rise to erythrocytes which are large and pale (**macrocytic**) or small (**microcytic**).

Certain factors are necessary for the production of mature red blood cells. These include iron and trace elements as well as vitamin C and folic acid. **Vitamin B$_{12}$** is also essential and is known as the **extrinsic factor**. These are all provided in the diet.

## Pernicious anaemia

However, a further substance known as **Castle's intrinsic factor**, found within the gastric juice produced by the stomach, is essential for the absorption of vitamin B$_{12}$ necessary in the diet. If this is not present, a condition known as **pernicious anaemia** will result where large pale immature red cells (macrocytic), unable to carry much oxygen, occur. Treatment is by giving regular B$_{12}$ injections.

## Iron deficiency anaemia

Iron deficiency anaemia is very common and occurs when there is insufficient iron or other necessary factors in the diet, or when there has been a loss of blood through haemorrhaging (bleeding), either severe or as a constant, slight loss, e.g. a slowly bleeding peptic ulcer. The condition of **menorrhagia** (heavy periods) is a common cause of this type of anaemia in women. The erythrocytes are pale (**hypochromic**) and small (microcytic).

## Leucocytes

These white cells are composed of two main types:

1. **Granulocytes (polymorphonuclear leucocytes):** 65–75% of white cells
2. **Non-granular leucocytes (mononuclear leucocytes):** 25–35% of white cells.

The life-span of white cells is approximately 3 weeks or less and is dependent on the state of infection in the body.

### Granulocytes (polymorphonuclear leucocytes)

These cells are manufactured in the bone marrow and are concerned with the defence of the body. They are mainly **phagocytes**, i.e. capable of changing their shape and ingesting (eating) bacteria and foreign matter. They are larger than the red cells but by changing their

## Blood cells

Average number
per cubic millimetre
of blood

**RED CELLS (Erythrocytes)**                                          5,000,000

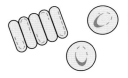

Biconcave discs
(contain no nucleus)

**WHITE CELLS (Leucocytes)**                                          8,000

Polymorphonuclear leucocytes
(or granulocytes)

Monocytes (mononuclear leucocytes
or non-granular leucocytes)

Lymphocytes
(large or small)

**PLATELETS OR THROMBOCYTES**                                          350,000

Fragmented cells

**Figure 22:** Blood cells

shape (**amoeboid action**) are able to squeeze out of the capillary walls to reach the tissues. Named after the stains which they will take up in the laboratory, they consist of three types:

- **Neutrophils** (60–70% of white cells)

- **Basophils** (0.5–2% of white blood cells)

- **Eosinophils** (2–4% of white blood cells).

The majority of phagocytes are neutrophils and their numbers increase greatly in response to bacterial infection.

#### Non-granular (mononuclear) leucocytes
These blood cells consist of:

- **Lymphocytes** (representing 20–30% of blood cells) and

- **Monocytes** (accounting for 4–8% of blood cells)

and are developed in the bone marrow and lymph tissue.

### Lymphocytes
These blood cells are concerned with immunity and when activated produce antibodies, so protecting the body from foreign materials e.g. viruses. These antibodies assist the other body defences to overcome infection. Lymphocytes form the majority of the non-granulocytes and are found in lymph tissue throughout the body.

### Monocytes
These blood cells are also concerned with immunity and are capable of phagocytic and amoeboid action. They work in close association with lymphocytes and their numbers are greatly increased in certain infective conditions, e.g. glandular fever.

### Thrombocytes
These are fragmented cells, with no nucleus, and are concerned with clotting. They are also manufactured in the bone marrow.

**Table 2:** Normal values of erythrocytes

| Abbreviation | Sex | Normal value |
|---|---|---|
| | | for meanings of the units used here, see Chapter 17 |
| Erythrocyte count | Female | **4.0–5.5** x10$^{12}$/l   **4.0–5.5** million/mm$^3$ |
| (RBC – red blood cells) | Male | **4.5–6.5** x10$^{12}$/l   **4.5–6.5** million/mm$^3$ |
| Haemoglobin | Female | **11.5–16.5** g/dl |
| (Hb) | Male | **13.5–18.0** g/dl |
| Mean cell volume | Female | **80–100** fl |
| (MCV) | Male | **80–100** fl |
| Mean corpuscular (cell) | Female | **30–36** g/dl of cells |
| haemoglobin concentration (MCHC) | Male | **30–36** g/dl of cells |
| Packed cell volume (PCV) | Female | **0.37–0.47** l/l   **37%** - **47%** |
| or Haematocrit (HCT) | Male | **0.40–0.54** l/l   **37%** - **54%** |

**NB:** There are variations of normal values with different laboratories.

## Clotting

The process of blood clotting requires many factors including **thrombocytes** (**platelets**). The clotting factors **prothrombin**, **fibrinogen** (manufactured in the liver) and **vitamin K** are essential.

Also necessary is **factor VIII**, a substance which is absent from the blood of patients suffering from **haemophilia**. Spontaneous bleeding occurs into joints with this condition. Factor VIII is given artificially by injection when necessary.

## Blood groups

These are genetically determined. There are many different groups. The main classification is the Landsteiner ABO type (agglutinin) present in the red cells.

- **Type A:** contains factor A in cells, anti-B in serum
- **Type B:** contains factor B in cells, anti-A in serum
- **Type AB:** contains factor A and B in cells, no anti-A or anti-B in serum.
- **Type O:** contains no factor in cells, anti-A and anti-B in serum.

Therefore the serum of group A blood, containing anti-B, will cause group B red blood cells to be destroyed and vice versa. The serum of group O blood will destroy A, B and AB. However, group AB blood will not react with any of the groups as it has no anti-factors in its serum to do so.

### The Rhesus factor

A further factor present in the plasma of the blood is the Rhesus factor (anti-D) present in 85% of the population. When present the type is known as **Rhesus positive** (Rh +ve). When absent it is known as **Rhesus negative** (Rh -ve).

The Rhesus factor must always be considered, particularly in the case of females, where the giving of Rhesus-positive blood to someone who is Rhesus negative, will cause antibodies (anti-factors) to be produced by the person's immune system. Subsequently, in pregnancy, these can damage the blood of the fetus if it is Rhesus positive.

### Compatibility

In a blood transfusion, if the blood given to a patient (**recipient)** from a **donor** contains a factor in the cells to which the patient's (recipient's) blood serum will react, the donor's blood will be destroyed, causing clumping together of the red cells (**agglutination**) which can be fatal. Therefore blood is normally 'cross-matched' for compatibility before transfusion is given. In extreme emergencies, the **'universal donor'** group is given, i.e. O Rhesus -ve, before any investigations are done.

In normal circumstances the same group as the recipient is given.

- **Group AB Rh +ve** is the universal recipient.
- **Group O Rh -ve is** the universal donor.

## Abbreviations

| | |
|---|---|
| **AIDS** | acquired immunodeficiency syndrome |
| **ALL** | acute lymphocytic leukaemia |
| **AML** | acute myeloid leukaemia |
| **APT** | activated prothrombin time |
| **APPT** | activated partial thromboplastin time |
| **BUN** | blood urea nitrogen |
| **CLL** | chronic lymphocytic leukaemia |
| **CML** | chronic myeloid leukaemia |
| **CO$_2$** | carbon dioxide |
| **ESR** | erythrocyte sedimentation rate |
| **FBC** | full blood count |
| **Hb** | haemoglobin (pigmented protein which carries oxygen) |
| **HDL** | high density lipoprotein |
| **Ig** | immunoglobulin |

| INR | international normalised ratio (prothrombin time) |
| LDL | low density lipoprotein |
| MCH | mean corpuscular haemoglobin |
| MCHC | mean corpuscular haemoglobin concentration |
| MCV | mean corpuscular volume |
| $O_2$ | oxygen |
| PCV | packed cell volume |
| RBC | red blood count |
| TIBC | total iron-binding capacity |
| WBC | white blood count |
| WBC & diff. | white blood count and different percentages present |

## Units used in biochemistry

| SI | international system (Système International) |
| IU or U | international unit |
| mmol | millimole |
| mmol/l | millimole per litre |
| nmol | nanomole |
| µmol | micromole |
| µg | microgram |
| g | gram |

## Terminology

| Coagulation | clotting of blood |
| Ery-, Erythro- | red |
| Gamma-globulin | plasma proteins which include antibodies |
| Haem-, Haemato- | stem for blood |
| Haemostasis | stopping bleeding |
| Immunoglobulin | plasma proteins which are antibodies |
| Leuco- | white |
| Thrombo- | clot |

*(see also Chapter 17 on pathology.)*

## Diseases and disorders

| Agranulocytosis | large decrease in number of white granulocytes (cells which fight against infection) |
| Anaemia | amount of oxygen carrying capacity is reduced due to either too few red blood cells or too little haemoglobin |
| Epistaxis | nose-bleed |
| Haemolysis | destruction of blood cells |
| Haemophilia A | hereditary disease caused by lack of clotting factor (VIII) in the blood |
| Haemophilia B | hereditary disease caused by lack of clotting factor (IX) in the blood |
| HIV | human immunodeficiency virus |
| Hypercholesterolaemia | raised blood cholesterol (lipid or fat levels) |
| Hyperlipidaemia | raised blood fat levels |
| Hypochromic anaemia | anaemia associated with pale, small red cells due to insufficient iron |
| Infectious mononucleosis | glandular fever – increase of white cells called monocytes present in blood |
| Leucocytosis | a normal increase of white blood cells in response to infection |
| Leucopenia | a decrease in the number of white blood cells in the blood |
| Leukaemia | a cancer of the blood – abnormal white cells increase |
| Pernicious anaemia | inability of body to manufacture normal red blood cells due to a missing factor |
| Polycythaemia | too many red and other blood cells present in the blood |
| Sickle-cell anaemia | anaemia associated with people of African ethnic origin, red cells have sickle shape |
| Thalassaemia | anaemia associated with people of Mediterranean origin |

## Procedures and equipment

**Cryoprecipitate**   use of very low temperatures to separate required factors from blood

**Paul-Bunnell test**   blood test for glandular fever

**Plasmapheresis**   taking blood from a donor, removing the required factor and returning the remainder to the donor's circulation

Chapter **5** | The cardiovascular system

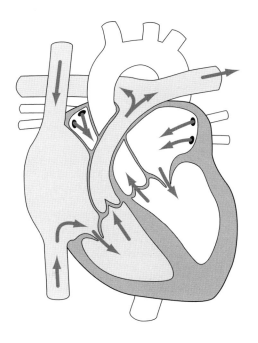

## Structure and function

The cardiovascular system consists of the heart and blood vessels, and is responsible for the transportation of blood throughout the body.

Organs forming the system are the:

- Heart

- Blood vessels

## The heart

### Structure

This heart is a hollow muscular organ, the size of the owner's fist, situated in the **mediastinal space** (between the lungs) of the **thoracic** (chest) cavity. It is tilted to the left and its base rests upon the diaphragm.

It is composed of three layers of tissue:

| | |
|---|---|
| **Pericardium** | a specialised fibrous sac, lined with serous membrane, covering the heart and preventing friction |
| **Myocardium** | composed of cardiac muscle forming the chambers and septum |
| **Endocardium** | a smooth endothelial lining which also forms the valves. |

The heart is a double pump. It consists of two thin-walled upper chambers known as **atria** and two thick-walled lower chambers known as **ventricles**, the left ventricle having the thickest wall. It is divided into left and right sides by a muscular septum. Blood contained in the left chambers has no communication with that in the right *(see Figure 23).*

### Valves of the heart

The upper and lower chambers are separated by non-return valves which prevent the backflow of blood – the **tricuspid valve** between the right chambers and the **bicuspid** or **mitral** valve between the left chambers.

### Specialised nerve supply to the heart

The **vagus nerve** supplies the heart as well as fibres from the **sympathetic chain** of the **autonomic nervous system (ANS)** (see Chapter 13).

There are also specialised areas of nerve fibres within the heart muscle. These are the:

- **sinu-atrial node** in the wall of the right atrium (pacemaker)

- **atrioventricular node** in the wall at the junction of the atria and ventricles

- **bundle of His** in the ventricular septum of the heart.

### Function

#### The cardiac cycle

The two upper chambers (atria) receive blood from the veins and, on contraction, force blood through the valves into the lower chambers (ventricles). This impulse is controlled by the sinu-atrial node. As the atria relax, blood is automatically sucked in from the attached blood vessels to refill these chambers.

As the atria relax, so the ventricles contract (at an impulse from the atrioventricular node, conducted down through the bundle of His), pumping blood into the attached arteries through one-way valves which guard their openings. The ventricles relax and the cycle recommences.

#### Blood flow

The right side of the heart contains deoxygenated blood, returned from the body via veins; the left side contains oxygenated blood returned from the lungs where gases have been exchanged. The left ventricle, the thickest walled chamber, pumps blood to the body via the main artery, the **aorta**.

### Heart sounds

Two sounds, which are produced by the closing of valves, can be clearly heard during the cardiac cycle: 'lubb' and 'dup'.

'**Lubb**' a long, dull sound is produced at the closing of the valves between the upper and lower chambers of the heart (**atrioventricular**

## The heart

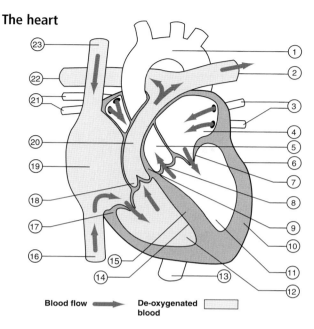

1. Aortic arch
2. Left pulmonary artery
3. Left pulmonary veins
4. Left atrium
5. Ascending aorta
6. Pericardium
7. Mitral valve
8. Aortic valve
9. Atrial septum
10. Myocardium
11. Left ventricle
12. Right ventricle
13. Descending aorta
14. Endocardium
15. Ventricular septum
16. Inferior vena cava
17. Tricuspid valve
18. Pulmonary valve
19. Right atrium
20. Pulmonary artery
21. Right pulmonary veins
22. Right pulmonary artery
23. Superior vena cava

Blood flow ➡ De-oxygenated blood ▭

**Figure 23:** The heart

valves), whilst '**dup**', a sharp, short sound is produced by the closing of the valves guarding the arteries arising from the ventricles (the **pulmonary valves** and **aortic valves**).

It is these sounds which are known as the heart sounds. Abnormality may be caused by disease of the heart valves (as in cases of **rheumatic fever**) and the sounds produced are then known as '**murmurs**'.

## Blood vessels

These form a completely closed system which transports blood, containing various substances, to and from the heart via all the tissues of the body.

They consist of:

- **Arteries** (*see Figure 24*)
- **Veins** (*see Figure 25*)
- **Capillaries**

### Arteries

Arteries, varying in size, are vessels travelling from the heart and (apart from the **pulmonary artery** travelling to the lungs which contains de-oxygenated blood) contain oxygenated blood. They contain muscle and elastic tissue in their walls to allow for contraction and relaxation with the contraction of the heart. They have a very smooth lining to prevent clotting. The smallest arteries are known as **arterioles**.

### Veins

There are more veins than arteries in the body. Veins, varying in size, carry deoxygenated blood (apart from the **pulmonary veins** containing oxygenated blood) returning to the heart. They have a similar structure to arteries, but the walls are thinner and much less elastic (Figure 26). If a vein is cut it collapses, but an artery remains open and spurts blood rhythmically. Veins possess one-way valves to prevent backflow of blood. It is these which become damaged in the condition of **varicose veins**. The smallest veins are known as **venules**.

## Main arteries of the body (carrying blood away from the heart)

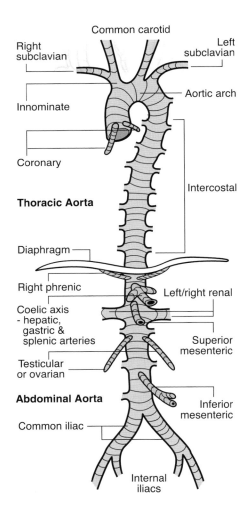

**Figure 24:** Main arteries of the body

## Capillaries

These are fine, hair-like vessels, consisting of one-cell-thick coats. It is from these structures, because they are only one cell thick, that fluid (**tissue fluid**) containing oxygen, nutrients and other substances, is able to flow into the tissues, so supplying the individual cells with their requirements.

These blood vessels are the only ones where substances are able to leave the blood stream. Large proteins remain behind in the blood vessels, as they are too large to pass through the capillary walls. These proteins enable some of the fluid to be attracted back into the venous capillaries by osmosis. The remaining fluid (lymph) is returned to the circulation via the lymphatic system (see Chapter 6).

### Main blood vessels:

| | |
|---|---|
| **Aorta** | main artery of the body, stems from the left ventricle to supply the body with oxygenated blood |
| **Pulmonary artery** | takes blood to the lungs for oxygenation and removal of carbon dioxide |
| **Superior vena cava** / **Inferior vena cava** | main veins of the body returning blood from the body to the right atrium |
| **Pulmonary veins** | return oxygenated blood to the left side of the heart for distribution to the body via the aorta. |

### Blood circulation

| | |
|---|---|
| **Systemic** | supplies the main body; the main artery is the **aorta** from which other large arteries arise; all organs have their own blood supply |
| **Pulmonary** | supplies the lungs for oxygenation of the blood and removal of carbon dioxide – oxygenated blood is returned to the left atrium |

**Portal** supplies the liver and is concerned with the transport of food substances from the intestine for assimilation by the liver; the liver has two blood supplies from the hepatic artery and the portal vein.

## Blood pressure (arterial)

This is the force, or pressure, that the blood is exerting against the walls of the blood vessels in which it is contained. This pressure varies during the cardiac cycle.

### Systolic pressure

This is the pressure felt when the ventricles of the heart are contracting and pumping blood through the arteries via the main aorta. This is also known as the **systole**. It is the higher reading.

### Diastolic pressure

This is the pressure felt when the heart chambers are at rest as the heart relaxes. This is also known as the **diastole**. It is the lower reading.

### Factors affecting normal blood pressure:

- **Cardiac output** – the pumping of the heart
- **Volume** of the blood circulating
- **Peripheral resistance** of the blood vessels – the **calibre** (diameter) of small arteries away from the centre of the body – this is also affected by hardening and narrowing caused by age and fatty deposits (**atherosclerosis**)
- **Elastic recoil** of large arteries
- **Viscosity** (thickness) of the blood.

## Pulse

This is a wave of distension and recoil, which can be felt in the wall of an artery as it passes over a bone near the surface of the body. It reflects the pressure transmitted from the aorta at the beating of the heart.

## Main veins of the body (carrying blood back to the heart)

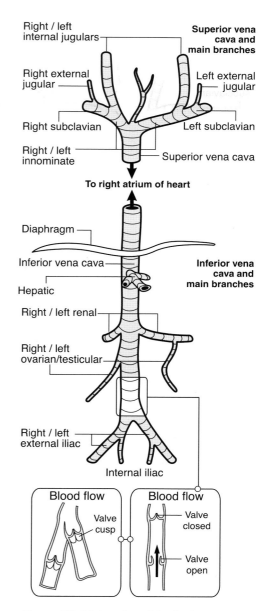

**Figure 25:** Main veins of the body

## Normal pulse range
### (number of beats per minute)

| | |
|---|---|
| In the newborn ........................... | **140** |
| Infants ...................................... | **120** |
| Children at 10 years .............. | **80 - 90** |
| Adults ..................................... | **60 - 80** |
| | (average 72) |

Emotion, exercise, age and health will all affect the pulse rate.

## Abbreviations

| | |
|---|---|
| **AS** | aortic stenosis |
| **ASD** | atrial septum defect |
| **ASHD** | arteriosclerotic heart disease |
| **AST\*** | aspartate transaminase (cardiac enzyme) |
| **BP** | blood pressure |
| **CABG** | coronary artery bypass graft |
| **CABS** | coronary artery bypass surgery |
| **CAD** | coronary artery disease |
| **CCF** | congestive cardiac failure |
| **CCU** | coronary care unit |
| **CHF** | congestive heart failure |
| **CPK\*** | creatine phosphokinase (cardiac enzyme) |
| **CPR** | cardiopulmonary resuscitation |
| **CVP** | central venous pressure |
| **CVS** | cardiovascular system |
| **DVT** | deep vein thrombosis |
| **EBT** | electron beam tomography, a way of scanning the heart |
| **ECG** | electrocardiogram (records the electrical impulses of the beating of the heart muscle) |
| **EOF** | end organ failure, e.g. kidney failure, caused by high or very low blood pressure |
| **GOT\*** | glutamic-oxaloacetic transaminase (cardiac enzyme) |
| **HCM** | see HoCM |
| **HI** | hypodermic injection |
| **HoCM (or HCM)** | hypertrophic (obstructive) cardiomyopathy, a genetic disease of the heart muscle which tends to show itself during development in adolescence |

## Structure of artery and vein

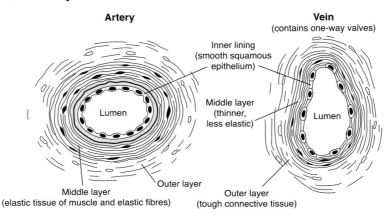

**Figure 26:** Structure of artery and vein

48

| | |
|---|---|
| **HS** | heart sounds |
| **ICU** | intensive care unit |
| **IM** | intramuscular injection |
| **ITU** | intensive therapy unit |
| **IV** | intravenous injection |
| **LD\*** | lactate dehydrogenase (cardiac enzyme) |
| **MI** | Myocardial infarction (wedge-shaped area deprived of its blood supply) |
| **MOF** | Multiple organ failure, e.g. all major organs do not work properly, caused by septicaemia, toxic shock syndrome etc. |
| **NT-pro BNP** | blood test for heart failure, enables early diagnosis |
| **PAT** | paroxysmal atrial tachycardia |
| **PTCA** | percutaneous transluminal coronary angioplasty |
| **PVC** | premature ventricular contraction |
| **SADS** | sudden adult death syndrome |
| **TC** | total cholesterol (LDLs and HDLs) |
| **TMR** | transmyocardial revascularisation |
| **TOE** | trans-oesophageal echocardiography: a procedure where a scan of the heart is performed with the equipment used, placed into the gullet (oesophagus). The computerised picture is produced by the bouncing back of sound waves. Used particularly in the diagnosis of hyper-trophic cardiomyopathy and other heart conditions |
| **VSD** | ventricular septal defect |

\* These enzymes also indicate metabolism of other organs

## Terminology

| | |
|---|---|
| **Angi/o** | stem for blood vessel |
| **Arteri/o** | stem for artery |
| **Blood pressure** | normally referring to the force of blood felt against the artery walls on the contraction and relaxation of the left ventricle (chamber of heart), measured in millimetres of mercury (mmHg) |
| **Cardi/o** (Coron/o) | stem for heart |
| **Cardiology** | study of the heart |
| **Diastole** | the relaxation phase of the heart cycle where chambers fill with blood – this is the lower reading of blood pressure |
| **Endocardi/o** | stem for endocardium, lining of the heart |
| **Myocardi/o** | stem for myocardium, muscle layer of the heart |
| **Pericardi/o** | stem for pericardium, outer covering of the heart |
| **Phleb/o** (Ven/o) | stem for vein |
| **Pulse** | a wave of distension and relaxation felt where an artery crosses a bone near the surface of the body |
| **Sinus rhythm** | the heart beating in normal rhythm |
| **Systole** | the contraction phase of the cardiac cycle – the force felt when the left ventricle contracts, forcing blood through the aorta to supply the body with its blood supply |
| **Vascular** | referring to blood vessels. |

## Diseases and disorders

| | |
|---|---|
| **Aneurysm** | a weakness in the wall of an artery (can cause ballooning and rupture) |

| | |
|---|---|
| **Angina pectoris** | pain in the chest and left arm caused by insufficient blood to the heart muscle, usually on exertion or excitement |
| **Angioma** | tumour of blood vessels, usually capillaries |
| **Arrhythmia** | abnormal rhythm of the heart |
| **Arteriosclerosis** | hardening of an artery |
| **Arteritis** | inflammation of an artery |
| **Atheroma** | fatty deposits in the wall of an artery |
| **Atherosclerosis** | narrowing (with fatty deposits) and hardening of an artery |
| **Atrial fibrillation** | disorder of the heart beat, no co-ordination between atria and ventricles |
| **Bradycardia** | an abnormally slow heart beat |
| **Cardiac arrest** | cessation of the heart beat |
| **Cardiac asthma** | breathlessness caused by right-sided failure of the heart, usually at night |
| **Carditis** | inflammation of the heart |
| **Coronary occlusion** | a sudden blocking of an artery supplying the heart muscle, e.g. thrombosis (formation of a blood clot) |
| **Coronary thrombosis** | a blocking of an artery by a blood clot in the coronary (heart) circulation |
| **Cyanosis** | blueness of the skin and mucous membranes due to lack of oxygen |
| **Diastolic murmur** | abnormal sound heard during relaxation phase of the cardiac cycle |
| **Dyspnoea** | laboured or difficult breathing |
| **Embolism** | sudden obstruction of a blood vessel by an embolus |
| **Embolus** | a detached and travelling particle of fat, air or blood clot |
| **Endocarditis** | inflammation of the lining of the heart (endocardium) |

| | |
|---|---|
| **End organ failure (EOF)** | e.g. kidney failure, caused by high or very low blood pressure |
| **Fibrillation** | a quivering of the heart chambers, an ineffective action of pumping blood |
| **Haemorrhoids** | varicose veins of the rectum |
| **Hypertrophic (obstructive) cardiomyopathy (HoCM)** | a genetic disease resulting in abnormal heart muscle |
| **Hypertension (hyperpiesis)** | high blood pressure |
| **Intermittent claudication** | painful condition of the leg caused by lack of blood supply |
| **Mitral incompetence** | disordered function of the mitral valve of the heart (between the left chambers of the heart) |
| **Mitral stenosis** | narrowing of the mitral valve |
| **Multiple organ failure (MOF)** | e.g. all major organs do not work properly, caused by septicaemia, toxic shock syndrome etc. |
| **Myocardial infarct** | death (necrosis) of a wedge-shaped area of heart tissue when the artery supplying it becomes blocked |
| **Myocarditis** | inflammation of the muscle of the heart |
| **Occlusion** | blockage of blood vessel |
| **Oedema** | excess fluid in the tissues |
| **Palpitations** | rapid forceful beating of heart of which the patient is aware |
| **Pancarditis** | inflammation of all structures of the heart |
| **Patent ductus arteriosus** | failure of the ductus arteriosus (artery bypassing lungs in fetus) to close at birth |
| **Pericarditis** | inflammation of the outside covering of the heart |
| **Phlebitis** | inflammation of a vein |
| **Phlebolith** | stone in a vein (calcium deposits) |

| | |
|---|---|
| **Pulmonary stenosis** | narrowing of the valve between the right ventricle and pulmonary artery |
| **Systolic murmur** | abnormal sound heard during contraction phase of cardiac cycle |
| **Tachycardia** | a rapid heart beat |
| **Thrombo-phlebitis** | inflammation of the wall of a vein causing a blood clot to form (thrombus) |
| **Thrombosis** | a condition where a thrombus has formed |
| **Thrombus** | a blood clot in a blood vessel |
| **Varices** | varicose veins |
| **Varicose veins** | presence of thickened and twisted veins caused by incompetent valves |
| **Ventricular fibrillation** | a quivering of the ventricles of the heart instead of contracting forcefully. |

## Procedures and equipment

| | |
|---|---|
| **Angio-cardiography** | demonstration of heart and major blood vessels using an opaque medium injected into the circulation |
| **Angiogram** | special X-ray of arteries using radio-opaque medium (dye which shows up in X-rays) |
| **Angioplasty** | reshaping or forming a blood vessel |
| **Aortograph** | recording of a pulse on a graph demonstration of aorta by use of opaque medium |
| **Arteriotomy** | cutting into an artery |
| **Auscultation** | listening to sounds for diagnostic purposes, usually with a stethoscope |
| **Cardiac catheterisation** | a fine hollow tube (catheter) is inserted into heart chamber to measure |

## Stent

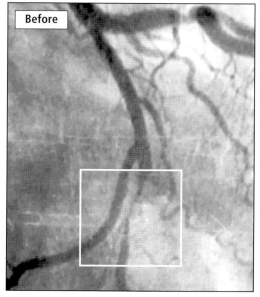
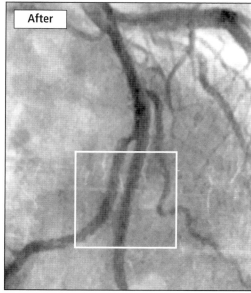

**Figure 27:** Before and after x-rays of a stent insertion *(with kind permission of Peter Woodford)*

| | |
|---|---|
| | gases and pressure/radio-opaque dye is introduced |
| **Defibrillation** | restoring the heart rhythm to normal sinus rhythm by means of electrical shock from defibrillator |
| **Electron beam tomography (EBT)** | a way of scanning the heart |
| **Electrocardio-gram (ECG)** | records the electrical impulses of the beating of the heart muscle |
| **Endarterectomy** | surgical removal of deposits (e.g. fat, blood clots) from the lining of arteries |
| **Exercise tolerance test** | test (ECG) on the heart during exercise |
| **Haemorrhoid-ectomy** | surgical removal of haemorrhoids |
| **Injection of varicose veins** | treatment of varicose veins – an injection is given of a substance which will cause the vein to sclerose, i.e. seal up |
| **Intravascular thrombolysis** | an agent which destroys/dissolves clots is infused into the blood vessels to clear a blood clot (thrombus) |
| **Ligation of varicose veins** | surgically tying off parts of a varicose vein to divert the blood supply through healthier veins |
| **Pacemaker** | referring to:<br>a) an artificial implant of an electrical mechanism to replace the damaged sinu-atrial node<br>b) the sinu-atrial node of specialised nerve tissue in the wall of the right atrium which initiates the contraction of the heart |
| **Percutaneous transluminal coronary angioplasty** | a procedure where an occluded (blocked) blood vessel is dilated using a ballon catheter; guidance is provided by a monitor which shows the position of the catheter within the body by fluoroscopy |

| | |
|---|---|
| **Phlebotomy** | cutting into a vein |
| **Phonocardi-ography** | the heart sounds of the cardiac cycle (contraction and relaxation of the chambers) are displayed as graphic images on a monitor; an ECG is displayed simultaneously |
| **Sphygmoman-ometer** | instrument used for measuring blood pressure |
| **Stent** (see figure 27) | small instrument/structure inserted into the blood vessel to keep it open in cases of lack of blood to an organ (ischaemic heart disease, etc.) |
| **Stethoscope** | instrument used for listening to sounds of the body |
| **Stripping of varicose veins** | surgical procedure where varicose veins are removed |
| **Thallium scan** | procedure of injecting radioactive thallium to demonstrate the condition of the blood vessels (coronary arteries) supplying the heart muscle (see Chapter 21 on Miscellaneous Tests: Electrocardiography) |
| **Transmyocardial revascularisation** | a procedure where smal holes are made in the cardiac muscle in order to stimulate growth of new blood vessels to increase blood supply to damaged heart muscle |
| **Valvectomy** | surgical removal of a valve |
| **Valvotomy** | cutting into a valve, by custom referring to the heart |
| **Varicotomy** | cutting into a varicose vein |
| **Venepuncture** | insertion of a needle into a vein |
| **Venesection** | cutting down into a vein for purposes of transfusion or insertion of drugs |
| **Venogram** | X-ray of a vein using an opaque medium. |

Chapter **6** | The lymphatic system

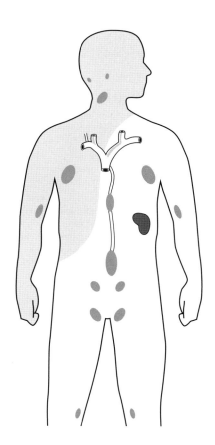

## Function

The lymphatic system is a transport and defence system.

**Lymph** is the remains of **tissue fluid** after it has passed through the tissues from the capillaries and given up its nutrients and gases to the cells. It has gathered waste products and is returned to the circulation via the lymphatic system.

## Structure

The lymphatic system consists of the following (*see Figure 28*):

- **Lymph**
- **Lymph capillaries**
- **Lymph vessels**
- **Lymph nodes (or glands), superficial and deep**
- **Main lymph ducts**
- **Specialised lymph glands.**

### Lymph capillaries

These are similar in structure to the blood capillaries, but start in the tissue spaces and are open-ended tubes; they are not continuous.

### Lymph vessels

These are similar in structure to veins, but have many more valves in their walls giving a beaded appearance.

### Lymph nodes or glands

These act as filters between the returning lymph fluid and the vessels, trapping debris and bacteria, and are part of the defence system of the body. Cancer cells are also filtered here, but unfortunately some of these cells manage to reach the main blood stream and secondary deposits of these malignant cells occur in distant tissues (**metastases**).

They also manufacture some types of white blood cells (**lymphocytes** and **monocytes)**.

## The lymphatic system

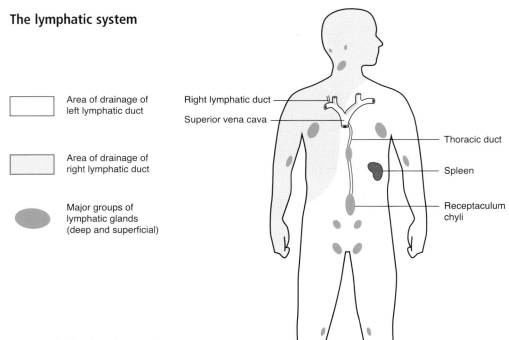

Area of drainage of left lymphatic duct

Area of drainage of right lymphatic duct

Major groups of lymphatic glands (deep and superficial)

Right lymphatic duct

Superior vena cava

Thoracic duct

Spleen

Receptaculum chyli

**Figure 28:** The lymphatic system

## Main lymph ducts

These consist of:

- **Right lymphatic duct**
- **Thoracic duct**

The right lymphatic duct drains lymph from the right upper trunk, head and right arm.

The thoracic duct receives lymph from the rest of the body. It also receives fat absorbed from the **ileum** of the small intestine.

The contents of both of these ducts empty into the main veins of the body for circulation.

## Specialised lymph glands

These include:

- **Tonsils** and **adenoids**
- **Peyer's patches** in the ileum
- **Appendix** in the large intestine
- **Spleen** in the abdominal cavity.

They act as defence mechanisms and also manufacture some types of white blood cells (**lymphocytes**).

**Peyer's patches** become infected in cases of **typhoid fever**.

The **spleen** also controls the volume and quality of blood circulating, destroys worn out red blood cells and produces **antibodies**.

## Terminology

| | |
|---|---|
| **Aden/o** | stem for gland (any) |
| **Antibody** | an immunoglobulin protein which is produced in response to the presence of an antigen or foreign protein, specific to the antigen. The production of antibodies is essential to immunity and the overcoming of infections such as measles, etc |
| **Antigen** | a substance which is capable of producing sensitivity/immunity of the body |

| | |
|---|---|
| **Antitoxins** | these neutralise poisons produced by micro-organisms |
| **Lymph/o** | stem for lymph |
| **Lymph** | fluid draining from the tissues to be returned to the circulation |
| **Lymphangi/o** | stem for lymph vessels |
| **Lymphocyte** | white blood cell which is manufactured in lymphatic tissue and fights infection by producing antibodies and antitoxins |
| **Splen/o** | stem for spleen |

## Diseases and disorders

| | |
|---|---|
| **Adenitis** | inflammation of a gland |
| **Adenoma** | tumour of glands |
| **Anasarca** | widely spread oedema |
| **Ascites** | free fluid in the peritoneal cavity |
| **GVHD** | graft versus host disease (in transplants) |
| **Hodgkin's disease** | malignant disease of the lymphatic system caused by a virus |
| **HVGD** | host versus graft disease |
| **Infectious mononucleosis** | glandular fever |
| **Lymphadenoma** | tumour of lymph gland |
| **Lymphangitis** | inflammation of lymph vessels |
| **Lymphocythaemia** | excessive number of lymphocytes in the blood |
| **Lymphocytopenia** | deficiency of lymphocytes in the blood |
| **Metastasis (pl. metastases)** | secondary deposit(s) of malignant cells from a primary tumour or source (usually through the lymph channels) |
| **Oedema** | free fluid in the tissues (fluid is not draining back to circulation) |
| **Splenitis** | inflammation of the spleen |
| **Splenomegaly** | enlargement of the spleen |

## Procedures and equipment

| | |
|---|---|
| **Adenectomy** | surgical removal of a gland |
| **Lymphangiogram** | special X-ray of the lymph vessels with an opaque dye |
| **Paracentesis abdominis** | drawing off of free fluid from the abdominal/peritoneal cavity |
| **Paracentesis thoracis** (or **thoracentesis**) | drawing off of fluid from the chest cavity (thorax) |
| **Paracentesis tympani** | drawing off of fluid from the middle ear |
| **Splenectomy** | surgical removal of the spleen |
| **Splenogram** | special X-ray of the spleen using opaque dye |

Chapter **7** | The respiratory system

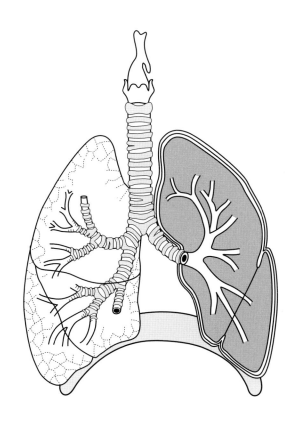

## Function

The respiratory system is concerned with the vital function of external respiration, the exchange of gases – taking in oxygen from the air and the excretion of carbon dioxide and water vapour as waste products.

## Structure

The structure of the respiratory system consists of the following organs:

- **Nose**
- **Nasopharynx** } upper respiratory tract
- **Larynx**

- **Trachea**

- **Bronchi** (two)
- **Bronchioles** } lower respiratory tract
- **Alveoli**
- **Lungs**

### Nose

The nose is made up of bone and cartilage and is connected to the **sinuses** (spaces of air). Its function is to receive, moisten, warm and filter air. It is also the organ of the sense of smell which is closely linked with taste (see Chapter 14).

### Pharynx

This extends from the back of the nose to the larynx, and the **nasopharynx** is the area at the back of the nose. The **eustachian tube** from the middle ear enters here. Both air and food pass through the pharynx.

### Larynx

The larynx *(see Figure 29)* is also known as the **voice box** as it contains the **vocal cords** *(Figure 30)*, two delicate folds of membrane which vibrate to produce sound.

The larynx is composed of several irregular-shaped cartilages:

- **Epiglottis**
- **Thyroid cartilage**
- **Arytenoid cartilages** (two)
- **Cricoid cartilage**

The **thyroid cartilage**, also known as the **Adam's apple** is found at the anterior of the larynx. The cricoid cartilage is shaped like a signet ring, whilst the **arytenoid cartilages** are attached to the vocal cords.

The entrance to the larynx, known as the **glottis**, is guarded by a flap of cartilage called the **epiglottis**. This structure prevents food or fluid passing into the air passages. This occurs automatically by a reflex action when the person is conscious. *However, in a state of unconsciousness this reflex does not occur and blockage of the airway can easily result.*

## The larynx

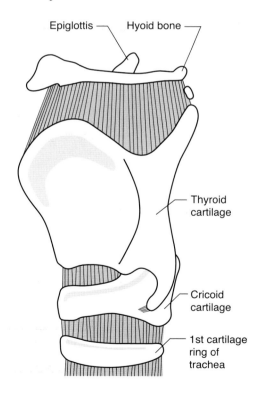

**Figure 29:** The larynx (lateral view)

## Vocal chords of the larynx

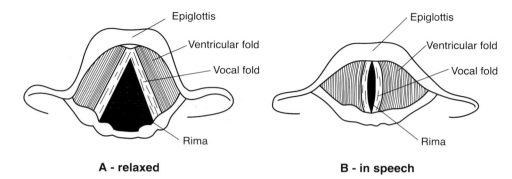

**A - relaxed**     **B - in speech**

**Figure 30:** Vocal chords of the larynx

### Trachea

This is known as the **windpipe** and is continuous with the larynx and extends to the bronchi. It is composed of several C-shaped rings of cartilage, which keep the structure open to allow air to pass down into the lungs.

### Bronchi

These are two short tubes, the right and left bronchi, continuous with the trachea and containing cartilage and muscle. The bronchi enter the lung at an area known as the **hilum**. The bronchi divide into numerous branches known as **bronchioles** – smaller tubes of similar structure to the bronchi, but which contain more muscle tissue in their walls. These take air to the delicate air sacs at their terminations known as **alveoli**.

### Lungs

These are two pink, spongy, cone-shaped organs lying in the thoracic cavity (the chest), one either side of the heart and great blood vessels. The base of each lung rests upon the **diaphragm** and the apex lies just below the level of the **clavicle** (collar-bone). The right and left lungs consist of lobes, covered in a serous membrane known as the **pleura**. The right lung, which is larger, has three lobes, the left lung has two. These are further divided into **lobules**, each being complete in itself, and including blood vessels, lymphatic vessels, elastic connective tissue, bronchioles and alveoli (*Figure 31*).

### Alveoli

These are tiny, delicate, one-cell-thick air sacs surrounded by a capillary network from the pulmonary circulation. This membrane is moist and it is only here that the exchange of gases occurs. All other parts of the respiratory tract or airway convey air to the air sacs for this vital purpose.

## Ventilation

This consists of **inspiration** (breathing in) and **expiration** (breathing out). The muscles of respiration are essential for this process; these are the **diaphragm** and the **intercostal muscles** (between the ribs).

### Inspiration

The chest cavity expands as the muscles of respiration contract, swinging the rib cage out and the diaphragm down. The action is similar to a pair of bellows and air (containing oxygen) is sucked in through the nose/mouth to fill the expanding lungs.

## Respiratory system

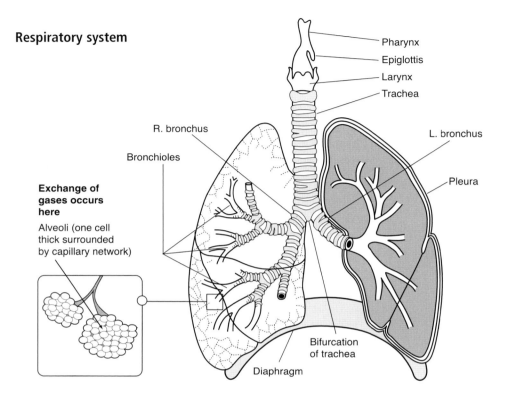

**Figure 31:** Respiratory system

## Expiration

When these muscles relax it has the opposite function to inspiration, decreasing the size of the chest cavity and forcing out expired air through the airway, removing waste gases (including carbon dioxide) and water vapour. Figures 32 and 33 show instruments designed for measuring peak expiratory flow.

## Air content

**Inspired air**  contains **21% oxygen** and **0.04% carbon dioxide**.

**Expired air**  contains **17% oxygen** and **4% carbon dioxide**.

In **cardiopulmonary resuscitation**, the presence of oxygen in the expired air provides sufficient oxygen for the patient's requirements. The higher level of carbon dioxide present can, in certain situations, also stimulate the **respiratory centre** in the brain to start spontaneous respiration

## Respiration

Breathing is an automatic process, although it can be controlled by the will. It is controlled by the respiratory centre in the brain which responds to the level of carbon dioxide in the blood. Oxygen is vital for every cell and the brain cells have the greatest requirement. If they do not receive a supply of oxygen for three to four minutes brain damage will occur and death will usually result. If the person is resuscitated after this time period, there is likely to be permanent damage to the brain.

## Exchange of gases

Pressure of oxygen in inspired air in the air sacs is high while the oxygen pressure within the capillary blood surrounding these sacs is low. Therefore the oxygen passes through the membrane into the blood, combining with the **haemoglobin** of the red cells to be carried back to the heart for distribution to the body.

Pressure of carbon dioxide in the air sacs is low, while the pressure of it within the capillary blood is high. Therefore carbon dioxide passes through the membrane into the air sac and is breathed out of the lungs on expiration.

## Respiration rate

The rate of respiration will vary with the individual, increasing with exercise, emotion, certain diseases and fever.

*Normal rate per minute*

| | |
|---|---|
| **Newborn** (first four weeks) | 40 |
| **Infants** (four weeks to one year) | 30 |
| **Children** (up to five years) | 24 |
| **Adults** | 12 – 18 |

## Abbreviations

| | |
|---|---|
| **AP** | artificial pneumothorax |
| **COAD** | chronic obstructive airway disease |
| **COLD** | chronic obstructive lung disease |
| **COPD** | chronic obstructive pulmonary disease |
| **CPR** | cardiopulmonary resuscitation |
| **FB** | foreign body |
| **IPPB** | intermittent positive pressure breathing |
| **LRTI** | lower respiratory tract infection |
| **NSCLC** | non-small cell lung cancer (slow growing type of lung cancer) |

| | |
|---|---|
| **PCP** | *Pneumocystis carinii* pneumonia (associated with AIDS) |
| **PE** | pulmonary embolism |
| **PEFR** | peak expiratory flow rate (see also vital capacity) |
| **PND** | paroxysmal nocturnal dyspnoea |
| **RD** | respiratory disease |
| **RDS** | respiratory distress syndrome |
| **SCLC** | small cell lung cancer (fast-growing, aggressive type of cancer also known as 'oat cell') |
| **SMR** | submucous resection (altering the structure of the nasal septum, i.e. cartilage division, or correcting crooked septum) |
| **SOB** | shortness of breath |
| **Ts & As** | tonsillectomy and adenoidectomy |
| **TB** | tuberculosis |
| **URI** | upper respiratory infection |
| **URTI** | upper respiratory tract infection |
| **VC** | vital capacity |

## Terminology

| | |
|---|---|
| **Adenoids** | specialised lymphatic tissue behind the nose (naso-pharynx) |
| **Bronchioles** | the smallest tubes of the lungs between the bronchi and the alveoli |
| **Bronch/o** | stem for bronchus(i) |
| **Bronchi/o** | stem for bronchioles (smaller tubes) |
| **Epiglottis** | flap of cartilage which guards the entrance of the glottis to prevent food being inhaled into the larynx (reflex action in the conscious person) |

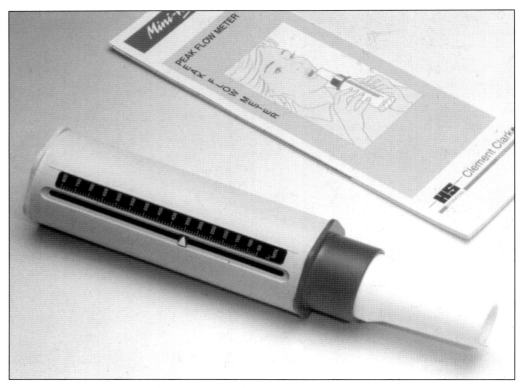

**Figure 32:** Mini-Wright standard range peak flow meter (for adults)
*Reproduced with kind permission from Clement Clarke International Ltd*

| | |
|---|---|
| **Laryng/o** | stem for larynx (voice box) |
| **Nasal** | referring to the nose |
| **Nas/o** | stem for nose. |
| **Pharyng/o** | stem for throat |
| **Pleura** | membrane covering lobes of lungs |
| **Pleur/o** | stem for pleura, covering of lungs |
| **Pneum/o** | |
| **(pneumon/o)** | stems for lungs |
| **Pnoe-** | stem for breathing |
| **Pulmon/o** | stem for lung |
| **Rhin/o** | stem for nose |
| **Tonsill/o** | stem for tonsils |
| **Trache/o** | stem for trachea (windpipe) |

| | |
|---|---|
| **Vital capacity** | amount of air which can be breathed out on a forced expiration following a forced inspiration (as on a peak expiratory flow meter) |

## Diseases and disorders

| | |
|---|---|
| **Apnoea** | cessation of breathing |
| **Asphyxia** | lack of oxygen in the blood and thus in the tissues |
| **Asthma** | inflammatory disease of the bronchial tubes due to hypersensitivity to foreign proteins (allergy) resulting in narrowing of airway as the result of bronchial constriction |

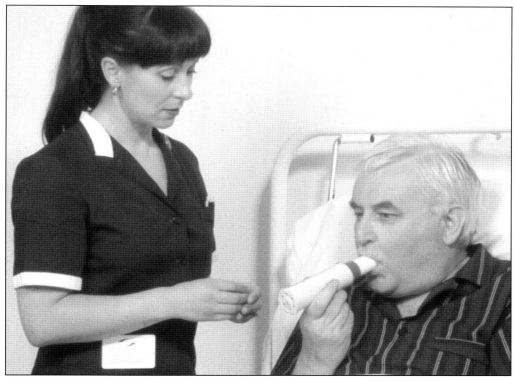

**Figure 33:** Peak flow meter in use
*Reproduced with kind permission from Clement Clarke International Ltd*

| | |
|---|---|
| **Atelectasis** | failure of the lungs to expand, e.g. at birth, or collapse of the alveoli (air sacs) |
| **Bronchiectasis** | over dilatation of the bronchioles due to fibrous tissue |
| **Bronchitis** | inflammation of the bronchial tubes |
| **Cheyne–Stokes respiration** | irregular breathing with periods of cessation of breathing (apnoea) and overbreathing (hyperventilation); this is due to change in pH of the blood passing through respiratory centre in the brain resulting from levels of urea build up in body as |

| | |
|---|---|
| | kidneys fail – this usually results in death |
| **Cor pulmonale** | right ventricular heart failure caused by lung disease |
| **Coryza** | the common cold |
| **Crêpitations** | fine crackling which can be heard |
| **Cyanosis** | blueness of the skin and mucous membranes due to lack of oxygen |
| **Dyspnoea** | difficulty in breathing |
| **Epiglottitis** | inflammation of the epiglottis |
| **Epistaxis** | nose-bleed |
| **Haemoptysis** | coughing up of blood from the lungs, usually bright red and frothy |

| | |
|---|---|
| **Hypoxia** | insufficient oxygen in the blood |
| **Laryngeal stridor** | harsh sounds on inspiration – can be due to spasm |
| **Laryngitis** | inflammation of the larynx |
| **Laryngostenosis** | constriction (narrowing) of the larynx |
| **Lobectomy** | surgical removal of a lobe of lung |
| **Nasal polyp** | pedunculated tumour of the lining of the nose (tumour with a stalk) |
| **Non-small cell lung cancer (NSCLC)** | less aggressive and slower growing type of lung cancer |
| **Oat cell** | small cell lung cancer (SCLC) fast-growing, aggressive type of cancer |
| **Orthopnoea** | only able to breath when sitting upright |
| **Pharyngitis** | inflammation of the throat (pharynx) |
| **Pleurisy (pleuritis)** | inflammation of the pleura, with effusion, producing fluid |
| **Pleurodynia** | Pain in the intercostal muscles of the chest |
| **Pneumonia (pneumonitis)** | inflammation of the lungs |
| **Pneumothorax** | air in the pleural cavity causing collapse of lung |
| **Pulmonary emphysema** | abnormal distension of the alveoli (air sacs) of the lungs in chronic respiratory disease, e.g. bronchiectasis |
| **Pulmonary empyema** | presence of pus in the pleural cavity |
| **Râle** | abnormal rattling sound heard – present in bronchitis and pneumonia |
| **Rhinitis** | inflammation of the nose |
| **Rhinorrhoea** | discharge from the nose |
| **Rhonchi** | abnormal sounds in the bronchial tubes on listening with a stethoscope (auscultation) |

| | |
|---|---|
| **Sinusitis** | inflammation of the lining of the cavities of the nasal and skull bones |
| **Sleep apnoea** | periods of cessation of breathing during sleep, particularly in men |
| **Small cell lung cancer** | fast-growing, aggressive type of cancer also known as 'oat cell' |
| **Spontaneous pneumothorax** | collapse of the lung spontaneously |
| **Stertorous** | noisy breathing, as in snoring, due to obstruction, e.g. tongue falling to back of throat |
| **Tachypnoea** | rapid breathing, as in pneumonia |
| **Tonsillitis** | inflammation of the tonsils (specialised lymphoid tissue) |
| **Tracheitis** | inflammation of the trachea |
| **Tuberculosis** | an infection of the lung or other organs by the bacteria tubercule bacillus (unfortunately this is increasing) |

## Procedures and equipment

| | |
|---|---|
| **Adenoidectomy** | surgical removal of the adenoids |
| **Antral puncture** | puncture of the antrum (sinus) in the maxillary bone of the face through the nose in order to drain pus and washout the cavity (antral washout) |
| **Artificial pneumothorax** | collapse of the lung by the deliberate introduction of air into the chest cavity |
| **Auscultation** | listening to sounds with a stethoscope |
| **Bronchogram** | special X-ray of the bronchial tubes using an opaque medium |
| **Bronchoscopy** | examination of the bronchi with a lighted instrument |

| | |
|---|---|
| **Heaf test** | skin test for tuberculosis |
| **Intubation** | introduction of a tube into air passages to allow air into the lungs (as in anaesthesia) |
| **Kveim test** | skin test for sarcoidosis |
| **Laryngectomy** | surgical removal of the larynx |
| **Laryngoscope** | a lighted instrument used for examination of the larynx |
| **Laryngoscopy** | examination of the larynx with a lighted instrument |
| **Lobectomy** | surgical removal of a lobe of the lung |
| **Mantoux test** | skin test for tuberculosis |
| **Pharyngoscopy** | examination of the pharynx with a lighted instrument |
| **Pneumonectomy** | surgical removal of the lung |
| **Rhinoplasty** | reshaping the nose |
| **Rhinoscopy** | examination of the nose with a lighted instrument |
| **Spirogram** | measurement of respiratory movements with a special machine – spirograph |
| **Tine test** | skin test for tuberculosis |
| **Tracheostomy** | making an artificial opening into the trachea (allowing air to enter the bronchi and lungs to relieve obstruction to breathing) |
| **Tracheotomy** | cutting into the trachea |
| **Underwater seal drainage** | the removal of air from the chest (thoracic) cavity by the insertion of a tube placed under water in a special drainage bottle |

Chapter **8** | The digestive (gastrointestinal) system

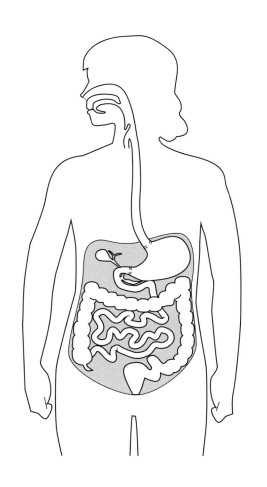

## Function

This system is concerned with the intake, breakdown and absorption of food substances for use and storage by the body cells.

Food is taken into the mouth, chewed, mixed with saliva and formed into a **bolus** which, on swallowing, is passed into the **oesophagus**. From here it travels through the remainder of the alimentary canal by means of **peristalsis** (alternate waves of contraction and relaxation of the muscular walls of the hollow organs). It mixes with the various digestive juices, secreted from glands situated in the lining of the stomach and small intestine. These juices contain enzymes which allow the chemical process of digestion to occur. Other substances are also received into the small intestine for this purpose, from the liver and pancreas, via ducts.

### Digestion

This is both:

**physical**
by means of chewing (mastication), peristalsis and churning (by muscular action of the stomach and intestinal walls) which reduce the food to smaller particles,

and

**chemical**
by the presence of chemicals, including substances known as **enzymes**. These allow chemical changes to occur enabling more simple compounds to be absorbed through the lining of the organs, especially in the ileum of the small intestine where most food substances are absorbed.

## Structure

The following organs form the system and are known as the **alimentary canal** (*see Figure 34*):

- **mouth** or **buccal cavity**
- **oral pharynx** (throat)
- **oesophagus** (gullet)
- **stomach**

- small intestine:

    **duodenum**

    **jejunum**

    **ileum**

- large intestine:

    **caecum**

    **appendix**

    **ascending colon**

    **transverse colon**

    **sigmoid colon**

    **rectum**

    **anus**

### Oesophagus

This is a strong muscular tube, situated in the thoracic cavity, extending from the pharynx above to the stomach below. It penetrates the diaphragm at its junction with the stomach.

### Stomach

This is the most dilated part of the alimentary canal, containing numerous glands, secreting enzymes and also mucus to protect its own tissues from digestion.

**Gastric juice** is produced, which includes enzymes, starting the digestion of protein, and hydrochloric acid aiding digestion. Absence of hydrochloric acid is common in **pernicious anaemia**.

The stomach is guarded at the junction to the oesophagus by a weak sphincter muscle (**cardiac sphincter**). At its junction with the duodenum is a stronger sphincter known as the **pyloric sphincter**. These regulate the entrance and exit of, the now liquid, food substances known as **chyme**.

### Sphincter muscles

A sphincter muscle consists of a ring of circular muscle which guards the entrance or exit of certain structures of the body. By its contraction or relaxation it controls the passage of various substances.

## Digestive system

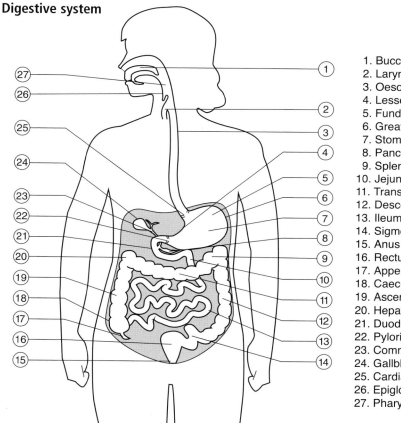

1. Buccal cavity
2. Larynx
3. Oesophagus
4. Lesser curvature
5. Fundus
6. Greater curvature
7. Stomach
8. Pancreatic duct
9. Splenic flexure
10. Jejunum of small intestine
11. Transverse colon
12. Descending colon
13. Ileum
14. Sigmoid colon
15. Anus
16. Rectum
17. Appendix
18. Caecum
19. Ascending colon
20. Hepatic flexure
21. Duodenum
22. Pyloric sphincter
23. Common bile-duct
24. Gallbladder
25. Cardiac sphincter
26. Epiglottis
27. Pharynx

**Figure 34:** The digestive system

### Small intestine

This consists of the **duodenum**, **jejunum** and **ileum**, each of which contributes to the mechanical and chemical digestion of food substances.

Numerous tiny projection-type structures, known as **villi**, are found in the lining of the small intestine, the most numerous being found in the ileum. It is through these specialised structures that most of the food substances reach the blood stream and fats, as fatty acids (**lipids**), are absorbed directly into the **lymphatic system** as **chyle**.

### Ileocaecal reflex

Whenever food or liquid is swallowed and passes into the stomach, a reflex action occurs known as the ileocaecal reflex. This involves the passing of the liquid food substances from the last part of the ileum of the small intestine, into the **caecum** through the **ileocaecal valve**, a one-way valve.

### Large intestine

This is also known as the **colon**. It consists of a long muscular tube, starting at the caecum, to which the **appendix** is attached, extending to the **anus** below. It is concerned with the reabsorption of water, mineral salts and vitamins, and the breakdown of indigestible matter (cellulose from plants) into faeces. At the act of defecation this is eliminated from the body via the anus. The anus is guarded by a voluntary sphincter muscle.

Certain vitamins, e.g. **vitamin K**, are manufactured here by the action of bacteria, naturally present in the bowel. Treatment with extended courses of oral antibiotics interfere with this function.

## Accessory organs of digestion

These consist of the following structures:

- **teeth**
- **tongue**　⎤
- **salivary glands**　⎦ in the mouth

- **pancreas**
- **liver**　⎤
- **gallbladder**　⎦ in abdominal cavity

### Teeth

There are 32 **permanent teeth** and 20 **primary** or **deciduous teeth** which are replaced in childhood and adolescence by the permanent or **secondary teeth**.

### Tongue

The tongue, also involved in speech and perception of taste (see Chapter 14), is concerned with formation of a **bolus** (a ball of food mixed with saliva), which is moved to the back of the pharynx and swallowed (**deglutition**), travelling into the oesophagus. Difficulty with swallowing is known as **dysphagia**.

### Salivary glands

The salivary glands secrete **saliva** which starts the digestion of cooked starches.

### Pancreas

The pancreas is a gland producing **insulin**. It secretes **pancreatic juice** containing several enzymes which are carried via ducts to the duodenum where it aids in the digestion of proteins, starches and sugars.

### Liver

The liver secretes bile which emulsifies fat ready for digestion and absorption. There are many other functions of the liver, including:

- The removal of nitrogen from proteins which are to be eliminated from the body (**deamination**)

- The breakdown of drugs and poisons ready for excretion by the kidneys (**detoxification**)

- Production of numerous enzymes

- Production of clotting factors, including **prothrombin**, **fibrinogen** and anti-clotting factor **heparin**

- Storage of essential vitamins, including **vitamins A**, **B**, **D** and **K**

- Storage of **iron** from worn out blood cells, and the conversion of pigments into bile pigments (**bilirubin**) which colour the faeces in which they are excreted

- Breakdown of many fatty acids (**desaturation**) ready for storage or use by the body

- Conversion and storage of glucose ready for release into the blood stream

- Production of heat for distribution via the blood stream to the rest of the body – the numerous chemical reactions occurring in the body produce heat.

### Gallbladder

The gallbladder is an elongated sac located below the liver. It stores and concentrates bile which it receives from the liver via ducts, ready for release into the duodenum of the small intestine to mix with other enzymes secreted by the intestinal walls.

## Abbreviations

| | |
|---|---|
| **ABC** | aspiration, biopsy, cytology |
| **abdo** | abdomen/abdominal |
| **Ba E** | barium enema |
| **Ba M** | barium meal |
| **BM** | bowel movement |
| **BO** | bowels open |
| **D&V** | diarrhoea and vomiting |
| **DU** | duodenal ulcer |
| **ERCP** | endoscopic retrograde cholangiopancreatography |
| **GI** | gastrointestinal |
| **GORD** | gastro-oesophageal reflux disease |
| **GU** | gastric ulcer |
| **HCl** | hydrochloric acid |
| **Hp** | *helicobacter pylori* (bacteria responsible for gastric ulcers) |
| **IBS** | irritable bowel syndrome |
| **IUC** | idiopathic ulcerative colitis |
| **IVC** | intravenous cholangiography |
| **LIF** | left iliac fossa |
| **LIH** | left inguinal hernia |
| **LLQ** | left lower quadrant |
| **LUQ** | left upper quadrant |
| **N&V** | nausea and vomiting |
| **NG** | new growth/nasogastric (tube) |
| **OGD** | oesophago-gastroduodenoscopy |
| **ORD** | oesophageal reflux disease |
| **PR** | per rectum |
| **PU** | peptic ulcer |
| **RIF** | right iliac fossa |
| **RIH** | right inguinal hernia |
| **RLQ** | right lower quadrant |
| **RUQ** | right upper quadrant |
| **UC** | ulcerative colitis |
| **UGI** | upper gastrointestinal |

## Terminology

| | |
|---|---|
| **Abdomino/o** | stem for abdomen |
| **An/o** | stem for anus |
| **Appendic/o** | stem for appendix |
| **Caec/o** | stem for caecum |
| **Chol/e** | stem for bile |
| **Cholangi/o** | stem for bile/biliary vessels |
| **Cholecyst/o** | stem for gallbladder |
| **Choledoch/o** | stem for common bile duct |
| **Col/o** | stem for colon (large intestine) |
| **Dent/o** | tooth |
| **Duoden/o** | stem for duodenum |
| **Gastr/o** | stem for stomach |
| **Gingiv/o** | stem for gums |
| **Gloss/o** | stem for tongue |
| **Hepat/o** | stem for liver |
| **Herni/o** | stem for hernia/rupture/protrusion |
| **Ile/o** | stem for ileum (part of small intestine) |
| **Jejun/o** | stem for jejunum |
| **Lapar/o** | stem for abdominal wall/flank |
| **Odont/o** | tooth |
| **Oesophag/o** | stem for oesophagus |
| **Pancreat/o** | stem for pancreas |
| **Phag/o** | swallow/eat |
| **Proct/o** | rectum |
| **Pylor/o** | part of stomach (pylorus) |
| **Rect/o (proct/o)** | stem for rectum |
| **Sial/o** | stem for salivary glands |
| **Sigmoid/o** | stem for sigmoid colon |
| **Stomat/o** | stem for mouth |
| **Atresia** | without a natural opening |
| **Biliary** | concerning bile |
| **Caries** | dental disease |
| **Deciduous teeth** | primary/first teeth (20) |
| **Orthodontal** | concerned with the correction of dentition (teeth) |
| **Orthodontist** | specialist in correction of teeth |
| **Permanent teeth** | secondary teeth (32) |

## Diseases and disorders

**Achlorhydria**   absence of hydrochloric acid secretion in the stomach

**Acholia**   absence of bile

**Adhesions**   fibrous tissue formation causes abnormal joining of two organ surfaces

**Anal fissure**   painful crack in the mucous membrane of the anus

**Anorexia**   loss of appetite

**Anorexia nervosa**   loss of appetite due to emotional states

**Appendicitis**   inflammation of the appendix of the intestine

**Ascites**   free fluid in the peritoneal cavity

**Barrett's oesophagus**   disease of the gullet where, in response to reflux of acid stomach contents, similar tissue to that which lines the stomach has grown to line the gullet (metaplasia). Danger of cancer arising from this condition

**Cholecystitis**   inflammation of the gallbladder

**Choledo-cholithiasis**   condition of stones in the bile duct

**Cholelithiasis**   condition of stones in the gallbladder

**Cirrhosis**   hardening of an organ, usually the liver

**Coeliac disease**   disease in which the protein gluten is not properly broken down – characterised by fatty stools (steatorrhoea) and failure to gain weight when it occurs in early childhood

**Colic**   spasmodic waves of pain due to contraction of muscles in tubular organs

**Colitis**   inflammation of the colon

**Crohn's disease**   chronic inflammation of the last part of the ileum (small intestine)

**Diverticulitis**   inflammation of a pouch formation in the lining of the intestine

**Diverticulum**   an abnormal pouch formation in the lining of a hollow organ, e.g. intestine

**Faecal vomiting**   present when all bowel movements have ceased – obstruction, paralytic ileus – vomit consists of liquid faeces

**Fistula**   abnormal communication between two organs or an organ with the skin

**Gastritis**   inflammation of the stomach

**Gastroenteritis**   inflammation of the stomach and intestine

**Gingivitis**   inflammation of the gums

**Haematemesis**   vomiting of blood from the stomach

**Haemorrhoid-ectomy**   surgical removal of haemorrhoids

**Haemorrhoids**   varicose veins of the rectum ('piles')

***Helicobacter pylori***   bacteria which live and reproduce in the gastric secretions of the stomach and may cause gastric ulcers

**Helminthiasis**   infestation with intestinal worms

**Hepatitis**   inflammation of the liver

**Hepatoma**   malignant tumour of the liver

**Hepatomegaly**   enlargement of the liver

**Hernia**   abnormal protrusion of an organ or structure through a weakness in a muscle

**Hiatus hernia**   protrusion of the stomach wall through a weakness in the diaphragm – allows regurgitation of acid contents

**Icterus**   Jaundice

**Intestinal obstruction**   an acute abdominal emergency – contents of intestine are unable to pass along due to obstruction, e.g. strangulated hernia

| | |
|---|---|
| **Intussusception** | the pushing of one part of the intestine into the lumen (space) of another part immediately adjacent to it; causes obstruction – common in children – an acute abdominal emergency |
| **Malocclusion** | badly aligned teeth when closing mouth |
| **Malnutrition** | deficiency of quantity or quality of food eaten |
| **McBurney's point** | area on the abdominal wall in the right iliac fossa where pain is felt when pressure is applied when diagnosing appendicitis |
| **Melaena** | black, tarry stools due to presence of digested blood (bleeding occurring) |
| **Metaplasia** | type of cells that have grown beyond the area where they are usually found |
| **Occult blood** | hidden blood, not visible to the naked eye (in stools) |
| **Oesophagitis** | inflammation of the oesophagus (gullet) |
| **Paralytic ileus** | no bowel sounds heard with stethoscope indicating no movement (peristalsis) |
| **Periodontal** | area around the tooth |
| **Peritonitis** | inflammation of the peritoneum (the membrane covering and nourishing the abdominal organs) |
| **Pilonidal sinus** | an abnormality consisting of an infolding of skin containing hair over the coccygeal area which has formed a space (sinus) and can become infected |
| **Plaque** | tartar upon the teeth causing caries etc. |
| **Proctalgia** | pain in the rectum |
| **Pyloric stenosis** | narrowing of the pyloric sphincter of the stomach (muscle fibres fail to relax sufficiently to allow passage of food from stomach into duodenum) – causes projectile vomiting, common in first-born male babies |
| **Pyorrhoea** | discharge of pus from the tooth cavity |
| **Steatorrhoea** | abnormal fatty stools |
| **Stomatitis** | inflammation of the mouth |
| **Strangulated hernia** | an acute abdominal emergency in which a portion of the alimentary canal protrudes through the muscle and becomes constricted, losing its blood supply – without intervention, gangrene will occur |
| **Ulcerative colitis** | chronic inflammatory disease of the colon which causes diarrhoea, blood and mucus in the stools |
| **Volvulus** | twisting of intestine upon itself, causing obstruction |

## Procedures and equipment

| | |
|---|---|
| **Abdominoperineal excision** | surgical removal of rectum and part of colon and a colostomy created |
| **Anastomosis** | surgical joining of two hollow organs |
| **Appendicectomy** | surgical removal of the appendix |
| **Barium enema** | X-ray where barium compound (opaque medium) is inserted into the bowel via the rectum for diagnostic purposes |
| **Barium meal** | as above, but taken by mouth |
| **Barium swallow** | as above, but the swallowing process is also screened |
| **Cholecystectomy** | surgical removal of the gallbladder |
| **Colectomy** | surgical removal of all or part of the colon |
| **Colostomy** | making an artificial opening of the colon onto the abdominal wall |

**Endoscopic retrograde cholangio-pancreatogram**    special X-ray of gall-bladder and pancreas using fluorescent dye which is inserted into ampulla of Vater ducts from duodenum using a duodenoscope with a catheter attached. It allows investigation of bile and pancreatic ducts and their contents. Cytology and biochemistry tests are performed

**Endoscopy**    examination of a hollow organ with a lighted flexible tube – fibre optics

**Extraction**    removal of (e.g.tooth)

**Gastrectomy**    surgical removal of the stomach

**Gastrojejunostomy**    anastomosis (joining together) the stomach and jejunum having removed or bypassed the duodenum; similar anastomosis terms follow this form

**Gastroscope**    lighted instrument used to examine the stomach

**Gastroscopy**    examination of the stomach with a lighted instrument

**Gastrostomy**    an artificial opening into the stomach, usually for feeding purposes

**Gastrotomy**    cutting into the stomach

**Herniorrhaphy**    surgical repair of a hernia

**Ileostomy**    making an artificial opening of the ileum onto the abdominal wall

**Laparoscopy**    examination of the abdomen with a lighted instrument through the abdominal wall

**Laparotomy**    incision into the abdominal wall for exploratory purposes

**Oesophagectomy**    surgical removal of the oesophagus

**Proctoscope**    lighted instrument for examination of the rectum

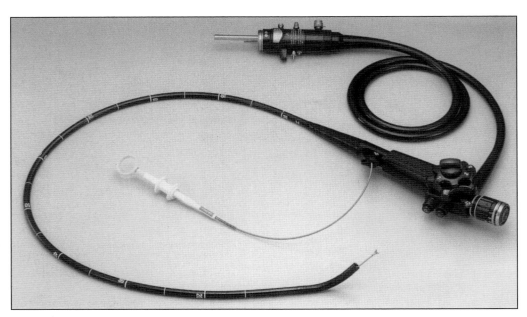

**Figure 35:** A gastrointestinal fibrescope

*Reproduced with kind permission from Keymed (Medical and Industrial Equipment) Ltd*

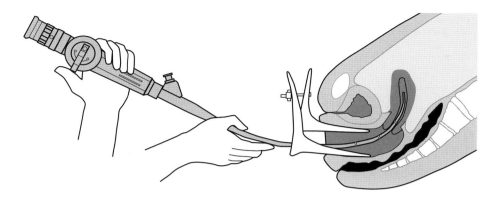

**Figure 36:** Hysteroscopy *Reproduced with kind permission from Keymed (Medical and Industrial Equipment) Ltd*

| | |
|---|---|
| **Proctoscopy** | examination of the rectum with a lighted instrument |
| **Ramstedt's operation** | cutting into tight muscle fibres of pyloric sphincter of stomach and reshaping the stomach wall (for pyloric stenosis in babies) |

## Endoscopy

Endoscopy is the examination of a canal or hollow organ with a lighted instrument (*Figures 35 and 36*). The conventional **endoscope** is rigid and non-flexible which has been widely replaced by the flexible fibre-optic variety. The

**Table 3:** Examples of endoscopies

| Procedure | Examination | Description |
|---|---|---|
| **Oesophagoscopy** | Oesophagus | Use of oesophagoscope for visual examination of oesophagus or removal of foreign body. |
| **Gastroscopy** | Stomach | Visual examination of stomach using a gastroscope inserted via the mouth and oesophagus. Biopsy and aspiration are performed. |
| **Duodenoscopy** | Duodenum (part of small intestine) | Visual examination of duodenum via mouth, oesophagus and stomach. Biopsy and aspiration are performed. |
| **Colonoscopy** | Large intestine | Visual examination of colon via rectum using a colonoscope. Polyps may be removed and a biopsy performed. |
| **Sigmoidoscopy** | Sigmoid area of large intestine | Visual examination of the sigmoid colon via the rectum using a sigmoidoscope. Polyps may be removed and a biopsy performed. |
| **Proctosigmoidoscopy** | Rectum and sigmoid area | Visual examination using proctoscope or sigmoidoscope. Polyps may be removed and a biopsy performed. |
| **Endoscopic retrograde cholangiopancreatography** | Bile and pancreatic ducts | X-ray by insertion of dye into ampulla of Vater via catheter attached to endoscope inserted into duodenum. |

endoscope is inserted into a hollow organ or tube such as the alimentary canal. Visual examination is performed and photography, biopsy and aspiration are carried out in appropriate cases *(Table 3)*.

Commonly, an **oesophagogastroduodenoscopy** (**OGD**) is performed which examines all three areas of the alimentary canal. Any lesion or abnormality can be seen and samples can be taken for histology.

## Other common endoscopies

| Procedure | Examination of |
|---|---|
| **Laryngoscopy** | larynx (voice box) |
| **Tracheoscopy** | trachea (windpipe) |
| **Bronchoscopy** | bronchial tubes |
| **Laparoscopy** | lower abdominal cavity via the umbilicus (also used for biopsy of ovaries and female sterilisation) |
| **Colposcopy** | vagina |
| **Culdoscopy** | through the recto-uterine pouch of pelvic peritoneum (pouch of Douglas) to view pelvic cavity |
| **Hysteroscopy** | cavity of uterus |
| **Cystoscopy** | bladder |
| **Retinoscopy** | retina of eye |
| **Rhinoscopy** | nasal cavities |
| **Otoscopy** | ear canal |

Chapter **9**

# The urinary system

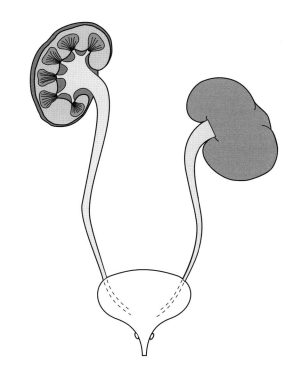

The urinary system is concerned with the removal of waste products from the body and the maintenance of correct water and **electrolyte** (ion) levels.

## Function

The kidneys remove the nitrogenous content from the protein food substances which have not been utilised by the body, after they have been broken down for excretion by the liver (deamination). Protein cannot be stored by the body. Drugs and toxins are also removed in this way.

The kidneys act as filters and also selectively secrete and reabsorb substances from the blood to maintain the correct balance of salts, water and other substances. This is an example of **homeostasis**, whereby the body is kept in the correct state for functioning. A sufficiently high blood pressure is necessary for this to occur and any prolonged condition of extreme **hypotension** (abnormally low blood pressure) can cause permanent damage to the kidneys.

## Structure

It comprises the following organs (*see Figure 37*):

- Two **kidneys**
- Two **ureters**
- **Bladder**
- **Urethra**

### Kidneys

Kidneys are brown/purple bean-shaped vascular organs which are divided into **lobules.** They lie on the posterior part of the abdominal cavity deeply embedded in fat, and are surrounded by a capsule consisting of an outer portion, the **cortex**, and an inner portion, the **medulla**. The medulla shows striations called **pyramids**; these project into the **pelvis of the kidney** which is continuous with the **ureter**. On the upper pole of each kidney is the **adrenal** or **supra-renal** gland.

### Microscopic structure of kidneys

The complex structures forming the kidneys are called **nephrons**, of which there are approximately 1 million in each. A nephron consists of a structure called a **Malpighian body** (in which **filtration** occurs) and various tubules, where substances are either secreted from or reabsorbed into the blood. Nephrons have a very rich blood supply.

### Nephron

The nephron consists of the following microscopic structures:

- **Glomerulus**, collectively known as Malpighian body or **glomeruli** apparatus
- **Bowman's capsule**
- **First convoluted tubule (proximal)**
- **Loop of Henle**
- **Second convoluted tubule (distal)**
- **Collecting tubule**

### Malpighian body or glomeruli apparatus

A Malpighian body, also known as the glomeruli apparatus, consists of the **glomerulus** and a cup-shaped tubular structure called the **Bowman's capsule**. The glomerulus consists of a tuft of capillaries tightly packed into the Bowman's capsule, which is the expanded commencement of a 'uriniferous' or **kidney tubule**.

The small arteries leading into the glomerulus (**afferent vessels**) are wider than the arteries leaving the glomerulus (**efferent vessels**), thus back-pressure arises to allow filtration of substances from the blood to occur in the Bowman's capsule.

### Tubules

The first convoluted tubule (**proximal tubule**) is coiled and continuous with the Bowman's capsule, the loop of Henle which dips down into the medulla of the kidney, and the second convoluted tubule (**distal tubule**) which joins the collecting tubule, also situated in the medulla.

## Urinary system

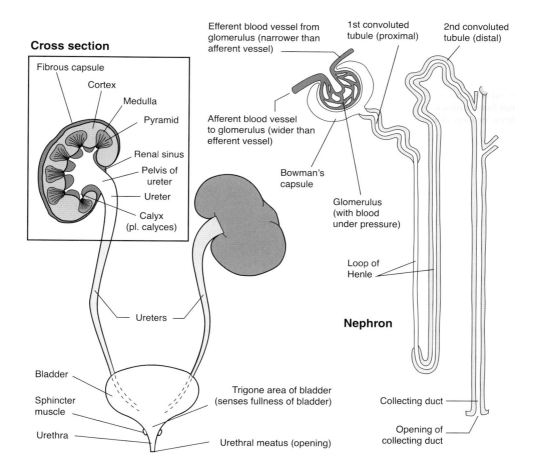

**Cross section**

Fibrous capsule
Cortex
Medulla
Pyramid
Renal sinus
Pelvis of ureter
Ureter
Calyx (pl. calyces)

Efferent blood vessel from glomerulus (narrower than afferent vessel)

1st convoluted tubule (proximal)

2nd convoluted tubule (distal)

Afferent blood vessel to glomerulus (wider than efferent vessel)

Bowman's capsule

Glomerulus (with blood under pressure)

Loop of Henle

**Nephron**

Ureters

Bladder
Sphincter muscle
Urethra

Trigone area of bladder (senses fullness of bladder)

Urethral meatus (opening)

Collecting duct

Opening of collecting duct

**Figure 37:** The urinary system

The collecting tubule terminates at a cup-shaped structure called the **calyx** (plural **calyces**) which opens into the pelvis of the kidney.

The Malpighian bodies and convoluted tubules are found in the **cortex** of the kidney where they are richly supplied with blood.

*Formation of urine*

Urine is formed by the following processes:

- **Filtration** – Non-selective
- **Secretion** – Selective
- **Reabsorption**

## Filtration

Filtration is a non-selective process which takes place in the Malpighian bodies. Water, salts, glucose, **urea**, **uric acid** and toxins are filtered from the blood in the glomerulus into the Bowman's capsule (pressure in the glomerulus is high due to the efferent arteries being narrower than the afferent vessels). The capillary walls are more permeable than those elsewhere in the body. The fluid produced in the Bowman's capsule by this pressure is known as **filtrate**.

## Secretion

Secretion occurs mainly in the first and second convoluted tubules. Special secretory cells line the tubules and **selectively** secrete substances from the blood which are at a high level, e.g. glucose in cases of **diabetes mellitus**. Foreign substances such as drugs and toxins will also be secreted. Similarly, any waste products of metabolism which have not already been filtered will be secreted into the tubules.

## Reabsorption

Harm would occur if all the fluid, salts and food substances (such as glucose) filtered from the blood were allowed to leave the body. Specialised cells **selectively** reabsorb the necessary factors. In the loop of Henle most of the water is reabsorbed and the salt balance is restored mainly in the second convoluted tubule. The **'renal threshold'** (whereby the level of various substances retained or excreted by the kidneys is governed by the requirements of the body) is another example of homeostasis.

Hormones influence reabsorption; **aldosterone** secreted by the adrenal cortex stimulates the sodium/potassium reabsorption or secretion by the second convoluted tubule. The action of the pituitary hormone, **anti-diuretic hormone (ADH)**, influences the amount of water reabsorbed.

After all these processes the end product is urine which is acid in reaction. This passes to the collecting tubules and then into the pelvis of the kidney. Approximately 1 litre of urine is secreted in 24 hours.

## Kidney damage

Any damage or disease to the kidney will obviously affect the processes of filtration, secretion and reabsorption, resulting in many beneficial factors, such as the **protein albumin** being lost from the body. Not all harmful substances and waste products will be excreted. If the damage is sufficient, then the resultant renal failure may require **dialysis** (the removal of waste products by artificial means) or a kidney transplant.

## Erythropoietin and renin

The kidneys also secrete a hormone known as erythropoietin which affects the production of red blood cells. In patients on permanent dialysis these red blood cells can become depleted, causing anaemia. The hormone **renin** is also produced by the kidneys and helps to maintain blood pressure. It acts by converting one of the blood proteins into **angiotensin** which causes constriction of the arterioles, thus raising blood pressure.

# Pelvis of the kidney

The dilated portion of the kidney, which acts as a funnel for the collection of the secreted urine from the tubules, is known as the pelvis of the kidney. Urine passes through this on its way to the ureters.

# Ureters

These are two muscular tubes which convey urine from the kidneys to the bladder. They are joined obliquely to the base of the bladder at an area known as the **trigone**.

## Bladder

This is a hollow, pear-shaped muscular sac where urine is stored before micturition (passing of urine) through the urethral **meatus** (opening). It is capable of great expansion and rises in the abdomen as it fills. Micturition is a reflex action which, after infancy, is normally controlled at will. In **incontinence** this property is lost.

Normal content of the bladder is approximately 150 ml, but it can hold up to 350-400 ml. A **sphincter muscle** guards the bladder opening.

## Urethra

This is a muscular tube through which the urine is passed to the outside of the body. It is short in the female - one to two inches in length – and seven to eight inches in the male. It is guarded by a **sphincter muscle**.

## Composition of urine

Normal urine has the following composition: straw-coloured acid fluid pH 5-7, containing –

| | |
|---|---|
| **Water** | 96% |
| **Solids** | 2% salts |
| **Nitrogenous products** of urea and uric acid | 2% |
| **Creatinine** – waste product of cell metabolism | |

## Abbreviations

| | |
|---|---|
| **AGN** | acute glomerulonephritis |
| **BNO** | bladder neck obstruction |
| **CAPD** | continuous ambulatory peritoneal dialysis |
| **C&S** | culture and sensitivity (to grow any micro-organisms and determine the antibiotic to which they are sensitive) |
| **CSU** | catheter specimen of urine |
| **EMU** | early morning urine |
| **ESL** | extracorporeal shock-wave lithotripsy |
| **GU** | genitourinary |
| **HPU** | has passed urine |
| **HNPU** | has not passed urine |
| **KUB** | kidney, ureter, and bladder (X-ray) |
| **MSU** | midstream specimen of urine |
| **NAD** | no abnormality detected/demonstrated |
| **NOAD** | no other abnormality demonstrated |

| | |
|---|---|
| **IVP** | intravenous pyelogram |
| **IVU** | intravenous urogram |
| **pH** | acid/alkaline balance |
| **RGP** | retrograde pyelogram |
| **UA** | urinalysis |
| **UTI** | urinary tract infection |
| **VCU** | voiding cystourethrogram |
| **VCUG** | voiding cystourethrogram |

## Terminology

| | |
|---|---|
| **Cyst/o** | stem for bladder |
| **Glomerul/o** | stem for glomerulus (part of nephron) |
| **Nephr/o** (pyel/o, ren/o) | stem for kidney |
| **Pyel/o** | stem for pelvis of kidney |
| **Ur/o** | stem for urine |
| **Ureter/o** | stem for ureter |
| **Urethr/o** | stem for urethra |
| **Urin/o** | stem for urine |
| **-uria** | suffix for condition of urine |
| **Genitourologist** | specialist in the treatment of sexually transmitted diseases |
| **Glomerulus** | small tuft of capillaries found within Bowman's capsule, forming part of the nephron |
| **Micturition** | the act of passing urine |
| **Urologist** | specialist in diseases of the urinary system |
| **Urology** | study of the urinary system |

## Diseases and disorders

| | |
|---|---|
| **Albuminuria** | the abnormal presence of albumin in the urine (protein) |
| **Anuria** | suppression of urine secretion from the kidneys – renal failure |
| **Bilirubinuria** | presence of bile pigments in the urine |
| **Biluria** | presence of bile salts in the urine |

| | |
|---|---|
| **Cystalgia** | pain in the bladder |
| **Cystitis** | inflammation of the bladder |
| **Cystocele** | protrusion of the bladder, usually into the vaginal wall |
| **Cystolithiasis** | condition of stones in the bladder |
| **Diuresis** | increase in the production of urine |
| **Dysuria** | difficulty/pain in passing urine |
| **Enuresis/ eneuresis** | bedwetting |
| **Glomerulo- nephritis** | any of a group of kidney diseases involving the glomeruli |
| **Glycosuria** | presence of glucose in the urine |
| **Haematuria** | presence of blood in the urine |
| **Hydronephrosis** | backlog of urine in the pelvis causing pressure and damaging the kidney |
| **Incontinence** | inability to control the passing of urine or faeces |
| **Ketonuria** | presence of acetone in the urine |
| **Nephritis** | inflammation of the kidney |
| **Nephrolith** | a kidney stone (calcium salts) |
| **Nephrolithiasis** | the condition of stones in the kidney |
| **Nephropathy** | degenerative disease of the kidney |
| **Nephrosis** | disease of the kidney |
| **Nephrotic syndrome** | extensive signs and symptoms of kidney disease; can be caused by a variety of disorders, usually glomerulonephritis |
| **Nocturnal enuresis /eneuresis** | bedwetting at night |
| **Oliguria** | scanty production of urine |
| **Papilloma** | a simple benign tumour of the bladder lining – can become malignant |
| **Phenylketonuria (PKU)** | presence of abnormal breakdown of protein in urine in hereditary disease of PKU; screened for at birth as causes mental deficiency if not treated |
| **Polydipsia** | excessive thirst |
| **Polyuria** | passing large amounts of urine |
| **Pyelitis** | inflammation of the pelvis of the kidney |
| **Pyelonephritis** | inflammation of the kidney and its pelvis |
| **Pyuria** | presence of pus in the urine |
| **Renal calculus** | kidney stone |
| **Renal colic** | severe spasmodic pain caused by presence of kidney stones in the renal system (kidneys or tubules) |
| **Renal failure** | the kidneys fail to produce sufficient urine to remove waste substances from the blood |
| **Urethral stricture** | narrowing of the urethra |
| **Uraemia** | high levels of urea (the waste part containing nitrogen) in the blood |
| **Ureteritis** | inflammation of the ureters |
| **Ureterolith** | stone in the ureter |
| **Ureterolithiasis** | condition of stones in the ureters |
| **Urethritis** | inflammation of the urethra |
| **Urethrocele** | protrusion of the urethra, usually into the anterior vaginal wall |

## Procedures and equipment

| | |
|---|---|
| **Catheterisation** | the withdrawal of urine from the bladder by the insertion of a catheter (fine hollow tube) into the urethra |
| **Continuous** | removing toxins and waste |

**ambulant peritoneal dialysis (CAPD)** products from the body in kidney failure by passing the peritoneal fluid through a bag (containing chemicals) attached to the abdomen

**Cystectomy** surgical removal of the bladder

**Cystoscope** instrument used to examine the bladder

**Cystoscopy** examination of the bladder with a lighted instrument

**Dialysis** artificial filtration of the blood to remove waste products by machine or by chemical means (peritoneal dialysis)

**Extracorporeal shock-wave lithotripsy** see lithotriptor

**Intravenous pyelogram** special X-ray demonstrating the shape and condition of the kidneys, ureters and bladder by intravenous injection of an opaque dye into the veins of the arm

**Lithotripsy** the breaking up of kidney stones (calculi) by a lithotriptor

**Lithotriptor** a machine which is used to break up stones by use of shock waves (pieces are then passed in the urine)

**Micturating cystogram** special X-ray of the bladder when passing urine to demonstrate any weakness in muscles

**Micturition** act of passing urine

**Nephrectomy** surgical removal of the kidney

**Nephrotomy** cutting into the kidney

**Peritoneal dialysis** artificial removal of waste products from the blood by means of passing peritoneal fluid from the abdominal cavity through a chemical (externally)

**Retrograde pyelogram** special X-ray of the kidney pelvis ureters and bladder by the insertion of fine catheters via the urethra and insertion of an opaque dye

**Ureterotomy** cutting into the ureter

**Voiding cysto-urethrogram** see micturating cystogram. Urethra is also demonstrated.

Chapter **10** | The skin

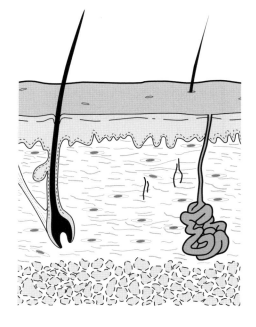

The skin is a vital organ which covers the whole of the body surface and is continuous with the mucous membranes.

## Structure

It is composed of (*see Figure 38*):

- **Epidermis**

- **Dermis**

- Appendages of **hair** and **nails**

### Epidermis

This is the uppermost layer of the skin and consists of several layers of stratified squamous epithelial-type cells. The top layers have no nucleus and are flattened and scaly. This is known as the horny layer or **keratin scales**. They are constantly being rubbed away and shed. These areas are thicker in various areas of the body which have to withstand friction and pressure, e.g. soles of feet.

The bottom layer of the epidermis, known as the **Basal (Malpighian) layer**, is the germinative layer from which these cells originate. It is here that the pigmentation (**melanin**), which gives rise to the colour of the skin, is found. There are no blood vessels in this layer and it is nourished by **lymph**.

### Dermis

This is the layer found beneath the epidermis. It is composed of dense connective tissue containing elastic fibres and numerous structures:

- **blood vessels**

- **sensory nerve endings**

- **hair follicles** attached to small muscles

- **sweat glands**

- **ebaceous glands**

**Blood vessels** are numerous and are concerned not only with nourishment and delivery of vital substances to the skin, but also with the control of body temperature.

**Sensory nerve endings** are concerned with the relay of messages to the brain concerning touch, pressure, pain and temperature changes.

### Sweat glands

These are concerned in the production of **sweat**, which excretes waste substances of water and salts from the body and also aids in the control of body temperature by loss of heat through **evaporation**.

### Sebaceous glands

These produce a substance known as **sebum** which keeps the skin and hairs supple. Blockage of the duct of the gland produces a condition known as a **sebaceous cyst**.

### Appendages

The hairs and nails are found in the dermis but are really outgrowths of the **epidermal** layer, as are sweat and sebaceous glands. Nails are protective and are outgrowths of the horny layer of the epidermis.

Beneath the dermis is a **subcutaneous layer** of connective tissue containing fat which helps to prevent heat loss.

## Function

### Control of body temperature

This is one of the main functions of the skin and is under the control of the brain. Special cells in the brain centre are triggered by the temperature of the blood flowing through it which, when the body temperature is becoming too hot, cause dilatation of the blood vessels in the skin, thus bringing more blood closer to the surface of the body. Sweat glands are stimulated to produce more sweat, excreting it through the pores onto the body surface where it evaporates.

**Evaporation** is a very efficient form of heat loss. **Radiation**, **convection** and **conduction** from the body surface also contribute to loss of body heat.

# Structure of the skin

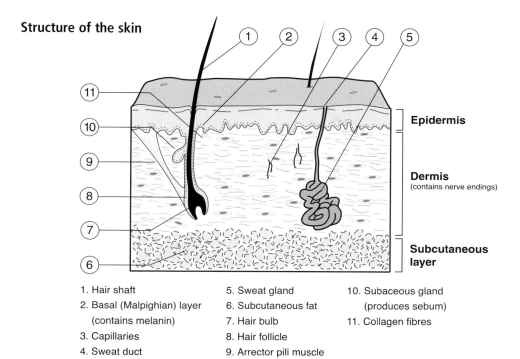

1. Hair shaft
2. Basal (Malpighian) layer (contains melanin)
3. Capillaries
4. Sweat duct
5. Sweat gland
6. Subcutaneous fat
7. Hair bulb
8. Hair follicle
9. Arrector pili muscle
10. Subaceous gland (produces sebum)
11. Collagen fibres

**Figure 38:** Structure of the skin

Conversely, blood vessels constrict causing a transfer of blood to the centre of the body (core) and less heat is lost. Small muscles attached to hairs make them erect and cause 'goose pimples' which are an attempt to produce heat and allow hairs to trap air to provide insulation of the body, when it is cold. This is a remaining reflex from a more primitive form of life in evolution, when the body was covered in hair.

The average body temperature is 37°C, but varies during the day being lower in the morning.

## Summary of other functions

- **Protection** by preventing micro-organisms entering the body and causing infection

- **Preservation** of body fluid

- **Conveys sensations** of touch, temperature, pain and pressure to the brain

- **Produces sweat** and excretes waste products by this action

- **Produces sebum**

- Converts a substance known as **ergosterol**, present in skin, to **vitamin D** in the presence of ultraviolet light in sunshine. This vitamin is necessary for healthy bones and teeth

- It is capable of **absorbing** some drugs, e.g. anti-inflammatory drugs

- It gives origin to the **hair** and **nails** which continue to grow for a short time after death

## Abbreviations

| | |
|---|---|
| DLE | disseminated lupus erythematosus |
| SLE | systemic lupus erythematosus |

## Skin lesions

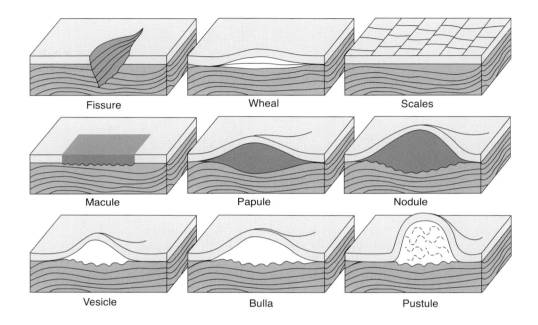

Fissure    Wheal    Scales

Macule    Papule    Nodule

Vesicle    Bulla    Pustule

**Figure 39:** Skin lesions *Redrawn after Glylys BA (1995) Medical Terminology: A Systems Approach, 3rd edn. FA Davis.*

## Terminology

| | |
|---|---|
| **Cutane/o** | skin |
| **Derma/to** | stem for skin |
| **Hidr/o** | sweat |
| **Kerat/o** | stem for scaly, horny |
| **Onych/o** | stem for nail |
| **Pil/o** | hair |
| **Trich/o** | stem for hair |
| **Ungu/o** | nails |
| **Dermatologist** | medical specialist of skin diseases |
| **Percutaneous** | through the skin (infusions) |
| **Subcutaneous** | under the dermis layer of the skin |

## Diseases and disorders (see *Figure 39*)

| | |
|---|---|
| **Abscess** | collection of pus in a cavity |
| **Acne rosacea** | skin disease due to thinning of the skin producing acne- like spots – can be caused by excessive use of steroid skin applications |
| **Acne vulgaris** | skin disease – inflammation of sebaceous glands causing papules (red spots) and pustules to form – common in adolescence |
| **Bullae** | large (fluid containing) blisters |

| | |
|---|---|
| **Carcinoma of the skin** | |
| **Basal cell** | cancer of the basal layer |
| **Melanoma** | cancer of the pigmented layer (invasive) |
| **Squamous cell** | cancer of the middle layer of the epidermis (invasive) |
| **Cellulitis** | inflammation of the sub-cutaneous layer of the skin |
| **Chancre** | an ulcer-type sore – primary stage of syphilis |
| **Comedone** | blackhead |
| **Contusion** | bruise – bleeding beneath the skin |
| **Cyst** | membrane – encapsulated sac containing fluid or other materials |
| **Decubitus ulcer** | bed sore (pressure sore) |
| **Dermatitis** | inflammation of the skin |
| **Dermatosis** | disease of the skin |
| **Dermoid cyst** | cyst present at birth containing embryonic materials – skin, nails, teeth etc; usually found in the ovary |
| **Eczema** | inflammatory skin disease due to allergy, usually against food; common in flexures of skin |
| **Erosion** | rubbing away of tissues |
| **Erysipelas** | acute contagious condition of the skin causing pain, fever and local inflammation of skin, usually on the face (caused by haemolytic streptococcus bacteria) |
| **Erythema** | reddening of skin |
| **Excoriation** | injury worsened by act of friction (scratching) |
| **Exfoliation** | scaling of skin tissue in layers |
| **Fissure** | a split or cleft |
| **Folliculitis** | inflammation of a hair follicle |
| **Furuncle** | a boil – an infection of the tissue around a hair follicle |
| **Haemangioma** | birth mark (e.g. port wine type) |

| | |
|---|---|
| **Herpes simplex** | virus causing skin infection, usually cold sores |
| **Herpes zoster** | painful shingles skin eruption along nerve path due to chicken pox virus |
| **Hidrosis** | sweating |
| **Hirsuitism** | excessive amount of body hair |
| **Hives** | (also known as urticaria) weal-type spots due to allergy, as in nettle rash |
| **Hyperhidrosis** | excessive production of sweat |
| **Hyperkeratosis** | thickening of the horny layer of the skin |
| **Impetigo** | acute contagious disease producing pustules and scabs |
| **Keloid scar** | overgrowth of scar tissue |
| **Lesion** | any abnormal change in tissue |
| **Lupus erythematosus** | inflammatory dermatitis characterised by 'butterfly' lesion over nose and cheeks; may become widespread and destroy vital tissues |
| **Macule** | spot or discolouration of skin not raised above the surface, e.g. measles rash |
| **Malignant melanoma** | virulent cancerous invasive type of melanin- (pigment-) producing cells |
| **Melanoma** | pigmented mole of melanin-producing cells |
| **Morbilliform** | describing a type of rash – similar to measles rash |
| **Naevus** | birth mark |
| **Nodule** | a small node (protuberence or swelling) |
| **Onychogryphosis** | thickened deformed nails |
| **Pachydermatous** | thickened skin |
| **Papilloma** | simple tumour (not malignant) |
| **Papule** | spot – small raised solid elevation |
| **Paronychia** | infection of a nailbed (whitlow) |

| | |
|---|---|
| **Pediculosis** | infestation with lice |
| **Pemphigus** | blister-like eruptions which can be acute or chronic |
| **Petechiae** | small purplish patches under skin due to fluid escaped from small blood vessels – can be sign of recent asphyxiation or pressure |
| **Prodromal rash** | a fleeting rash which appears before the true rash of an infectious disease |
| **Pruritus** | irritation of the skin |
| **Psoriasis** | chronic skin disease characterised by scaly patches of unknown cause |
| **Pustule** | pus-filled small elevation of the skin |
| **Roseola** | a rose-coloured rash as in secondary syphilis |
| **Scabies** | infestation with the parasite scabies mite producing itching and soreness |
| **Scales** | compact layers of epithelial tissue shed from the skin |
| **Seborrhoea** | overactivity of the sebaceous glands which produce excessive sebum |
| **Tinea pedis** | athlete's foot |

| | |
|---|---|
| **Trichosis** | any abnormal state of hair |
| **Ulcer** | an open sore of skin or mucous membranes |
| **Urticaria** | nettle rash, an allergic reaction |
| **Vesicle** | small fluid-filled blister |
| **Vitiligo** | patchy white depigmentation of the skin |
| **Wart (verucca)** | an epidermal tumour of viral origin, or any benign hardening |
| **Wheal** | an acute reaction of the skin in nettle rash/urticaria/hives |
| **Xeroderma** | abnormally dry skin |

## Procedures and equipment

| | |
|---|---|
| **Débridement** | surgical cleaning of wounds by removing dead tissues |
| **Dermatology** | scientific study of the skin |
| **Dermatome** | instrument used to cut very thin layers of skin for skin grafting |
| **Escharectomy** | removal of scar tissue |
| **Escharotomy** | dividing burn-scar tissue (to prevent scarring) |

Chapter **11**

# The female reproductive system, pregnancy and childbirth

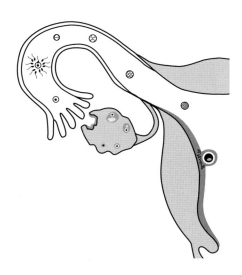

## Introduction

This chapter is concerned with women's reproductive health. It is presented in two sections:

### Gynaecology:

The branch of medicine that deals with disorders of the female reproductive system

### Obstetrics:

The branch of medicine that deals with **pregnancy**, **childbirth** and the **puerperium** (the first six weeks after giving birth)

---

**Note on spelling: Fetus or foetus**

In recent years, **'fetus'** has become the accepted UK spelling in medical and scientific publishing and has been adopted in this text. However, readers should be aware that some organisations prefer to use the old spelling **'foetus'**.

Candidates for examinations should find out which spelling is preferred by their examiners. If in doubt, candidates should make it clear that they recognise both spellings.

---

# Gynaecology

## The female reproductive system

### Structure

The female reproductive system is concerned in the reproduction of the species (*see Figures 40 and 41*). It is composed of both internal and external organs.

#### Internal organs

- Two **ovaries**
- Two **fallopian tubes**
- **Uterus**
- **Vagina**

situated in the pelvic cavity

*Ovaries*

The ovaries, situated in the pelvic cavity, are the female **gonads** and produce **ova** (eggs) after **menstruation** starts (**menarche**). They are under the influence of the hormones from the **pituitary gland** and produce the female sex hormones **oestrogen** and **progesterone** at different stages of the menstrual cycle.

Oestrogen is responsible for the development of the female sexual characteristics, while progesterone, produced in the second phase of the menstrual cycle, supplements the action of oestrogen by thickening the lining of the uterus ready for the possible implantation of a fertilised egg. Progesterone also stimulates the breasts, preparing them for **lactation**. The female is born with all the eggs (immature) present at birth. Normally only one egg (**ovum**) ripens and is released each month.

At the **menopause** (**climacteric**), egg production and hormonal secretion cease, although the adrenal gland cortex continues to influence the production of sex hormones at a lower level.

*Fallopian tubes*

These are situated one each side of the uterus, and attached to the ovaries by fine, finger-like strands. They are composed of muscle and are hollow tube-like structures which carry the released ovum along into the uterus ready for embedding, or shedding if fertilisation has not occurred. **Fertilisation** occurs when the male **spermatazoon** fuses with the ovum in the fallopian tube.

# Female reproductive system

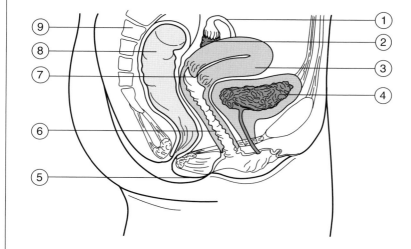

1. Fallopian tube
2. Ovary
3. Uterus
4. Bladder
5. Perineum
6. Vagina
7. Cervix
8. Rectum
9. Vertebrae

**Figure 40:** The female reproductive system (side view)

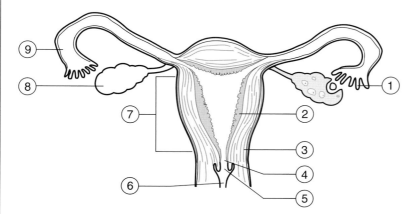

1. Fimbria
2. Endometrium (lining of uterus)
3. Myometrium
4. Cervical canal
5. Cervical os
6. Vagina
7. Uterus
8. Ovary
9. Fallopian tube

**Figure 41:** Female reproductive system (front view)

*93*

### Uterus

This consists of a muscular pear-shaped hollow organ partially covered in a layer of membrane known as the **peritoneum**. It normally slopes forwards (**anteverted**).

The three layers are the:

- **peritoneum**
- **myometrium**
- **endometrium**

The neck of the uterus is known as the **cervix** and protrudes into the **vagina** which envelopes it.

The endometrium, the lining of the uterus, is under the influence of the female hormones and is the site for the embedding of the fertilised ovum. If fertilisation and embedding do not occur, the lining is shed in monthly menstruation.

### Vagina

This is a muscular tube-like structure of vascular, **erectile tissue** extending from the cervix of the uterus above to the **vulva** externally below. Its function is for the deposit of the male spermatazoa, a passage way for menstruation and the birth of a baby. Its walls are convoluted to allow for expansion.

### External organs

Collectively these are known as the vulva (*see Figure 42*). They consist of the:

| | |
|---|---|
| **Bartholin's glands** | two glands, one in each of the labia minora providing a secretion lubricating the vestibule |
| **Clitoris** | a rudimentary penis of erectile tissue (becomes engorged with blood) |
| **Hymen** | thin membrane guarding the entrance to the vagina |
| **Labia majora** | large outer lips |
| **Labia minora** | smaller inner lips |
| **Mons veneris** | pad of fat upon the pubis |
| **Perineum** | area of skin and muscle extending from the vagina to the anus (in the male the area from the scrotum to the anus) |
| **Vestibule** | opening containing entrance to vagina and urethral meatus (opening) |

## External genital organs

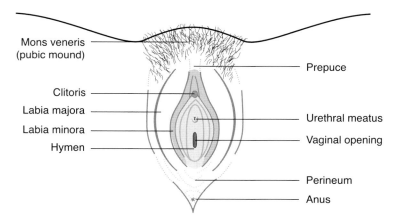

**Figure 42:** The external genital organs

# The breast

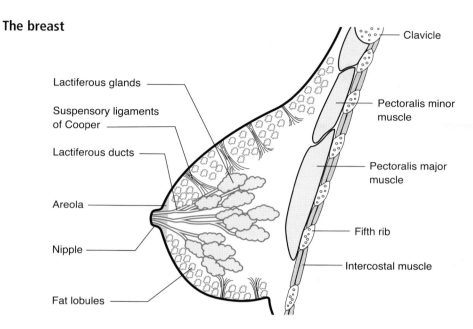

Lactiferous glands

Suspensory ligaments of Cooper

Lactiferous ducts

Areola

Nipple

Fat lobules

Clavicle

Pectoralis minor muscle

Pectoralis major muscle

Fifth rib

Intercostal muscle

**Figure 43:** The female breast

## The breasts

The breasts, or **mammary glands**, are the accessory glands of the female reproductive system. They are rudimentary in the male. Their function is to produce milk for feeding the newborn baby.

### Development

At puberty they enlarge and develop in the female, being under the influence of the female hormones. In pregnancy they increase in size and are stimulated ready to produce milk following delivery. They atrophy in old age.

### Structure

The milk-secreting glands are found in **lobes** grouped together in **lobules**, separated by fibrous connective and fatty tissue. Each lobule opens into tubules, known as **lactiferous ducts**, which unite to form the main ducts terminating at the **nipple** (*see Figure 43*).

### Hormone influence

The influence of the female hormones, **oestrogen** and **progesterone**, secreted by the ovaries at puberty and the start of menstruation, causes the enlargement and development of the breasts ready for future suckling.

In pregnancy, the production of progesterone by the **placenta** also influences further enlargement and development.

**Prolactin (LTH)**, a hormone secretion of the anterior part of the **pituitary gland**, stimulates the production of milk. **Oxytocin**, from the posterior part of the pituitary gland, stimulates the **ejection** (or let down) of milk from the breast. Suckling encourages more milk to be produced.

### Milk

This is a complete food for the newborn and is the most suitable nourishment for the human baby, having the correct proportions of nutrients.

Cow's milk contains a larger proportion of protein which is not easily digestible, being very complex. Numerous **antibodies** produced by the mother are also present and help to prevent infection occurring in the baby.

## Colostrum

During the latter part of pregnancy, a yellowish clear fluid, known as **colostrum**, containing sugar and protein, is produced. The milk production does not normally occur until the second or third day following birth. This substance provides nourishment and also acts as an **aperient** to remove secretions present in the newborn's intestine.

## The menstrual cycle (28 days)

This is the monthly cycle, occurring regularly in females every 26 days to 30 days throughout the child bearing period (approximately 36 years in total). Stimulated by changes in the concentration of hormone production, it is concerned with the release of the **ovum** and the preparation of the woman's womb (**uterus**) for **conception**.

The menstrual cycle (*see Figure 44*) can be divided into the:

- **Proliferative phase**
- **Ovulation**
- **Secretory phase**
- **Menses**

## Proliferative phase (10 days)

This is under the influence of the **anterior pituitary hormone**, known as the **follicle stimulating hormone (FSH)**, which stimulates an immature follicle (**graafian follicle**) in the ovary to mature and ripen, resulting in the release of an egg (**ovum**), ready for fertilisation. Oestrogen is produced by the follicle, which stimulates the rapid growth (**proliferation**) of the lining of the womb (**endometrium**).

## Ovulation

The egg (ovum) is released from the ripened follicle of the ovary, on approximately the 14th day from the first day of the last menstrual period. There is a corresponding rise in body temperature just before this occurrence. Sometimes there is a small amount of blood shed at this time, which can irritate the tissues and cause some women regular monthly pain.

The ovum is wafted into the **fallopian tube** (**oviduct**), by the movement of the specialised, **ciliated epithelium**, lining the tubes. One egg is usually released each month from the onset of periods (**menarche**) to the menopause (**climacteric**).

## Secretory phase (14 days)

This phase is under the influence of the anterior pituitary hormone known as the **luteinising hormone, (LH)** in the second part of the menstrual cycle. This hormone stimulates the follicle to develop into the **corpus luteum** (yellow body), which then begins to secrete the hormone, progesterone.

This second phase is concerned with preparing the lining of the womb for the implantation of the embryo and supplying the correct environment for the embryo to grow. Under the influence of progesterone, numerous glands begin to secrete watery mucus, which is thought to assist the **spermatazoa** in their passage through the uterus to reach the fallopian tubes, to fertilise the ovum. There is a similar increase in the secretion of mucus from the glands in the **cervix** (neck of the womb) and the fallopian tubes.

The ovum probably remains able to be fertilized for only about 8 to 12 hours; the spermatazoa capable of doing so, for about 24 hours, although they may survive for several days.

## The menses (4 days)

If the ovum is not fertilized, the corpus luteum in the ovary, withers and stops producing progesterone. The sudden drop in the levels of this hormone causes the **shedding** of the lining of the womb, as a **period** (the **menses**). The corpus luteum withers and eventually becomes scar tissue upon the surface of the ovary.

### Hormone control

The hormones of the menstrual cycle are governed by feed back mechanisms of **homeostasis**, in that as levels rise there is a corresponding drop in the hormone stimulating its production and vice versa. Overall, hormone production is governed by the part of the brain known as the **hypothalamus** (see Chapter 15 on the endocrine system).

## The menstrual cycle

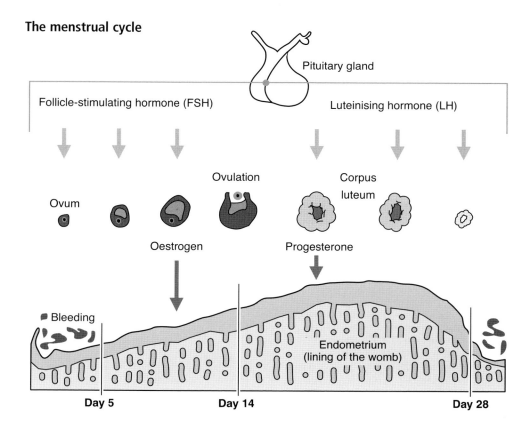

**Figure 44:** The menstrual cycle

# Obstetrics

## Pregnancy, childbirth and puerperium (the first six weeks after giving birth)

### Stages of pregnancy

The stages of development in pregnancy include:

- **Gamete**
- **Fertilisation**
- **Zygote**
- **Conception and implantation**
- **Embryo**
- **Fetus**

### Gonads

This is the proper name given to the sex organs which produce the **sex cells**, i.e. the **ovum** in the female and **spermatazoon** (plural: **spermatazoa**) in the male. The female gonads are the **ovaries**; the male gonads are the **testes**.

### Gamete

This is the name given to the primitive sex cell, i.e. the egg or ovum in the female and the spermatazoa in the male. By process of reduction division (**meiosis**) the nucleus of each gamete contains only 23 single **chromosomes**. One of these will be the sex chromosome.

The chromosome from the ovum will always be an **X chromosome**. The chromosome from the male spermatazoon may be an **X** *or* **Y chromosome**. If the ovum is fertilised by sperm carrying a Y chromosome the fetus will be **male (XY chromosomes)**; if with an X it will be **female, (XX chromosomes)**. It is therefore the male spermatazoon, which determines the sex of the developing fetus.

### *Zygote*

This is the name given to the **fertilised egg**. Only one spermatazoon is able to penetrate each egg.

### Fertilisation

During **intercourse**, the male spermatazoa are deposited into the vagina at ejaculation. Fertilisation occurs in the **fallopian tube** (**oviduct**), when the successful spermatazoon, having travelled up through the **cervix** into the **uterus** and then the fallopian tube, penetrates the egg (ovum) and invades its nucleus, causing the mixing of the 23 single chromosomes of each gamete (i.e. ovum and spermatazoon) to form 23 pairs. It is this mixing of the genetic material, which makes each person unique.

On fertilisation many changes occur in the zygote and a hollow ball of cells is formed known as a **morula** (mulberry). These contain the **stem** cells. They divide into approximately 100 cells, by the time **implantation** occurs. They differentiate to form two distinct layers:

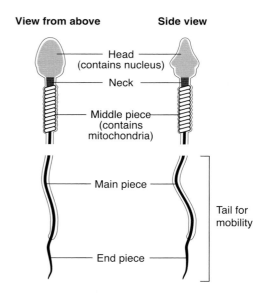

**Figure 45:** Spermatazoa

- the outer layer, which burrows into the uterine lining and will form the **choroid, placenta** and **amnion**;

- and the inner one divides again into three layers, to form the tissues and organs of the developing fetus.

At the time of **implantation** this ball of cells is known as a **blastocyst**.

## Conception and implantation

This occurs when the fertilised egg (ovum) embeds in to the lining of the uterus (**implantation**).

## Corpus luteum

If **conception** occurs, the **corpus luteum** (see the menstrual cycle earlier in this chapter) of the ovary continues to produce the hormone **progesterone**, which helps to maintain the pregnancy until the placenta is fully formed and able to produce sufficient of its own **chorionic gonadotrophic hormone (HCG)**. It is this substance which forms the basis of chemical pregnancy testing. (An early morning urine sample will show a greater concentration of this substance). A negative test is not necessarily proof of non-pregnancy. It is the influence of these hormonal changes, which prepare the mother's body for child birth.

## Embryo

The embedded fertilised egg is known as the **embryo** for the first 8 weeks of the pregnancy.

## Fetus

At 8 weeks of pregnancy the embryo starts to resemble a human being, having all its rudimentary organs and is now known as a **fetus**.

## Fertilisation, conception and implantation

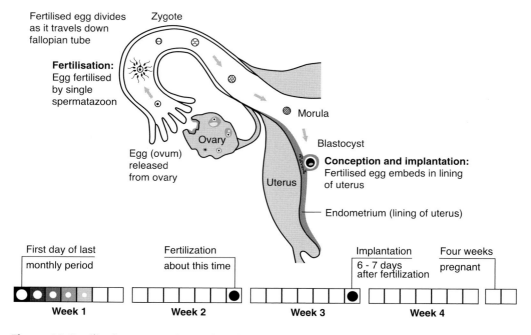

**Figure 46:** Fertilisation, conception and implantation

## The duration of pregnancy (gestation)

The duration of pregnancy is normally 40 weeks. The **expected date of delivery** or **confinement** (**EDD** or **EDC**), is calculated from the first day of the last menstrual period. Nine months plus 7 days is added, to estimate the relevant due date.

## The developing embryonic membranes

The structures of the developing membranes consist of:

- **Chorion**
- **Placenta**
- **Umbilical cord**
- **Amnion**
- **Germinative layer of blastocyst** forming the embryo

### Chorion

The **chorionic membrane** is the outermost layer of the **blastocyst**. By producing numerous finger-like projections (**villi**) where it comes into contact with the lining of the womb (**decidua**), the chorion allows **implantation** of the fertilized egg and the formation of the **placenta**. In later pregnancy, the lower part of the chorionic layer, which has not formed the placenta, fuses with the adjacent **amnion**. In the earliest days of pregnancy it is the chorion which starts to produce the hormone **HCG (human chorionic gonadotrophic hormone)** which acts upon the **corpus luteum** in the ovary and maintains the continuing production of oestrogen and progesterone.

### Placenta (complete at 3 months)

The placenta passes **nutrients**, **antibodies** and **oxygen** from mother to fetus. It also removes waste products in the form of **toxins**, **urea** and **carbon dioxide**

It acts as a barrier for some diseases and drugs from passing from mother to fetus, (although many smaller molecules of substances and micro-organisms, will pass through into the fetus).

The placenta (*see Figure 47*) continues to produce certain hormones – large amounts of oestrogen and progesterone as well as human chorionic gonadotrophic hormone (HCG) which maintain the pregnancy. This is essential for the pregnancy to continue and causes the changes to the mother's body, including the preparation of the breasts for milk production.

### Umbilical cord (containing Wharton's jelly)

The umbilical cord links the fetus to the placenta. It supports two arteries and a vein which transfer blood to and from the fetus. The blood circulation of mother and fetus never actually mix, as there is a thin membrane separating the maternal and fetal parts of the placenta (*see Figure 47 and Figure 54*).

### Amnion

The **amnion** is the term used to describe the **amniotic sac** (the "bag" around the fetus) and the **amniotic fluid** that surrounds the fetus.

#### Amniotic sac

The inner layer of cells of this sac form the **amniotic layer** which supports a bag of fluid in which the fetus develops and is cushioned. It also helps to prevent infection

#### Amniotic fluid

The **amniotic fluid** surrounding the fetus, consists of **water**, **salts**, **fat** and **fetal urine**. It absorbs fetal waste products and is also the medium in which the fetus swallows and learns to breathe. The fluid cushions and protects the fetus; maintains temperature and pressure around the fetus; and gives the fetus freedom of movement.

### The germinative layer of the blastocyst

Following implantation, the inner layer of the blastocyst divides into three layers from which all the body organs form:

- **Ectoderm**    forming the skin (**epidermis**), **nails**, etc. and also the **brain** and **nervous system**
- **Mesoderm**    forming **dermis**, **connective tissue**, **muscle**, **blood**, **cardiovascular** and

lymphatic tissue and most of the urogenital system

- **Endoderm**    forming **lining of gut**, **lining of respiratory tract**, and **glands** including the **liver** and **pancreas**

## Damage

Any damage to the embryo by **drugs** (e.g. a**l**cohol, prescribed drugs or **nicotine**), or **viral infection**, (e.g. rubella) at this early stage will be devastating, as so many organs will be affected. The results of the **thalidomide** disaster, are remembered as a cautionary tale of human vulnerability.

It should also be noted that all the ovum or sperm of the developing fetus, are present in a primitive form before birth, so that future generations may be affected by damage to the present yet unborn fetus.

## Trimesters

The pregnancy is divided into three three-month periods:

- **First trimester** – the first three months
- **Second trimester** – the middle three to six months
- **Third trimester** – the last three months

The development of the embryo and fetus is shown in Figure 48.

## The placenta, amnion and chorion

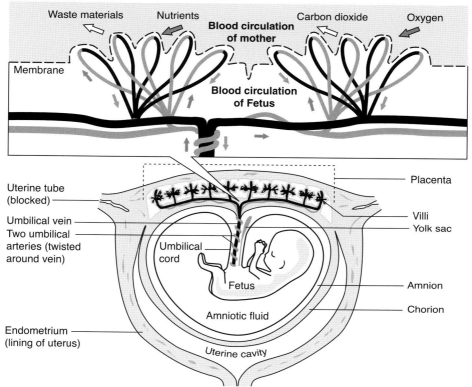

**Figure 47:** The placenta, amnion and chorion

## Stages of embryonic and fetal development

Weeks: 4-5    Size: 4 mm long

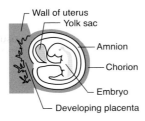

Development:

Rudimentary organs are already forming in the **embryo** but the mother is only just aware that she might be pregnant (**gravid**)

Weeks: 6-7    Size: 8 mm long
(crown to rump)

Development:

Limb buds are forming and dimples where the ears and eyes will be

Weeks: 8-9    Size: 17 mm long

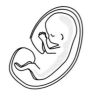

Development:

Major internal organs are developing, including the heart; the face is forming and a mouth and tongue are apparent; recognisable as a human being, it is now known as a **fetus**

Weeks: 10-14    Size: 56 mm long

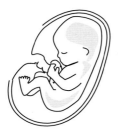

Development:

All organs are formed; from now on the fetus will grown and mature; the heart beat is strong and can be detected by ultrasound; movement is occuring but is not yet felt by the mother

**Figure 48:** Stages of embryonic and fetal development

Weeks: 15-22    Size: 16 cm long

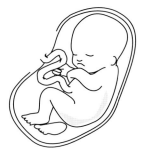

Development:

Hair and eyebrows begin to grow; eyelids remain closed; lines on skin are forming and nails are growing; movement is usually felt by the mother (known as **quickening**).

At 22 weeks, the fetus is covered with **lanugo**, a very fine hair which may be an aid to controlling body termperature. The fetus is termed **previable** as it is unlikely to survive if it is born at this stage

Weeks: 23-30    Size: 24 cm long

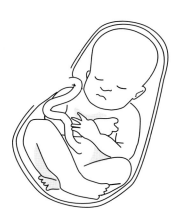

Development:

The fetus is now moving vigorously; it responds to touch and sound. Loud noise may make it kick. It is swallowing **amniotic fluid** and passing small amounts of **urine** into fluid. Hiccups occur and fetus is developing a pattern of waking and sleeping. The heart beat can be heard through a stethescope. The fetus is covered in a white, greasy substance known as **vernix**, which may be to protect the fetal skin. This usually disappears before birth.

At 24 weeks the fetus is legally **viable**, i.e. it is considered capable of survival. If pregnancy terminates at this stage, it is considered to be a **premature birth** or **still birth** (rather than a miscarriage or abortion. Registration of the birth is required.)

At 26 weeks the eyelids open and the eyes will be blue at this stage

**Figure 48:** Stages of embryonic and fetal development (continued)

## Stages of embryonic and fetal development

Weeks: 31-40   Size: 31 cm long;
Weight:  4 kg in weight at 36 weeks

Development:

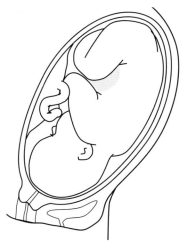

The fetus consolidates and grows plumper. Both the lanugo and vernix begin to disappear. Usually by 32 weeks the head is downwards, ready for birth. The crown of the head will move down into the pelvis some time prior to birth and is termed to be **engaged**, (**vertex presentation**). Occasionally, this does not occur until labour has commenced. If the presentation is bottom downwards, it is known as a **breech**. In the male the **testes** descend into the **scrotum** (which is necessary for the sperm to be kept at a temperature below that of the abdominal cavity, where they develop)

**Figure 48:** Stages of embryonic and fetal development (continued)

## Height of the fundus

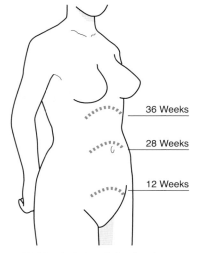

36 Weeks

28 Weeks

12 Weeks

As the fetus develops so the top part of the uterus (**fundus**) rises in the abdominal cavity (*see Figure 49*). Towards the last month, when it reaches the level of the rib cage, the mother finds some difficulty in breathing easily

### Braxton Hicks contractions

These are episodes of light, painless, irregular tightening of the uterus during pregnancy. They commence at the end of the first trimester and increase in duration and intensity by the third trimester.

**Figure 49:** The height of the fundus

## Multiple pregnancy

### Identical twins (uniovular)

These develop when a fertilised ovum divides into two to form two fertilised eggs with exactly the same chromosomes. These grow and develop sharing one placenta (*see Figure 50*). They will be the same sex and appear alike.

### Non-identical twins (binovular)

These develop from two completely separate ovum, fertilised by two different sperm. They have separate placenta (*see Figure 51*). Their chromosomes are completely different and children will have individual appearances. They may be different sexes.

### Triplets and other multiple pregnancies

In triplets, they may be identical, having arisen from one fertilised egg or identical twins with a separate third non-identical fetus. With the current use of fertility drugs, several eggs may be released from the ovaries, resulting in completely separate fertilisations. Triplets, quads, quins and sextuplets are not as rare as previously, although carrying these multiple pregnancies to full term is uncommon.

# Birth (parturition)

This is known as **labour** and normally commences as the result of hormone changes. The levels of oestrogen and progesterone decrease and a hormone **oxytocin** is released from the **posterior lobe** of the **pituitary gland**, causing contractions of the uterus to begin.

## Stages of labour

There are three stages of labour:

**Stage One**
from expulsion of **mucus plug** to the dilation of the neck of the womb (cervix) until (fully dilated) approximately 10cm (**cervical effacement**)

**Stage Two**
the **contractions** of pushing out the fetus until **crowning** and **expulsion** (**birth**) of the baby

**Stage Three**
the expulsion of the placenta known as the **afterbirth**

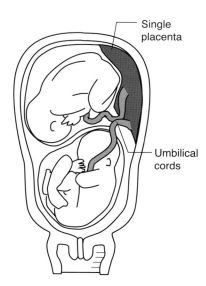

**Figure 50:** Uniovular (identical) twins share one placenta

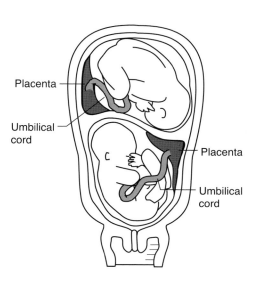

**Figure 51:** Binovular (non-identical) twins have separate placentas

## Presentation of the fetus

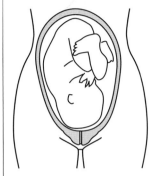

ROL: right occipitolateral
(ROT: right occipitotransverse)

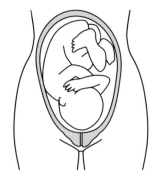

ROP: right occipitoposterior

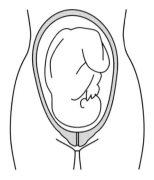

ROA: right occipitoanterior

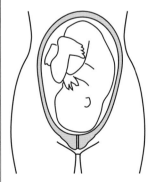

LOL: left occipitolateral
(LOT: left occipitotransverse)

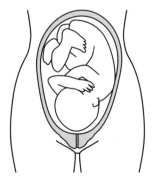

LOP: left occipitoposterior

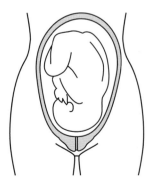

LOA: left occipitoanterior

**Figure 52:** The fetus may present in different positions

### Stage one

Stage one may last for up to 24 hours in a first birth. The plug of blood-stained **mucus** within the cervix is expelled and is known as a **show**. Usually the **waters (amniotic sac)** break. **Contractions** commence. They vary in length and severity and are concentrated on the cervix dilating. The last part of this stage is known as the **transitional** stage. The fetus may present (be positioned) in a number of ways (*as shown in Figure 52*).

### Stage two

Stage two is the most intense part of birth and contractions change their character, so that the mother pushes hard, and the fetus's head moves down the birth canal (**vagina**) until it **crowns** or is showing. The fetal skull bones are not fused and so they are able to move and overlap, changing the shape of the head, enabling it to adapt and squeeze through the cervix.

Contractions are frequent, usually every two or three minutes. If the area from the vagina to the anus (**perineum**) is not elastic enough or the baby is large, the skin is cut to prevent tearing (**episiotomy**). This stage usually lasts one or two hours.

As soon as the baby has cried and is breathing regularly, the umbilical cord is clamped, cut and tied off. **Apgar readings** (*see Table 4*) of the baby's condition are performed which are important indications of the baby's overall condition. These are recorded in the permanent notes for future reference. This is highly relevant, should the child develop any condition which may have been caused by deprivation of oxygen at birth etc.

The baby is given to the mother to hold as soon as possible after the birth, in order to encourage **bonding** (and breast feed if she has planned to do so). The act of breast feeding stimulates more oxytocin to be released, which causes contractions of the uterus which in turn helps to prevent bleeding.

**Stage 1** Dilation of the cervix

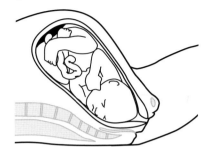

**Stage 2** Expulsion of the fetus

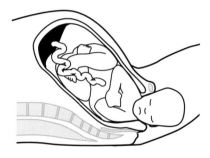

**Stage 3** Expulsion of the placenta (afterbirth)

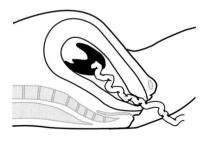

**Figure 53:** The three stages of birth

**Table 4:** The Apgar scores

| Apgar Score | Score 0 | Score 1 | Score 2 |
|---|---|---|---|
| **1. Heart rate** | Absent | Below 100 | Over 100 |
| **2. Respiratory effort** | Absent | Irregular, slow or weak | Lusty cry, good chest movement |
| **3. Muscle tone** (in all four limbs) | Limp | Poor tone, some movement | Active resistance, strong movement |
| **4: Reflex irritability** (response to flicking soles of feet) | No response | Slight withdrawal | Vigorous withdrawal of leg, strong cry |
| **5. Colour** (in white babies) | Blue or pale | Body pink, extremities blue | Completely pink |

**Total scores**

*Stage three*

Stage three is the **expelling of the placenta** after the baby's birth. An injection of **ergometrine** is usually given, intramuscularly, which makes the uterus contract. This is intended to prevent the risk of bleeding (**post-partum haemorrhage**). The placenta is carefully examined and weighed to ensure it is intact and there is none remaining in the uterus, which would increase the risk of infection (**puerperal sepsis**). Blood loss is also measured carefully.

(Some mothers copy the action of animals in eating the placenta, following birth, although generally they ensure that it is cooked!! It is highly nutritious and also contains high levels of hormones, which probably help the mother overcome the sudden drop in hormone levels which occurs after birth).

## Circulation of the fetus

The circulation (cardiovascular system) in the fetus (*see Figure 54*) is different from that post-birth. The main differences in fetal circulation are structures which bypass the blood supply to the lungs and liver. The maternal circulation carries out the main functions of those organs by supplying oxygen to the fetus and removing waste products.

There are three main differences in fetal circulation:

- **Ductus arteriosis**

- **Foramen ovale** (oval hole)

- **Ductus venosis**

## Ductus arteriosis

Found between the **left pulmonary artery** (from the lung) and the **aorta** (main artery), preventing blood from going to the, as yet, non-functioning lungs.

## Foraman ovale

Found in the **septum** (dividing wall) of the upper heart chambers (**atria**).

## Ductus venosis

Found supplying blood from the **umbilical** to the main lower vein of the body (**inferior vena cava**), bypassing the liver.

## Changes at birth

At birth (**parturition**), when the baby breathes, the **foramen ovale** and **ductus arteriosis** close, so that normal circulation is established. In the case of **'blue babies'** or some **'hole in the heart babies'**, these changes do not occur. Oxygenated blood mixes with deoxygenated blood in the heart chambers, so depriving the child of its ability to obtain sufficient oxygen from the lungs. The umbilical cord, having been cut, gradually shrivels and after approximately 7 to 10 days falls away from the fetal abdomen.

## Pigmentation in pregnancy

The influence of the hormones in pregnancy, causes pigmentation of the **areola** of the breasts and also the **linea alba**, a line which is found on the abdominal wall. As pregnancy progresses, the pigmentation becomes more marked. Stretching of the skin produces stretch marks (**striae gravidarum**) on the abdomen and thighs. In dark skinned people, this can later become pigmented.

## Circulation of the fetus

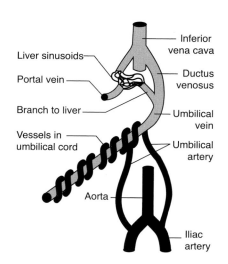
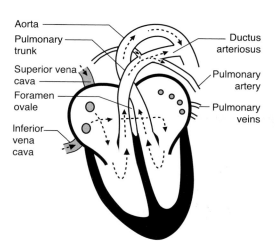

**Figure 54:** The circulation of the fetus

## Induced labour

This is when the mother is artificially stimulated to go into labour. It may involve the rupturing of the membranes of the **amnion** and the intravenous administration of **oxytocin**.

Reasons for induction are numerous but include overdue dates and medical concerns, including **toxaemia of pregnancy** where the mother's blood pressure rises rapidly, kidneys begin to fail and the life-threatening condition known as **eclampsia**, is developing. (**Caesarian section** may be required)

The signs and symptoms of toxaemia of pregnancy (**PET**) include:

- Retention of fluid producing free fluid in the tissues especially of the face and hands (**oedema**)

- Albumin in the urine (**albuminuria**)

- Rising blood pressure (**hypertension**)

## Post natal period (puerperium)

### Involution

This is the period of approximately six weeks following birth, in which the mother's reproductive tract returns to normal. The uterus shrinks quickly in the first two weeks.

The vaginal discharge (**lochia**), following birth (**post-partum**), persists for several weeks, during which it changes in colour and consistency:

- **Lochia rubra**    bloody discharge first 1-4 days

- **Lochia serosa**    pinkish brown watery (serous) discharge approximately from day 5-7

- **Lochia alba**    greyish white or colourless discharge approximately 1 to 3 weeks after delivery

## Neonatal period

This is the term used for the period of the first four weeks of life. The baby is known as the **neonate**.

## Ectopic pregnancy

If the fertilised egg implants itself in the fallopian tube, or even into the abdominal cavity itself, it is known as an **ectopic** pregnancy, i.e. in the wrong place. This is a life-threatening condition. As the pregnancy progresses and the products of conception grow, the tube itself ruptures. This would normally occur at about 6–8 weeks of pregnancy. Loss of blood and subsequent shock can cause the death of the mother.

There have been rare ectopic pregnancies that have gone to **term**, when the implantation has

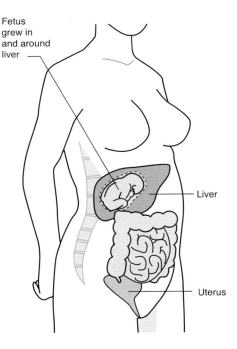

Fetus grew in and around liver

Liver

Uterus

**Figure 55:** A case of abdominal ectopic pregnancy. The baby was delivered successfully through surgery

taken place on the mother's liver or intestine (*see Figure 55*). Usually death is inevitable for the fetus, however, in 2003 a child was born alive after a complicated surgical procedure. The fetus had developed in and around the mother's liver but was delivered successfully through abdominal surgery.

## Epidural block

Some mothers are offered this procedure for the removal of pain in labour. An injection of **local anaesthesia** is injected into the **epidural space** of the **meninges** (membrane covering the brain and spinal cord). This prevents any messages of sensation travelling to the brain and gives total pain relief. There is an increased likelihood of a **forceps delivery** with this procedure as the woman does not recognise any impulse to push.

## Caesarian section

This is a surgical delivery where the womb is cut into (**hysterotomy**) and the fetus removed. It is performed when:

- The presentation of the fetus would make it impossible to deliver vaginally, e.g. some **breech** or **transverse** (laying across the womb) presentations (*see Figure 56*), where it has not been possible to manually turn the fetus in the womb

- There is indication that immediate removal is necessary, e.g. **fetal distress** shows that the fetus is in danger of immediate death. (Passing of a substance known as **meconium** by the mother vaginally would indicate this, as it consists of the contents of the fetal bowel).

- Danger of infection from mother's vagina to fetus during birth is also considered.

In recent years, caesarian sections have also been performed as a convenience for social reasons. (This practice is controversial).

The name is derived from the fact that Julius Caesar, the Roman Emperor was born in this fashion. The shape of the child's head, which has not been distorted by the pressure from the vaginal delivery, is a distinctive feature.

## Fetus in breech position

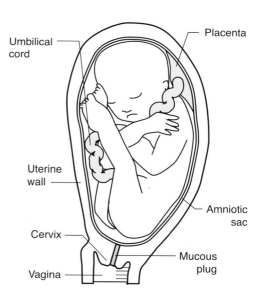

Umbilical cord

Placenta

Uterine wall

Cervix

Vagina

Amniotic sac

Mucous plug

**Figure 56:** The fetus in a breech position

## Weight gain during pregnancy

It is important that a woman's weight is monitored during her pregnancy to ensure that her weight gain is as expected. Excessive weight gain can lead to raised blood pressure and even eclampsia. Figure 57 shows the expected weight gain during pregnancy.

## Normal weight gain during pregnancy

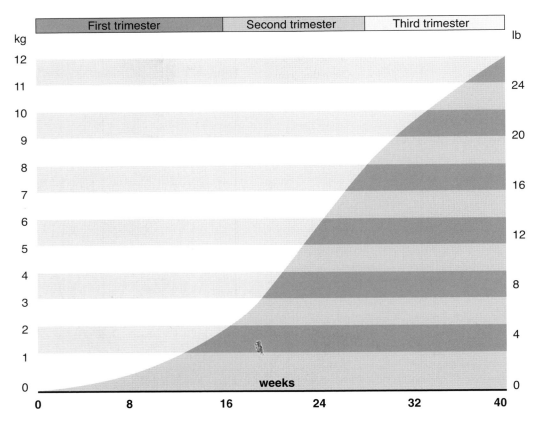

**Figure 57:** The normal rate of weight gain of the mother during pregnancy

## Abbreviations

| | | | | |
|---|---|---|---|---|
| **A&W** | alive and well | | **AIH** | artificial insemination by husband |
| **ab** | abortion | | | |
| **AFP** | alphafetoprotein (test for abnormality in fetus) in amniotic fluid or maternal blood | | **AN** | antenatal |
| | | | **APH** | antepartum haemorrhage |
| | | | **ARM** | artificial rupture of membranes |
| **AI** | artificial insemination | | | |
| **AID** | artificial insemination by donor | | **ART** | assisted reproductive technology |

| | |
|---|---|
| **BBA** | born before arrival |
| **BSO** | bilateral salpingo-oophorectomy (surgical removal of both fallopian tubes and both ovaries) |
| **BW** | birth weight |
| **CIN** | cervical intra-epithelial neoplasia (cervical precancer). It is graded from one to three depending on degree of abnormality |
| **COC** | combined oral contraceptive pill |
| **COHS** | controlled ovarian hormone stimulation |
| **CVS** | chorionic villus sampling (to detect fetal abnomalities) |
| **Cx** | cervix (neck of womb) |
| **D&C** | dilatation and curettage (scraping out of womb) |
| **DCIS** | ductal carcinoma in situ (a type of breast cancer) |
| **DUB** | dysfunctional uterine bleeding |
| **EDC** | expected date of confinement |
| **EDD** | expected date of delivery |
| **EMU** | early morning urine |
| **ERPC** | evacuation of retained products of conception |
| **EUA** | examination under anaesthetic |
| **FAS** | fetal abnormality syndrome |
| **FHH** | fetal heart heard |
| **FHNH** | fetal heart not heard |
| **FMF** | fetal movements felt |
| **G&A** | gas and air |
| **GIFT** | gamete intra-fallopian transplantation |
| **HPL** | human placental lactogen assay blood test (monitors health of placenta and fetus) |
| **HPV** | human papilloma virus |
| **HRT** | hormone replacement therapy |
| **HSV** | herpes simplex virus |

| | |
|---|---|
| **HVS** | high vaginal swab |
| **IUCD** | intra-uterine contraceptive device |
| **IUD** | intra-uterine device or intra-uterine death |
| **IUFB** | intra-uterine foreign body |
| **IVF** | in vitro fertilisation |
| **LMP** | last menstrual period |
| **LOA** | left occipitoanterior (position of fetus in uterus) |
| **LOL** | left occipitolateral (position of fetus in uterus) |
| **LOP** | left occipitoposterior (position of fetus in uterus) |
| **LOT** | left occipitotransverse – same as LOL (position of fetus in uterus) |
| **LSCS** | lower section caesarean section |
| **NAI** | non-accidental injury |
| **ND** | normal delivery |
| **NTDs** | neural tube defects (of the brain, spinal cord or meninges ) e.g. spina bifida |
| **PAP** | Papanicolaou smear (cervical smear test) |
| **PCB** | post-coital bleeding |
| **PCO** | see PCOS |
| **PCOS** | polycystic ovarian syndrome |
| **PET** | pre-eclamptic toxaemia |
| **PID** | pelvic inflammatory disease (also prolapsed intervertebral disc) |
| **PMB** | postmenopausal bleeding |
| **PMS** | premenstrual syndrome |
| **PN** | postnatal |
| **PNC** | postnatal clinic |
| **POD** | pouch of Douglas (fold of peritoneum lying behind the womb) |
| **POP** | progestogen only pill (contraceptive) |
| **PP** | placenta praevia |
| **PPH** | postpartum haemorrhage |
| **PV** | per vaginam |

| | |
|---|---|
| **RDS** | respiratory distress syndrome |
| **ROA** | right occipitoanterior (position of fetus in uterus) |
| **ROL** | right occipitolateral (position of fetus in uterus) |
| **ROP** | right occipitoposterior (position of fetus in uterus) |
| **ROT** | right occipitotransverse – same as ROL (position of fetus in uterus) |
| **RVS** | respiratory virus syndrome |
| **SB** | still birth |
| **SCAN** | suspected child abuse or neglect |
| **SCBU** | special care baby unit |
| **SI** | sexual intercourse |
| **SIDS** | sudden infant death syndrome |
| **STD** | sexually transmitted disease |
| **STYCAR** | standard tests for young children and retardates, developed by Sheridan to assess visual development |
| **TAH** | total abdominal hysterectomy |
| **TCRE** | transcervical resection of endometrium |
| **TOP** | termination of pregnancy |
| **TOP** | termination of pregnancy |
| **TSS** | toxic shock syndrome |
| **TUP** | tubal uterine pregnancy |
| **TV** | trichomonas vaginalis (infection of vagina causing frothy yellow discharge) |
| **TVH** | total vaginal hysterectomy |
| **USS** | ultrasound scan |
| **VI** | virgo intacto (virgin) |
| **Vx** | vertex (the crown of the head of the fetus) |
| **XX** | female sex chromosomes |
| **XY** | male sex chromosomes |
| **ZIFT** | zygote intra-fallopian transfer |

## Terminology

| | |
|---|---|
| **Colp/o** | stem for vagina |
| **Gest/o** | stem for pregnancy |
| **Gynaec/o** | stem for female |
| **Hyster/o** | stem for womb/uterus |
| **Mamm/o (mast/o)** | stem for breast |
| **Men/o** | stem for period |
| **Metr/o** | stem for womb/uterus |
| **Nat/o, /a** | stem for birth |
| **Oophor/o (ovari/o)** | stem for ovary |
| **Salping/o** | stem for fallopian tube |
| **Uter/o** | stem for womb |
| **Vagin/o** | stem for vagina |
| **Vulv/o** | stem for vulva |
| **-gravida** | suffix for pregnancy |
| **-para, -partum** | suffix for having given birth |
| **-tocia** | suffix for labour |
| **Amniotic membrane** | the innermost layer which encloses the fetus and produces amniotic fluid |
| **Antenatal care** | care given to both mother and fetus during pregnancy |
| **Anteverted uterus** | normal forward tilting of the womb |
| **Binovular twins** | derived from separate eggs (not identical – do not share genetic material |
| **Braxton Hicks contractions** | contractions felt in the womb during pregnancy from 16 weeks, which become more frequent towards full term |
| **Breech presentation** | presentation of the buttocks of the fetus during labour |
| **Chadwick's sign** | bluish coloration of vulva and vagina occurring after 6 weeks of pregnancy |
| **Chorionic membrane** | outer layer which forms the placenta |

| | |
|---|---|
| **Clone** | identical copy of a cell/ fertilised egg (genetically identical from a SINGLE cell) |
| **Cyesis** | pregnancy |
| **Embryo** | the developing fertilised egg (first eight weeks of development while all rudimentary organs are forming) |
| **Fetus** | the developing baby after embryo stage until birth |
| **Fundus of uterus** | the area of the uterus opposite its opening into the vagina (the top part) |
| **Gestation** | duration of pregnancy |
| **Goodell's sign** | softening of the cervix as a sign of pregnancy |
| **Grand multipara** | woman who has given birth to several children from different pregnancies |
| **Gravida** | pregnant woman |
| **Gynaecologist** | specialist in diseases of the female reproductive system |
| **Gynaecology** | study of the female reproductive system |
| **Hegar's sign** | softening of lower part of uterus at approximately 7 weeks of pregnancy |
| **in vitro** | in glass (test tube) |
| **Involution** | return of the womb to its normal size following the baby's birth |
| **Lactation** | production of milk |
| **Linea nigra** | pigmented line on abdomen in pregnancy |
| **Multigravida** | pregnant woman who has been pregnant more than once |
| **Multipara** | woman who has had more than one child |
| **Neonatal period** | the four-week period following the baby's birth (pertaining to the baby) |
| **Neonate** | first four weeks of a baby's life |

| | |
|---|---|
| **Nullipara** | woman who has never given birth |
| **Obstetrics** | medicine concerned with pregnancy and childbirth. |
| **Para 1** | see Primipara |
| **Parturition** | giving birth |
| **Placenta praevia** | the placenta is the presenting part for birth – antepartum haemorrhage occurs – caesarean section is essential in complete placenta praevia |
| **Presentation** | the part of the fetus which presents in the birth canal (vagina) |
| **Primigravida** | woman in her first pregnancy |
| **Primipara** | woman who has given birth to a first child |
| **Pudenda** | external genital area |
| **Puerperium** | period of six weeks for mother following the birth of baby |
| **Retroverted uterus** | backward tilting of the womb |
| **Trimester of pregnancy** | a three-month period of pregnancy, e.g. first three months |
| **Uniovular twins** | derived from one egg (identical twins) |
| **Viable** | capable of independent life (i.e. the fetus from 24 weeks of pregnancy) |

## Diseases and disorders

| | |
|---|---|
| **Amenorrhoea** | absence of menstruation |
| **Anaplasia** | highly malignant cells |
| **Antepartum haemorrhage** | abnormal bleeding from the womb before the birth |
| **Bartholin's abscess** | painful collection of pus in the Bartholin's glands of the vulva |
| **Bicornuate uterus** | abnormality where womb has two cavities |

**Caput succedaneum** soft swelling caused by free fluid (oedema) on the head of a newborn baby at, or shortly after, birth – disappears rapidly

**Carneous mole** pregnancy ceases and products of conception are retained in the womb

**Cervical erosion** erosion of the neck of the womb

**Cervical polyp** a stalk-like benign tumour in the cervix

**Cervicitis** inflammation of the neck of the womb

**Chlamydia** an infection of the vagina

**Chloasma** patchy brown pigmentation on face (like a mask) appearing in pregnancy due to hormone changes – also in women on contraceptive pill

**Chorion epithelioma** malignant tumour of chorionic (embryo) cells usually after formation of hyatidiform mole complication

**Conjoined twins** 'siamese twins' i.e. those that share an organ (organs)

**Crypto-menorrhoea** hidden menstruation – loss remains inside the womb due to an unbroken hymen

**Cystic fibrosis** inherited disease in which glandular tissue abnormal and, in particular, lung tissue becomes increasingly unable to function properly

**Cystocele** prolapse of the base of the bladder in women; causes bulging of the wall of the vagina

**Dermoid cyst** congenital (present at birth) sac containing embryonic tissue of hair, nails, teeth, skin etc.

**Down's syndrome** congenital condition in which there is often severe mental abnormality together with physical features of a mongoloid appearance, large tongue and stubby hands (abnormality of chromosome 21)

**Dysfunctional uterine bleeding** heavy menstrual bleeding which does not appear to have any anatomical cause

**Dysmenorrhoea** painful periods

**Dyspareunia** painful intercourse

**Dystocia** slow, difficult labour

**Eclampsia** a condition in which fits occur as blood pressure becomes extremely high (danger to both fetus and mother, see pre-eclampsia)

**Ectopic pregnancy** embedding of fertilised egg outside of the womb – usually in the fallopian tube

**Endometriosis** condition where lining of womb is found in other sites, e.g. colon or pouch of Douglas

**Fibroadenoma** a benign tumour composed of fibrous and glandular tissue

**Fibroid** a benign tumour composed of fibrous and muscle tissue found in the womb

**Fibromyoma** a fibroid (as above)

**Galactocele** milk cyst

**Gynaecomastia** enlargement of the male breast

**Hydatidiform mole** an intrauterine neoplastic mass

**Hydramnios** excessive amount of amniotic fluid

**Hyperemesis gravidarum** excessive vomiting during pregnancy

**Infertility** inability of woman to become pregnant or man to fertilise the ovum (does not mean sterility)

**Leucorrhoea** whitish vaginal discharge

| | |
|---|---|
| **Leukoplakia vulva** | chronic condition characterised by thick, hard, white patches on the vulva |
| **Lochia** | vaginal discharge following childbirth |
| **Malpresentation** | abnormal presentation of fetus for delivery |
| **Mastitis** | inflammation of the breast |
| **Mastodynia** | pain in the breast |
| **Meconium** | first fetal stools – if passed in the womb it is a clear indication of fetal distress in labour |
| **Menorrhagia** | excessive loss of blood during menstruation |
| **Metritis** | inflammation of the womb |
| **Metrorrhagia** | heavy bleeding not at the time of a period |
| **Metrostaxis** | persistent slight bleeding from the womb |
| **Miscarriage** | spontaneous abortion |
| **Munchausen syndrome by proxy** | a situation where a child or other person is deliberately made to appear ill or suffer injury so that the person responsible gains attention |
| **Oligohydramnios** | scanty amniotic fluid |
| **Polycystic ovarian syndrome** | an increasingly common condition in women in which there are multiple, enlarged follicles of the ovary, together with high levels of testosterone (male hormone). A cause of infertility and also linked with Diabetes Type II |
| **Polymenorrhoea** | frequent periods |
| **Post-partum haemorrhage** | bleeding following delivery |
| **Pre-eclampsia** | a condition during pregnancy where there is a raised blood pressure, albumin in the urine and oedema of the face and body (also known as toxaemia of pregnancy) – it precedes eclampsia |

| | |
|---|---|
| **Procidentia** | complete prolapse of womb into vagina through to the outside of the body |
| **Prolapse** | womb or vaginal wall protrudes into the vagina |
| **Pseudocyesis** | false pregnancy |
| **Puerperal psychosis** | severe mental illness following childbirth |
| **Puerperal sepsis** | infection of the genital tract and blood poisoning following childbirth |
| **Pyosalpingitis** | inflammation of the fallopian tube with pus formation |
| **Pyosalpinx** | presence of pus in the fallopian tube |
| **Rectocele** | prolapse of the rectum into the vaginal wall |
| **Salpingitis** | inflammation of the fallopian tubes |
| **Striae gravidarum** | silvery lines (red at first) on thighs and abdomen occurring due to pregnancy – 'stretch marks' |
| **Supernumerary nipples** | development of extra nipples (male or female) |
| **Teratogenic** | 'monster producing'– a virus or factor which is capable of producing deformities in the developing fetus, e.g. drugs/rubella |
| **Vaginismus** | involuntary spasm of the vagina preventing penetration during sexual intercourse |
| **Vaginitis** | inflammation of the vagina |

## Procedures and equipment

| | |
|---|---|
| **Abortion** | miscarriage or expulsion of the 'products of conception' from the uterus before 24 weeks: |
| *Criminal a.* | not within the legal definition; |
| *Induced a.* | intentional abortion; |

| | | | |
|---|---|---|---|
| **Incomplete a.** | parts of 'products of conception' are still remaining in the womb; | **Cordocentesis** | withdrawal of fetal blood for examination directly from the umbilical vein |
| **Inevitable a.** | profuse bleeding, cervix dilated – products are bound to be expelled; | **Cryopreservation** | preserving embryo, ova in cold storage |
| **Spontaneous a.** | naturally occurring abortion; | **Endometrial smear/biopsy** | following a small amount of local anaesthetic, a thin, hollow curette is inserted through the cervical opening and a small amount of uterine lining is removed for histology |
| **Threatened a.** | slight bleeding (cervix closed) | | |
| **Amniocentesis** | withdrawal of the amniotic fluid which surrounds the developing fetus for examination purposes, e.g. for Down's syndrome | | |
| **Amniography** | procedure of x-raying the pregnant uterus after contrast medium has been injected into the amniotic sac surrounding the fetus | **Epidural** | injection of anaesthesia into meninges of lumbar spine, used to remove pain of childbirth |
| | | **Episiotomy** | cutting the perineum (area between the vaginal opening and anus) to facilitate birth |
| **Apgar score/ rating** | an estimation of the state of the newborn baby one minute after birth and again five minutes later – respiration, colour, muscle tone, pulse and response are measured with a maximum score of 10 being awarded for a healthy condition | **Fetoscopy** | direct examination and pictures recorded of the fetus 'in utero' |
| | | **Fine needle aspiration** | aspiration of breast lump, etc. for cytological investigation |
| | | **Guthrie test** | blood test to detect phenylketonuria performed on newborn after establishment of feeding ('heel prick test') |
| **Ballottement** | passive fetal movements in response to tapping of lower uterus or cervix | **Hysterectomy** | surgical removal of the uterus which may be performed vaginally or by abdominal incision |
| **Caesarian section** | delivery of fetus through abdominal incision | | |
| **Chorionic villus sampling** | a sampling of cells from the chorion layer of the developing embryo for diagnostic purposes (can be done earlier than amniocentesis) | **Hysterotomy** | cutting into the womb |
| | | **Induction** | causing labour to begin by artificial means |
| | | **Lumpectomy (tilectomy)** | surgical removal of a tumour without removal of the breast itself |
| **Colporrhaphy** | surgical repair of vaginal wall prolapse | **Mammogram (mammography)** | an X-ray procedure examining breast tissue |
| **Cone biopsy** | cone-shaped portion of tissue removed from cervix for microscopic examination | **Mastectomy** | surgical removal of the breast |

**Maternal Serum Screening tests**  a group of blood tests which are used to check for substances linked with birth deformities

**Myomectomy**  surgical removal of fibroids

**Non-stress test**  a non-invasive test to detect fetal heart acceleration in response to fetal movement

**Nuchal translucency scan**  ultrasound test to show density of neck area in diagnosis of fetal abnormality for Down's syndrome

**Oestradiol – 17B**  blood test for ovarian function

**Oophorectomy**  surgical removal of the ovary – (bilateral oophorectomy – both ovaries).

**Oxytocin challenge test**  a stress test to evaluate fetal ability to withstand oxytocin (hormone) induced contractions

**Panhysterectomy**  surgical removal of womb and surrounding reproductive organs

**Pelvic ultrasound test**  passes ultrasound waves through the body to diagnose pelvic disease or examine a developing fetus for abnormalities

**Salpingectomy**  surgical removal of the fallopian tube(s)

**Salpingo-oophorectomy**  surgical removal of ovary and fallopian tube

**Salpingogram**  X-ray of the fallopian tubes

**Thermography**  investigation of the breast by measuring the heat of the tissues

**Tilectomy**  see Lumpectomy

**Version**  turning of a fetus to aid delivery

**Vibro-acoustic**  stimulation test - non-invasive test using vibration and sound to induce fetal activity

**Vulvectomy**  surgical removal of the vulva.

Chapter **12**

# The male reproductive system

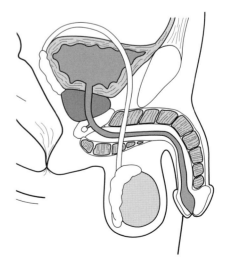

## Structure

The male reproductive system (*see Figure 58*) is composed of:

- Two **testes**
- Two **epididymes** } within the scrotum
- Two **vasa deferentia**
- Two **seminal vesicles**
- **Prostate gland**
- Two **ejaculatory ducts**
- **Bulbourethral (Cowper's) glands**
- **Penis** containing the **urethra**

### Testes

These develop within the abdominal cavity in the fetus, but prior to birth they descend through a canal known as the **inguinal canal** into the **scrotum**. They produce numerous **spermatazoa** (male sex cells) (*see Figure 45 in Chapter 11*) for fertilisation of the female **ovum**. Also produced are the male hormones known as **androgens**, the main one being **testosterone**, which are responsible for secondary male characteristics (hair distribution etc).

### Scrotum

The scrotum is a pouch of skin and specialised tissue lying outside the abdominal cavity and containing the **testis** and **epididymis**, together with the attached start of the **vas deferens**. It is essential that the developing spermatazoa are kept at a temperature lower than that within the abdominal cavity where the organs were first developed in fetal life. Unless this occurs the man will be infertile. The scrotum is lowered from and raised closer to the body, by special muscles dependent on the temperature of blood passing through the structure.

### Epididymes

These are situated upon the testes; here the immobile **spermatazoa** become mature and are stored.

### Vasa deferentia

Tubes through which the spermatazoa are released. These are cut in the operation of **vasectomy** to produce sterilisation of the male.

### Seminal vesicles

These contribute their own secretion to the **seminal fluid** which keeps the spermatazoa active and alive. Some spermatazoa are stored here ready for **ejaculation**.

### Ejaculatory ducts

These join the seminal vesicles to the urethra.

### Bulbourethral glands

These are also known as **Cowper's glands** and produce further secretions to the seminal fluid.

### Prostate gland

A gland the size of a walnut surrounding the junction of the vasa deferentia and urethra. It secretes a fluid making the spermatazoa more mobile and fertile. It commonly becomes enlarged in older men causing difficulty in passing urine due to constriction of the urethra.

### Urethra

This is a common passageway for both **seminal fluid** and **urine**. A **sphincter muscle** prevents both functions occurring at the same time.

### Penis

This is the male organ composed of **erectile tissue** and capable of becoming erect when distended with blood. The enlargement at its tip is known as the **glans**; the fold of skin protecting the opening of the urethra is known as the **foreskin** or **prepuce** and it is this area which is removed in the procedure of **circumcision**.

## Male reproductive system

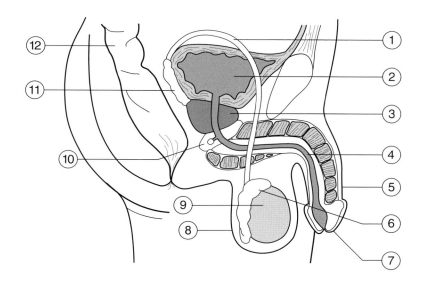

1. Vas deferens
2. Bladder
3. Prostate gland
4. Urethra
5. Penis
6. Epididymis
7. Prepuce
8. Scrotum
9. Testis
10. Cowper's gland
11. Seminal vesicle
12. Colon

**Figure 58:** The male reproductive system

## Abbreviations

| | |
|---|---|
| **HPV** | human papilloma virus |
| **PSA** | prostatic specific antigen (test for cancer of prostate) |
| **TUR** | transurethral resection (of prostate gland) |
| **TURB** | transurethral resection of bladder |
| **TURBT** | transurethral resection of bladder tumour |
| **TURP** | transurethral resection of prostate gland |

## Terminology

| | |
|---|---|
| **Andr/o** | stem for male |
| **Epididym/o** | stem for epididymis (fine tubules) |
| **Genit/o** | stem for genital |
| **Orchi(d)/o** | stem for testis |
| **Phall/o (pen/o)** | stem for penis |
| **Prostat/o** | stem for prostate gland |
| **Semin/o** | stem for semen |
| **Vas/o** | stem for vas deferens |

## Diseases and disorders

| | |
|---|---|
| **Balanitis** | inflammation of glans, penis and foreskin |
| **Ectopic testes** | testicles which are in the wrong place, i.e. not in the scrotum |
| **Epididymitis** | inflammation of the epididymis (tubules above the testis) |
| **Epididymo -orchitis** | inflammation of the epididymis and testis |
| **Epispadias** | opening of urethra on the upper side of penis |

| | | | |
|---|---|---|---|
| **Haematocele** | effusion of blood in area surrounding the testis | | be screened in order to eliminate the possibility of malignancy |
| **Hydrocele** | collection of fluid in the tunica vaginalis (membrane surrounding the testis) | **Suprapubic cystostomy** | incision above the prostate to allow drainage of the bladder |
| **Hypospadias** | opening of urethra is on the lower side of the penis | **Transurethral resection of prostate (TURP)** | surgical removal of the prostate through the urethra |
| **Impotence** | inability to have sexual intercourse, or the inability to have or maintain an erection of the penis (may have a physical or a psychological cause) | **Urethroplasty** | reshaping of the urethra |
| | | **Vasectomy** | surgical cutting/ removal of the vasa deferentia in order to produce sterility. |
| **Orchitis (orchiditis)** | inflammation of a testicle | | |
| **Phallitis** | inflammation of the penis | | |
| **Phimosis** | constriction of foreskin of penis preventing retraction of skin | | |
| **Prostatitis** | inflammation of the prostate gland | | |
| **Sterility** | inability to fertilise female egg (ovum) | | |
| **Urethritis** | inflammation of the urethra | | |
| **Varicocele** | dilatation of veins around the testis and vas deferens | | |

## Procedures and equipment

| | |
|---|---|
| **Circumcision** | surgical removal of part of foreskin |
| **Ileal conduit** | ureters are transplanted into the ileum (intestine) in order to discharge urine to bypass a tumour or following removal of bladder |
| **Orchidectomy** | surgical removal of a testicle |
| **Orchidopexy** | fixing of an undescended or rotating testicle into the scrotal sac |
| **Prostatic specific antigen test** | this is a screening blood test used to aid diagnosis of carcinoma of the prostate gland. Patients with prostatism (enlargement of the prostate gland) should |

Chapter **13**

# The nervous system

including the terminology

of mental health

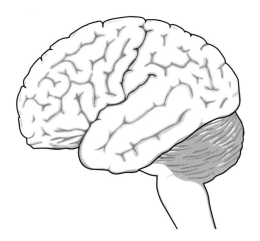

## Function

This is concerned with the rapid conduction and interpretation of messages in the form of electrical impulses from one part of the body to another. It also coordinates the activities of the body.

## Structure

The nervous system is made up of specialised tissue containing cells known as neurones, and is divided into three systems:

- **Central nervous system** (CNS)

- **Peripheral nervous system**

- **Autonomic nervous system** (ANS)

Nerve cells are known as **grey matter** and the fibres from them are covered in **myelin** (a fatty substance) are known as **white matter**. In the CNS, nerve cells, when damaged, are unable to regenerate themselves.

Messages can only travel in one direction along a nerve fibre.

### Motor nerves (efferent)

These convey messages from the brain to parts of the body to perform an action (*see Figure 59*).

### Sensory nerves (afferent)

These convey messages from the body to the brain with information about stimuli such as pain.

## Central Nervous System

This consists of the **brain** and **spinal cord**.

## Brain

The brain lies within the bony **cranium** of the skull. It is covered in a specialised membrane containing the blood vessels which supply oxygen and nourishment, known as the **meninges**, which also covers the spinal cord. The need for oxygen to reach every cell in the brain is critical. If deprived of oxygen for more than three to four minutes, these cells will die and death will occur.

## Motor neurone

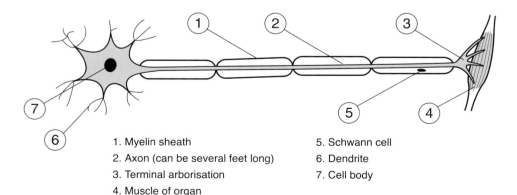

1. Myelin sheath
2. Axon (can be several feet long)
3. Terminal arborisation
4. Muscle of organ
5. Schwann cell
6. Dendrite
7. Cell body

**Figure 59:** A motor neurone

# The brain

1. Parietal lobe of cerebrum

2. Fissure of Rolando

3. Cerebrum

4. Occipital lobe of cerebrum

5. Cerebellum

6. Midbrain (hidden)

7. Pons varolii

8. Medulla oblongata

9. Brain stem

10. Temporal lobe

11. Fissure of Sylvius

12. Frontal lobe of cerebrum

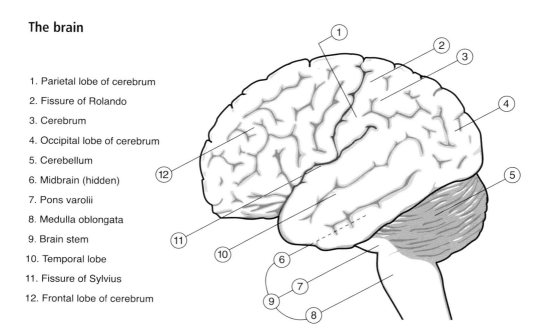

**Figure 60:** The brain

The brain consists of (*see Figure 60*):

- **Cerebrum**

- **Cerebellum**

- **Brain stem**

## Cerebrum

This forms the larger lobes of the brain and is divided into two **hemispheres** joined together with a bridge of white matter. The cerebrum contains the **higher centres** including those of intellect, consciousness, movement, sensory perception etc.

There are many specialised centres and the **convoluted surface**, together with numerous **fissures** (giving a larger surface area), contains **grey matter**, with **white matter** within the hemispheres. There are also specialised areas of grey matter deep within the hemispheres known as the **basal ganglia**. The **hypothalamus**, which controls the ANS, is situated here.

The **cerebrum** consists of numerous **lobes** which are named from the cranial bones beneath which they lie, i.e. **frontal, parietal, temporal** and **occipital**.

## Cerebellum

This also has two hemispheres joined together at the posterior portion. It is involved in the control of **muscle tone** and coordinates muscular movement as well as balance and equilibrium. Damage can cause **ataxia** (uncoordinated gait), tremor and loss of sense of balance.

## Brainstem

This consists of:

- **Midbrain**

- **Pons varolii**     — all interconnected

- **Medulla oblongata**

### Midbrain

This joins the two cerebral hemispheres to the **cerebellum** and the **pons varolii** below. It has specialised centres deep within it. All sensory impulses pass through this area.

### Pons varolii

This joins the **cerebellum** to the **midbrain** and **medulla oblongata** below.

### Medulla oblongata

This is continuous with the pons above and contains the **vital centres**, including the control of respiration, heart beat and the calibre of the blood vessels etc.

Damage to these centres is very serious and often causes death, e.g. fracture of the base of the skull. This area is continuous with the spinal cord below and passes through the **foramen magnum** (large hole) of the cranium.

It is in the medulla oblongata that the white nerve fibres, travelling to the spinal cord, cross over so that the left area of the brain controls the right side of the body and vice versa.

## Ventricles

Deep within the brain are spaces known as **ventricles**, which are continuous with each other and with the fine spinal canal in the spinal cord. **Cerebrospinal fluid** from the meninges circulates throughout these areas.

## Meninges

This is a very specialised membrane which covers both brain and spinal cord.

It is composed of three special layers:

1. **Dura mater** a hard, tough outer layer.

2. **Arachnoid mater** a vascular layer with many blood vessels.

3. **Pia mater** a soft layer closely attached to brain and spinal cord

### Functions

It has the following functions:

- **Supports** the delicate nervous tissue

- Acts as a **shock absorber**

- Maintains **uniform pressure** around it

- Provides **nourishment** and removes **waste products**

## Cranial nerves

The 12 pairs of cranial nerves arising from the brain, are sensory and motor.

- **Motor nerves** carry messages *from* the brain *to* the body

- **Sensory nerves** carry messages *to* the brain *from* the body

### List of cranial nerves

**Key:** (m) = motor
(s) = sensory

I **olfactory**
concerning sense of smell (s)

II **optic**
concerning sight (s)

III **oculomotor**
eye muscles (m)

IV **trochlear**
eye muscles (m)

V **trigeminal**
forehead and face (s)

VI **abducens**
eye muscles (m)

VII **facial**
facial expression (m)

VIII **auditory**
hearing and balance (s)

IX **glossopharyngeal**
tongue and pharynx (ms)

X **vagus (vagal)**
pharynx, trachea, heart, larynx, bronchi lungs, oesophagus, stomach, intestine (m & s)

XI **spinal accessory**
muscles of pharynx etc. (m)

XII **hypoglossal**
muscles of tongue (m)

## Spinal Cord

### Structure

This is continuous with the **medulla oblongata** above and extends to the level of the **second lumbar vertebra** below. It travels through the **neural canal** or **foramen** (hole) in the vertebrae which surround and protect it.

Unlike the brain, the grey matter of the spinal cord is found deep within it in an H-shaped pattern and the white matter distributed in the outer aspects. It is covered in **meninges** and has a small space through its centre, known as the **spinal canal**.

Arising from the spinal cord are the **peripheral nerves** of which there are 31 pairs, travelling to the various parts of the body, receiving and sending messages and interconnecting.

A group of nerve fibres (**white matter**) travelling together is known as a **plexus** and groups of cells (**grey matter**) as **ganglia**.

At the termination of the spinal cord (at the level of the second lumbar vertebra in the adult) numerous peripheral nerves give rise to the **cauda equina** (horse's tail) which supply the **lumbar-sacral** area (in the groin) and lower limbs (*see Figure 61*).

### Function

Its function is to relay messages to and from the body and also at different levels of the cord itself.

### Reflex action

This is the automatic reaction by the body to a stimulation. In a **reflex arc**, a message to the sensory area of the spinal cord is immediately relayed across the cord to the **motor area**, which in turn sends an impulse to a **motor organ**, e.g. a muscle. The original sensory message still travels to the appropriate part of the brain, but the resulting movement of the limb is started more quickly by the reflex action, i.e. the reaction of the body to a pin-prick of the arm is a reflex arc that moves the arm (*see Figure 62*).

## Spinal cord and peripheral nerves

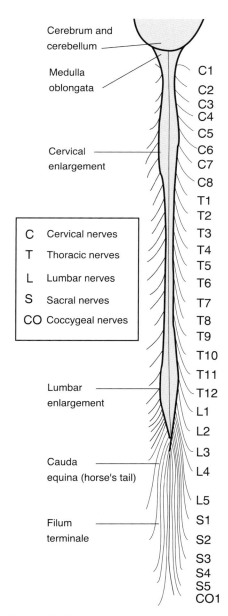

Cerebrum and cerebellum

Medulla oblongata

Cervical enlargement

| C | Cervical nerves |
| T | Thoracic nerves |
| L | Lumbar nerves |
| S | Sacral nerves |
| CO | Coccygeal nerves |

C1
C2
C3
C4
C5
C6
C7
C8
T1
T2
T3
T4
T5
T6
T7
T8
T9
T10
T11
T12
L1
L2
L3
L4
L5
S1
S2
S3
S4
S5
CO1

Lumbar enlargement

Cauda equina (horse's tail)

Filum terminale

**Figure 61:** The spinal cord and peripheral nerves

## Reflex arc

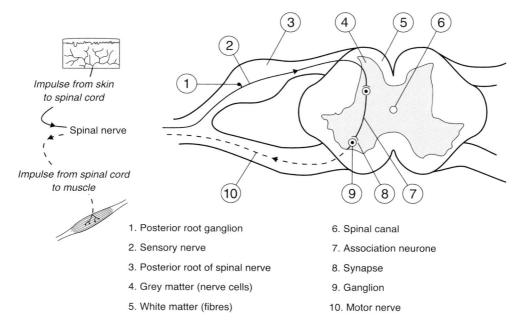

*Impulse from skin to spinal cord*

*Spinal nerve*

*Impulse from spinal cord to muscle*

1. Posterior root ganglion
2. Sensory nerve
3. Posterior root of spinal nerve
4. Grey matter (nerve cells)
5. White matter (fibres)
6. Spinal canal
7. Association neurone
8. Synapse
9. Ganglion
10. Motor nerve

**Figure 62:** The reflex arc

### Inhibition

This is where the resulting reflex action is overcome by the brain, e.g. picking up a very hot plate which is very expensive. The automatic dropping of the plate is overridden by the knowledge that it is expensive to replace.

## Peripheral nervous system

This consists of:

- 12 pairs of **cranial nerves**

- 31 pairs of **peripheral nerves**

The cranial nerves arise from the brain itself. The peripheral nerves stem from differing levels of the spinal cord and supply the body. They convey sensory and motor impulses to and from the brain and spinal cord, and also to different levels of the cord itself.

## Autonomic nerve supply

This is the system which controls the workings of the body organs and keeps the body in its correct state (**homeostasis**). It is not normally within the control of the will but is automatic.

It supplies all organs composed of **smooth muscle** as well as other organs, including the heart, blood vessels, respiratory system and eyes.

There are two sets of fibres to each organ which are known as the:

- **sympathetic chain**

- **parasympathetic chain**

These are controlled by a centre in the brain known as the **hypothalamus**. All systems work in conjunction with each other and the two sets of fibres work in harmony.

## Sympathetic chain

This set of fibres is stimulated to prepare the body for the 'fight or flight' response. When stimulated, it increases the heart rate and respiration, raises blood pressure, dilates the pupil of the eye and increases energy supplies as well as many other actions.

## Parasympathetic chain

This set of fibres has an inhibiting or resting action and has the opposite effect upon the body to the sympathetic chain. Its action slows the heart rate, decreases the breathing rate and increases digestion and secretion of saliva.

The **vagus nerve**, as part of the parasympathetic chain, supplies the heart and many of the major organs of the body.

# Abbreviations

## Nervous system: abbreviations

| | |
|---|---|
| **ANS** | autonomic nervous system |
| **BSE** | bovinespongiform encephalopathy ('mad cow' disease) |
| **CA** | chronological age |
| **CAT (CT)** | scan – computerised X-ray of layers of tissues |
| **CJD** | Creutzfeldt-Jacob disease |
| **CNS** | central nervous system |
| **CSF** | cerebrospinal fluid |
| **CVA** | cerebrovascular accident (stroke) |
| **DS** | disseminated sclerosis (old term for MS) |
| **DTs** | delirium tremens |
| **EEG** | electroencephalogram |
| **EMG** | electromyogram |
| **GA** | general anaesthetic |
| **GPI** | general paralysis of the insane |
| **IQ** | intelligence quotient |
| **LA** | local anaesthetic |
| **MA** | mental age |

| | |
|---|---|
| **MAOI** | monoamine oxidase inhibitors (antidepressants which require abstinence from certain foods, e.g. cheese - can cause bleeding in the brain) |
| **MND** | motor neurone disease |
| **MRI** | magnetic resonance imaging (see NMR) |
| **MS** | multiple sclerosis |
| **NMR** | nuclear magnetic resonance (scan) |
| **OCD** | obsessive compulsive disorder |
| **PVS** | persistant vegetative state: a continuing level of coma in head injuries where there appears to be no response. Can continue for years with patient on a life support machine |
| **REM** | rapid eye movements |
| **RT** | radiation therapy |
| **RTA** | road traffic accident |
| **SAH** | subarachnoid haemorrhage |
| **SOL** | space-occupying lesion (tumour, usually malignant, in the cranium) |
| **TENS** | transcutaneous electrical nerve stimulation |
| **TIA** | transient ischaemic attack (in the brain) |
| **TLE** | temporal lobe epilepsy (fits which originate in the temporal lobe of brain causing aura of taste, hearing, smell etc.) |
| **vCJD** | variant Creutzfeldt-Jacob disease |

## Mental health: abbreviations

| | |
|---|---|
| **ADD** | attention deficit disorder |
| **ADHD** | attention deficit hyperactivity disorder |
| **AIA** | allergy induced autism |
| **ANS** | autonomic nervous system |

| | |
|---|---|
| **AS** | autistic spectrum disorder |
| **ASD** | Asperger's syndrome disorder |
| **BP** | bipolar disorder |
| **DTs** | delirium tremens |
| **ECT** | electroconvulsive therapy |
| **GAD** | general anxiety disorder |
| **GPI** | general paralysis of the insane |
| **IQ** | intelligence quotient |
| **LD** | learning disability |
| **MA** | mental age |
| **MAOI** | monoamine oxidase inhibitor - antidepressant drug which must not be taken with certain foods or drugs eg: lentils, cheese etc (can cause death) |
| **OCD** | obsessive compulsive disorder |
| **PTSD** | post traumatic stress disorder |
| **SAD** | seasonal affective disorder (depression due to lack of light in winter) |
| **SSRI** | selective serotonin reuptake inhibitor (antidepressants which affect particular enzyme actions in brain) |
| **TCA** | tricyclic antidepressant (old type of antidepressant) |
| **TS** | Tourette's syndrome |

## Terminology

### Nervous system: terminology

| | |
|---|---|
| **Cephal/o** | stem for head |
| **Cerebell/o** | stem for cerebellum (part of the brain) |
| **Cerebr/o** | stem for cerebrum (part of the brain) |
| **Crani/o** | stem for cranium |
| **Encephal/o** | stem for brain |
| **Myel/o** | stem for spinal cord |
| **Neur/o** | stem for nerve |

| | |
|---|---|
| **Poli/o** | stem for grey matter |
| **Ventricul/o** | stem for ventricles of brain |
| **-kinesis** | suffix meaning movement |
| **-paresis** | suffix meaning weakness |
| **-phasia** | suffix meaning speech |
| **-plegia** | suffix meaning paralysis |
| **-somia** | suffix meaning body |
| **Cerebrospinal fluid** | fluid similar to plasma found in the meninges which nourishes the brain and spinal cord |
| **Dura mater** | outermost and thickest of the three meninges surrounding brain and spinal chord. |
| **Perception** | the interpretation and response of the nervous system to sensory stimuli |

### Mental health: terminology

| | |
|---|---|
| **Aut/o** | stem for self |
| **Neur/o** | stem for nerve |
| **Psych/o** | stem for mind / behaviour |
| **Schiz/o** | stem for split/diaphragm |
| **-mania** | suffix meaning frenzy, wild activity |
| **-phobia** | suffix meaning irrational fear |
| **-somia** | suffix meaning body |
| **Catharsis** | an outlet of repressed emotion |
| **Cognitive behaviour psychology** | a treatment which concentrates on changing behaviour instead of treating causes of a problem |
| **Cognitive therapy** | therapy concentrated on improving person's negative thinking, perceptions and attitudes |
| **Complex** | a pattern of behaviour which demonstrates an over-reaction to a problem |
| **Delusion** | false belief, usually associated with psychological illness, |

which cannot be altered despite logic and evidence to the contrary

**Perception**    the interpretation and response of the nervous system to sensory stimuli

**Psychiatrist**    medical doctor specialising in the treatment of mental illness

**Psychiatry**    the medical speciality concerning mental illness

**Psychoanalysis**    Freudian method of exploring the mind

**Psychologist**    not a medical doctor; qualified in study of the mind, and behaviour; can provide therapy but not drugs etc

**Psychology**    scientific study of behaviour

**Psychotherapy**    treatment by talking etc to relieve symptoms or resolve problems

## Diseases and disorders

### Nervous system: diseases and disorders

**Acute**    rapid onset

**Affective disorders**    those conditions which affect mood

**Akathisia**    restlessness that results in an inability to sit still

**Alzheimer's disease**    progressive dementia – caused by destruction of the neurones (brain cells)

**Amnesia**    loss of memory

**Anaesthesia**    loss of sensitivity and feeling (local) to a part or (general) throughout the body, causing loss of consciousness

**Anencephaly**    partial or complete absence of the bones of the rear of the skull and of the cerebral hemispheres of the brain

**Anorexia nervosa**    eating disorder characterised by refusal to eat – person has body image of obesity (common in teenage girls)

**Aphasia**    inability to speak caused by brain damage

**Apoplexy**    a stroke

**Ataxia**    uncoordinated gait (limp)

**Aura**    warning symptoms preceding epileptic seizure or migraine attack

**Autism**    absorption with the self – a condition in which the person is withdrawn into their own world, showing little response to events around them; it is a development disorder arising in early years of life and is characterised by significantly impaired social and language skills – several categories classified

**Babinski's sign**    reflex of the toe upwards instead of down – shows damage to central nervous system

**Bell's palsy**    paralysis of face muscles due to injury or disease of cranial nerve supplying face muscles (usually one-sided)

**Bovine spongiform encephalopathy**    see Creutzfeldt–Jacob disease

**Bulimia nervosa**    eating disorder characterised by eating 'binges' and self-induced vomiting

**Catatonia**    state of stupor, strange posture, outbursts of excitement – form of autism common in schizophrenia

**Causalgia**    severe burning-type pain caused by nerve injury

**Chorea**    involuntary contraction of muscles causing writhing movements (eg: St Vitus' dance)

**Chronic** long-term condition or frequently recurring

**Circadian rhythm** chemical and psychological variations over a 24 hour period

**Clonus response** the production of a series of muscle contractions in response to a stimulus which are only produced in the presence of CNS (central nervous system) disease

**Coma** complete unconsciousness – a level where there is no response on normal stimulation

**Complex** a pattern of behaviour which demonstrates an over-reaction to a problem

**Compression** pressure on the brain tissue due to swelling, blood clot or tumour

**Compulsion** insistent and repetitive need to behave in unreasonable or excessive way

**Concussion** limited period of unconsciousness caused by injury to the head

**Coning** pressure on brain forcing brainstem through foramen magnum

**Conversion** problems expressed as physical symptoms eg abdominal pain, panic attacks, paralysis etc.

**Convulsion** spasmodic contraction and relaxation of muscles in a fit

**Coprolalia** involuntary use of vulgar/foul language as in Tourette's syndrome

**Creutzfeldt-Jacob disease** a disease in which the brain tissue degenerates; linked with bovine spongiform encephalopathy (mad cow disease) it is now known to be transmitted to humans

**Delirium** mental excitement resulting from hallucinations, e.g. in state of high fever, alcohol consumption, or mental illness

**Delirium tremens** mental excitement due to chronic excessive alcohol intake, known as 'DTs'

**Diplopia** double vision

**Dysarthria** difficulty in articulation of speech due to nerve damage

**Dyskinesia** abnormal movements associated with side-effects of major tranquillising drugs

**Dyslexia** word blindness – inability to decipher words by the brain producing difficulty in reading, writing etc. by an individual with the intelligence to perform these tasks

**Dystonia** muscle spasms occurring in the tongue, jaw, eyes, neck; side-effect of some medications

**Encephalitis** inflammation of the brain

**Epilepsy** condition of suffering seizures, convulsions – abnormal electrical activity of the brain

**Familial** affecting more members of family than would be chance

**Fixation** an arrest in psychological development at a particular stage

**General paralysis of the insane** paralysis caused by the terminal effects of syphilis

**Glioma** malignant tumour of nerve support system

**Grand mal** epileptic attacks which include loss of consciousness and convulsions where the disturbance in electrical activity spreads across the various areas of the brain

| | |
|---|---|
| **Hallucination** | false perception without any true sensory stimuli – any sense may be involved, e.g. taste, hearing, sight etc. |
| **Hemianaesthesia** | loss of feeling of one side of the body |
| **Hemiparaesthesia** | heightened sensation of one side of the body |
| **Hemiparesis** | weakness of one side of the body |
| **Hemiplegia** | paralysis of one side of the body |
| **Herpes zoster** | shingles – painful infection along the nerve by the virus which causes chicken-pox |
| **Hydrocephaly** | 'water on the brain' – excess cerebrospinal fluid present due to a blockage in its circulation – skull enlarges in the baby |
| **Hyperkinetic** | overactivity of movement |
| **Hysteria** | a neurosis arising from psychological problems producing bodily symptoms, e.g. paralysis |
| **Idiopathic epilepsy** | epilepsy of unknown cause |
| **Jacksonian epilepsy** | epilepsy having a focal area – caused by an abnormality in that area of the brain, e.g. scar tissue. |
| **Kernig's sign** | inability to straighten leg at knee joint when thigh is flexed at right angles to the body – present in meningitis |
| **Libido** | sexual energy/ behaviour/drive |
| **Limbic system** | area of the brain concerned with the emotional control and memory |
| **Meningioma** | tumour of the meninges (covering of the brain and spinal cord) |
| **Meningism** | irritation of the meninges (covering of the brain and spinal cord) |

| | |
|---|---|
| **Meningitis** | inflammation of the meninges |
| **Meningocele** | protrusion of the meninges through the gap in the unfused vertebra of spina bifida |
| **Microcephaly** | having an abnormally small head |
| **Migraine** | headache, often one-sided, characterised by disturbance of vision, nausea, vomiting etc. caused by dilatation of the cranial arteries |
| **Monoplegia** | paralysis of one limb |
| **Motor neurone disease** | disease of the motor areas of the central nervous system causing paralysis – rapidly progressive |
| **Multiple sclerosis** | disease of central nervous system in which the myelin (fatty) sheath covering nerve fibres is destroyed and various functions are impaired, including movement. It is characterised by relapses and remissions |
| **Myelitis** | inflammation of the spinal cord |
| **Myelo-meningocele** | meningocele where the spinal cord is also protruding |
| **Narcolepsy** | compulsive sleeping (at any time) |
| **Neuralgia** | nerve pain (along the course of a nerve) |
| **Neuritis** | inflammation of a nerve |
| **Nystagmus** | involuntary rapid movements of the eyeballs |
| **Palsy** | paralysis |
| **Panic attacks** | present in anxiety states – body response produces rapid heart rate etc |

| | |
|---|---|
| **Paraplegia** | paralysis of both legs |
| **Paresis** | weakness |
| **Parkinson's disease** | damage to grey matter in the brain known as the basal ganglia; causes involuntary tremors of limbs etc. |
| **Perception** | the interpretation and response of the nervous system to sensory stimuli |
| **Petit mal** | type of epilepsy where the person momentarily loses concentration ('absences') |
| **Photophobia** | a fear of (or intolerance to) light |
| **Poliomyelitis** | inflammation of the grey matter of the spinal cord (infantile paralysis) |
| **Polyneuritis** | inflammation of many nerves |
| **Post-epileptic automatism** | a period following an epileptic fit when the person functions automatically and is unaware of their actions |
| **Quadriplegia (tetraplegia)** | paralysis of all four limbs |
| **Romberg's sign** | an inability to stand without swaying when the eyes are closed and the feet are together – sign of brain damage |
| **Sciatica** | pain along the sciatic nerve (down the back of the leg to the toe) |
| **Sinus thrombosis** | formation of blood clot in the brain sinuses (spaces in which the venous blood drains before entering the jugular veins) |
| **Spastic** | damage to motor area of brain producing increased muscle tone |
| **St Vitus' dance** | see Chorea |
| **Status epilepticus** | a continuous fit passing from one straight into another – very dangerous |
| **Stupor** | a level of consciousness – person not fully conscious but does respond to certain stimuli |
| **Subarachnoid haemorrhage** | bleeding between the layers of the meninges known as the pia mater and the arachnoid mater |
| **Subdural haematoma** | a blood clot between the layers of the meninges – the dura mater and the arachnoid mater |
| **Syncope** | fainting – temporary lack of blood to the brain |
| **Syphilis** | sexually transmitted disease which, in its final stages, produces damage to the central nervous system (CNS) |
| **Tabes dorsalis** | nerve damage to the (locomotor ataxia) spinal cord caused by the late stages of syphilis and giving rise to an abnormal gait |
| **Tardive dyskinesia** | side-effects of long term antipsychotic drugs; involuntary movements of face, etc. |
| **Tetraplegia** | (quadriplegia) paralysis of all four limbs |
| **Tic** | involuntary, rapid, recurrent stereotyped movement or vocalisation |
| **Tourette's syndrome** | neurological syndrome characterised by a tic disorder with mutiple muscle or vocal tics occurring in bouts. Involuntary use of foul language |
| **Tremor** | involuntary quivering of the muscles – inability to control them |
| **Trigeminal neuralgia** | inflammation of the Vth cranial nerve supplying three areas of the face; causes severe pain |
| **Vertigo** | dizziness |

## Mental health: diseases and disorders

**Acute** — rapid onset

**Advocate** — someone who speaks on behalf of the person

**Affective disorder** — term for mood disorder

**Affective psychosis** — major mental disorder in which there is serious disturbance of the emotions

**Agoraphobia** — a fear of open spaces or of leaving one's home

**Akathisia** — restlessness that results in an inability to sit still

**Alzheimer's disease** — progressive dementia – caused by destruction of the neurones (brain cells)

**Amnesia** — loss of memory

**Androphobia** — a fear of men

**Anhedonia** — incapable of experiencing pleasure from previously enjoyable activities

**Anorexia nervosa** — eating disorder characterised by severe weight loss as result of refusing to eat. Person thinks they are fat despite obvious thinness

**Anosognosia** — failure to recognise one's own condition or disease

**Anxiety** — apprehension, tension

**Anxiety disorder** — group of disorders characterised by overwhelming and persisting feelings of worry and fear which interfere with everyday life

**Arachnophobia** — a fear of spiders

**Asperger's disorder or syndrome** — thought to be related to autism, significantly impaired social interactions but patient is usually above average intelligence with no problems in language development

**Autism** — development disorder arising in early years of life; significantly impaired social and language skills – several categories classified

**Bipolar disorder** — mood disorder previously known as manic depression, characterised by extreme alternating moods of depression and mania (many different classifications by numbers)

**Borderline personality disorder** — group of persisting maladaptive patterns of deviant and social behaviour, lifestyle etc. not caused by psychotic illness

**Bulimia nervosa** — eating disorder characterised by recurrent bingeing and self-induced vomiting

**Catatonia** — state of stupor, strange posture, outbursts of excitement – form of autism common in schizophrenia

**Catharsis** — an outlet of repressed emotion

**Chronic** — long-term condition or frequently recurring

**Circadian rhythm** — chemical and psychological variations over 24 hr period

**Claustrophobia** — a fear of confined spaces

**Complex** — a pattern of behaviour which demonstrates an over-reaction to a problem

**Compulsion** — insistent and repetitive need to behave in unreasonable or excessive way

**Conversion** — problems expressed as physical symptoms eg abdominal pain, panic attacks, paralysis etc

**Coprolalia** — involuntary use of vulgar/foul language as in Tourette's syndrome

**Delirium** — mental excitement resulting from hallucinations, e.g. in state of high fever, alcohol consumption, or mental illness

**Delirium tremens** — mental excitement due to chronic excessive alcohol intake, known as 'DTs'

| | |
|---|---|
| **Delusion** | false belief that has no basis which cannot be changed despite obvious proof to the contrary |
| **Denial** | refusing to believe an unpleasant fact – a normal method of protection of the mind |
| **Depression** | mood disorder characterised by sadness, inability to experience pleasure, lack of energy, suicidal thought, guilt, indecisiveness, sleep disturbance etc |
| *Endogenous D* | caused by internal body factors, as in manic depression where there are alternating mood swings to intense euphoria |
| *Exogenous D* or *reactive D* | caused by events and environmental factors, e.g. bereavement or unemployment |
| *Involutional D* | caused by ageing process including menopause |
| **Dissociation** | disruption in integrated functions of consciousness, memory, perception etc. |
| **Doraphobia** | a fear of fur |
| **Dyskinesia** | involuntary muscle movement –side-effect of some medications |
| **Dyslexia** | word blindness learning disability |
| **Dysphoria** | unpleasant mood |
| **Dysthymia** | depression associated with imaginary illness |
| **Dystonia** | muscle spasms occurring in the tongue, jaw, eyes, neck: side-effect of some medications |
| **Echolalia** | parrot-like repetition of overheard words |
| **Euphoria** | exaggerated sense of well being |
| **Familial** | affecting more members of family than would be chance |

| | |
|---|---|
| **Fixation** | an arrest in psychological development at a particular stage |
| **Fugue** | period of altered awareness often associated with wandering, of which the person has no recall |
| **Gender dysphoria** | a belief that individual is the opposite gender i.e. a man a woman; a woman a man |
| **Haemophobia** | a fear of blood |
| **Hallucination** | false perception can be hearing, sight, touch, smell, taste, somatic (within the body): a psychosis |
| **Hydrophobia** | a fear of drinking |
| **Hypochondria** | an abnormality in which the person is pre-occupied with imaginary illnesses |
| **Hypomania** | mood characterised by unrealistic optimism, speech and activity |
| **Hysteria** | a neurosis arising from psychological problems producing bodily symptoms, e.g. paralysis |
| **Libido** | sexual energy/ behaviour/drive |
| **Limbic system** | area of the brain concerned with the emotional control and memory |
| **Mania** | abnormal elevation of the mood and over-activity – see bipolar disorder |
| **Manic depression** | a form of depression which is characterised by alternating mood swings of overactivity (mania) and sadness (depression) – a psychosis; see Depression, endogenous |
| **Melatonin** | hormone produced by the pineal gland in response to darkness, which induces sleep and depresses mood and mental ability |

| | | | |
|---|---|---|---|
| **Munchausen Syndrome by Proxy** | someone who draws attention to themselves by causing harm to others | | (i.e. psychotic) – unaware that they are ill; affects the whole personality – is often characterised by delusions, hallucinations, etc. |
| **Mysophobia** | a fear of dirt | **Psychosomatic** | bodily sensations produced from the mind |
| **Narcoleptic** | drug used to treat psychoses, i.e. an antipsychotic | **Rationalisation** | giving a reasonable explanation for behaviour which is in fact caused by a problem which the person cannot accept |
| **Neurosis** | a form of mental illness of which the (neurotic) patient has insight (awareness that they are ill), anxiety and depression. | | |
| | | **Schizoid** | split personality – being more than one personality (*not* 'as in schizophrenia') |
| **Nosophobia** | a fear of disease | | |
| **Nyctophobia** | a fear of darkness | **Schizophrenia** | a psychosis of unknown cause in which the person suffers delusions and hallucinations – thought processes are disordered; chronic disorder which commonly arises in teens |
| **Obsession** | recurrent, persistent and obtrusive ideas which is not removed by logic or reasoning | | |
| **Panic attack** | sudden periods of intense fear, discomfort etc. – chest pain breathlessness, dizzyness, sweating, nausea etc. | | |
| | | **Seasonal affective disorder (SAD)** | winter mood disorder caused by lack of light |
| **Panphobia** | a fear of everything | | |
| **Paranoia** | condition characterised by onset of delusions often of persecution | **Tardive dyskinesia** | side-effects of long term antipsychotic drugs; involuntary movements of face, etc. |
| **Perception** | the interpretation and response of the nervous system to sensory stimuli | | |
| | | **Tic** | involuntary, rapid, recurrent stereotyped movement or vocalisation |
| **Personality disorder** | group of persisting maladaptive patterns of deviant and social behaviour, lifestyle, etc. – not caused by psychotic illness | **Tourette's syndrome** | neurological syndrome characterised by a tic disorder with mutiple muscle or vocal tics occurring in bouts. Involuntary use of foul language |
| **Phobia** | irrational fear | | |
| **Phobophobia** | a fear of phobias | **Transference** | transferring strong emotions of love or hate onto another person, often the therapist or doctor |
| **Photophobia** | a fear of (or intolerance to) light | | |
| **Projection** | putting our own faults or behaviour onto another person | | |
| **Psychopath** | a person having no social conscience | **Trichophobia** | a fear of hair |
| **Psychosis** | mental illness in which the patient has no insight | **Xenophobia** | a fear of foreigners |

## Procedures and equipment

| | |
|---|---|
| **Cerebral angiogram** | X-ray demonstration of the blood vessels of the brain using an opaque dye |
| **Cisternal puncture** | same as lumbar puncture, but the needle is inserted into area at base of skull – used in investigation of cerebrospinal fluid (CSF) in children |
| **Craniotomy** | cutting into the bony cranium of the skull; used to relieve pressure etc |
| **Electro- encephalogram** | a tracing which records the electrical activity of the brain (used in diagnosis of epilepsy, tumours and other brain conditions) |
| **Electromyogram** | a tracing which records the electrical activity of muscles to show if there is any abnormality in the pattern of activity, both at rest and on movement |
| **Intrathecal** | injection directly into the meninges |
| **Lumbar puncture** | insertion of a needle into the meninges of the spinal cord to withdraw CSF for investigation |
| **Myelogram** | special X-ray using radio-opaque dye of the spinal cord |
| **Transcutaneous nerve stimulation** | a method of relieving chronic pain by electrical stimulation of other nerve endings |
| **Trephine** | instrument used for removing circular sections of tissue from skull area (trephining) |
| **Ventriculogram** | X-ray demonstration of the ventricles of the brain. This procedure is being replaced by CT and MRI scans |

Chapter **14**

# The sensory organs

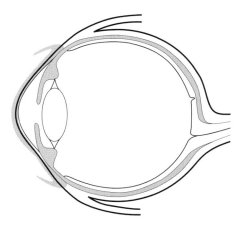

## Structure

The special senses of the body consist of sight, hearing, smell, taste, touch, temperature and pain. The receptors for these senses are found in the following sensory organs:

- **eye**          sight

- **ear**          hearing and balance

- **nose**         smell

- **tongue**       taste

- **skin**         touch, temperature and pain (dealt with in Chapter 10)

## The eye

The eye is the sensory organ of sight and is situated in the bony **orbit** of the skull which protects it. It receives messages which are conveyed to the brain for interpretation.

It consists of the following structures:

- **eyeball**

appendages:

- **eyebrows**

- **eyelids**

- **lacrimal apparatus** (for producing tears)

## Eyeball

The eyeball is almost spherical in shape and is embedded in fat. It is protected at the front by eyebrows, eyelids and lashes, and is composed of three layers:

- **sclera**

- **choroid**

- **retina**

It also contains the **lens** and fluids known as the **aqueous** and **vitreous humour** which **refract** (bend) the rays of light to focus upon the retinal layer and form an image very similar to that within a camera (*see Figure 63*).

## Sclera

This is the tough outer fibrous coat which helps to maintain the shape of the eyeball. Muscles are attached to it and the orbit, keeping it in place and enabling movement of the eyeball. The front part is covered in **conjunctiva**, a membrane which also lines the eyelids. At the front lies the **cornea** with which it is continuous.

## Choroid

This is the vascular layer attached to the sclera, forming the middle layer of the eyeball. At the front of the eyeball it is continuous with the **ciliary body**, a muscular organ from which the lens is suspended, and the **iris**.

The iris is a pigmented muscular body with a hole in its centre which forms the **pupil**, through which light rays enter to focus upon the **retina** (nervous layer).

It is capable of constricting and relaxing, so altering the size of the pupil which controls the amount of light entering the eye.

## Retina

This forms the inner layer of the eyeball and is attached to the choroid. It contains nerve fibres which are the origins of the **optic nerve** and include specialised light-sensitive structures known as **rods** and **cones**, which receive light and colour information for interpretation by the brain.

Rods receive sensations of light and dark, and are more numerous towards the front of the eye. Cones are concerned with sensations of colour. They are more numerous towards the back of the eyeball; red, green and blue are the prime colours for interpretation. **Colour blindness** arises from a lack or abnormality of these receptor cells.

The optic nerve, sheathed at the back of each eye, conveys the sensations from the retina to the **occipital** area of the brain for interpretation into sight. The nerve from each eye joins at an area known as the **optic chiasma**.

## The eyeball

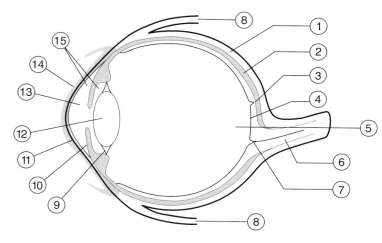

1. Sclera
2. Choroid
3. Macula (fovea)
4. Retina
5. Vitreous humour
6. Optic nerve
7. Optic disc (blind spot)
8. Rectus muscle
9. Suspensory ligaments
10. Iris
11. Cornea
12. Lens
13. Aqueous humour
14. Conjunctiva
15. Anterior/posterior chambers

**Figure 63:** The eyeball

### Macula (fovea)

This is an area of the retina where cones are most numerous and central vision most acute. It is immediately opposite the cornea.

### Optic disc

This is the area where there are no rods or cones present, and is at the back of the eye where the optic nerve leaves the eyeball. It gives rise to an area known as the **'blind spot'**, which is present in each field of vision. No sight is perceived from this area.

### Optic fundus

This is an area including the **optic disc**, which can be examined by use of an **ophthalmoscope**. Changes to the retina and evidence of effects of high blood pressure or raised intra-cranial pressure, can be viewed in this way, enabling early diagnosis in some cases.

### Muscles of the eyeball

There are three pairs attached to the sclera and the bony orbit, which enable movement of the eyeball. Normally the eyes move in unison which enables **binocular vision**. When the eyes move independently the condition produced is known as **strabismus** (squint). It is most important that any defect is diagnosed early in childhood as deficiency of sight can occur if treatment is delayed. Surgery and/or **orthoptic** exercises are used for correction.

### Refraction

This is the term used for the bending of the light rays. It is necessary to ensure that images are focused upon the retina for clear vision. Images are perceived as inverted and are correctly interpreted by the brain. It is because of this that, in conditions of cerebral disturbance such as strokes and head injuries,

## Visual paths

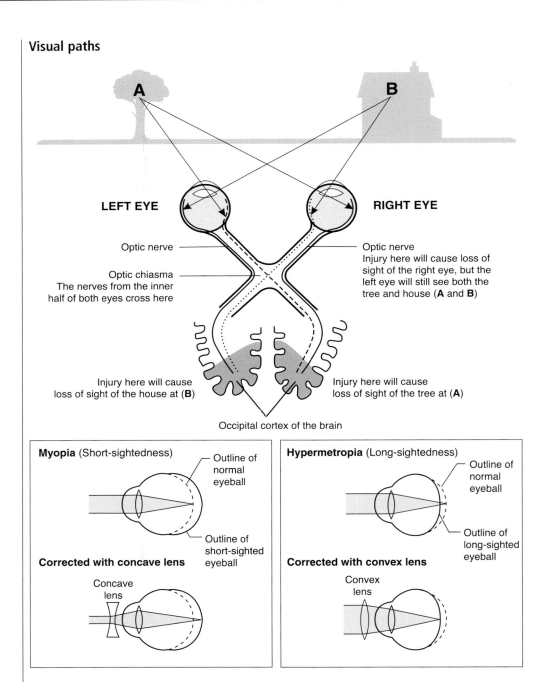

**A**

**B**

LEFT EYE

RIGHT EYE

Optic nerve

Optic chiasma
The nerves from the inner
half of both eyes cross here

Optic nerve
Injury here will cause loss of
sight of the right eye, but the
left eye will still see both the
tree and house (**A** and **B**)

Injury here will cause
loss of sight of the house at (**B**)

Injury here will cause
loss of sight of the tree at (**A**)

Occipital cortex of the brain

**Myopia** (Short-sightedness)

Outline of
normal
eyeball

Outline of
short-sighted
eyeball

**Corrected with concave lens**

Concave
lens

**Hypermetropia** (Long-sightedness)

Outline of
normal
eyeball

Outline of
long-sighted
eyeball

**Corrected with convex lens**

Convex
lens

**Figure 64:** Visual paths

vision is often disturbed. People who are **myopic** (short-sighted) tend to have a mis-shapen eyeball that is too long front to back, thus the images are in focus in front of the retina. The opposite of this is **hypermetropia** (long-sightedness) where a visual defect means the light rays come to focus behind the retina as a result of the eyeball being too long top to bottom (*see Figure 64*).

The structures involved in refraction are the:

- **Cornea**
- **Lens**
- **Aqueous humour**
- **Vitreous humour**

The cornea and lens, by their curvature, will bend light rays striking upon their surface.

## Aqueous humour

This is a water-like fluid situated within the **anterior** and **posterior** chambers at the front of the eyeball.

Rays of light will also be bent while travelling through this substance.

## Vitreous humour

This is a thick jelly-like substance which fills the posterior portion of the eyeball (situated behind the lens) ensuring it maintains its shape. Light travelling through this substance is further bent to achieve focusing of images.

## Pressure in the eyeball

In conditions of **glaucoma** where the aqueous humour fails to drain effectively, **intraocular pressure** is raised and damage to the retina occurs. In acute cases, urgent treatment is required to reduce this pressure if blindness is to be prevented.

## Accommodation

This is the ability of the eye to focus near objects upon the retina. This is achieved by the alteration in the shape of the lens and its

capsule by the constriction and relaxation of the **ciliary body** from which the lens is suspended. Ability to accommodate decreases with age as the elasticity of the lens and its capsule decreases.

## Lacrimal apparatus

This consists of structures which produce tears:

- **Lacrimal gland**
- **Lacrimal ducts**
- **Lacrimal sac**
- **Nasolacrimal duct**

Tears consist of a slightly alkaline, salty fluid. These have a slightly antiseptic action and also keep the eyeball moist. They are involved in the expression of emotion.

# The ear

This is the receptor organ of hearing and balance. Sound waves travel through the organ conveying messages to the brain for interpretation.

There are three main parts to the ear:

- **External ear**
- **Middle ear**
- **Inner ear**

## External ear

This consists of the **auricle** or **pinna**, attached to the side of the head, and the **auditory canal**. The pinna acts like an ear trumpet to receive sound waves and is composed of skin and elastic cartilage.

The auditory canal within the skull carries sound waves from the pinna to the eardrum (**tympanic membrane**) which separates it from the middle ear. It is lined with skin containing hair and modified glands, which produce wax (**cerumen**) to protect the delicate membrane. If excessive wax is produced, deafness can occur because of the obstruction to the eardrum, preventing vibration. This wax may be removed by **syringing**.

# The ear

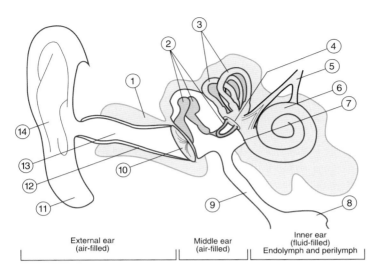

1. Temporal bone
2. Ossicles of:
   Malleus
   Incus
   Stapes
3. Semi-circular canals
4. Fenestra ovalis (oval window)
5. Auditory nerve
6. Cochlea
   (concerned with hearing)
7. Fenestra rotunda (round window)
8. Naso-pharynx
9. Eustachian tube
10. Tympanic membrane (eardrum)
11. Ear lobe
12. Cerumen (wax) producing cells
13. Auditory canal
14. Pinna

External ear
(air-filled)

Middle ear
(air-filled)

Inner ear
(fluid-filled)
Endolymph and perilymph

**Figure 65:** The ear

## Middle ear

This consists of a cavity within the temporal bone of the skull, filled with air and lined with mucous membrane. A canal known as the **eustachian tube** extends from the middle ear into the back of the nose (**naso-pharynx**) and it is through this, when swallowing occurs, that air is conducted, so ensuring an equal pressure between the external and middle ear.

Infection present in the nose or throat can easily spread to the middle ear, causing inflammation (**otitis media**), which in turn can cause **mastoiditis** (inflammation of the bone cells of the temporal bone of the skull). This can also lead to a brain abscess. It is for this reason that any infection must be treated as quickly as possible.

### Ossicles

These are three tiny bony structures named

from their shapes of **hammer** (**malleus**), **anvil** (**incus**) and **stirrup** (**stapes**). They are attached in a chain by ligaments, allowing them to vibrate causing the conduction of sound waves from the **tympanic membrane** into the inner ear.

The malleus is connected to the tympanic membrane and the stapes to the oval window (**fenestra ovalis**) of the inner ear. Each of these two ossicles is attached to the incus (*see Figure 65*).

## Inner ear

This is situated within the bony labyrinth of the temporal bone. It consists of numerous bony canals and cavities. It is lined with a membrane known as the **membranous labyrinth** and is filled with fluid. It communicates with the middle ear with which it is continuous.

It is composed of the following parts:

- **Vestibule**
- **Semicircular canals**
- **Cochlea**

### Vestibule

This forms the entrance to the inner ear and here the oval and round windows are situated, communicating with the middle ear.

### Semi-circular canals

These contain specialised structures which, upon movement of the fluid within the membranes, stimulate nerve endings which convey information concerning position of the head and position in space to the brain.

Disease within these structures can cause giddiness (**vertigo**) and loss of balance.

### Cochlea

This structure, within the membranous labyrinth, contains the **organ of Corti**, the true organ of hearing. It is coiled like a snail around a tiny bone.

Within it are numerous specialised nerve endings which convey the effect of sound waves received along the **auditory nerve** for interpretation by the **temporal lobe** of the brain (cerebrum).

### Interpretation of sound

The round window bulges outwards as vibration is conducted through the oval window from the stapes, so maintaining the correct pressure of the fluid in the inner ear. In blast injuries these windows may perforate. Sensations of volume, pitch and harmony are perceived due to fluctuations in pressure.

## The nose

The sense of smell is received by specialised nerve fibres in the mucous membrane of the nasal cavities and is conveyed to the brain via the **olfactory nerve** for interpretation (*see Figure 66*).

## The nose

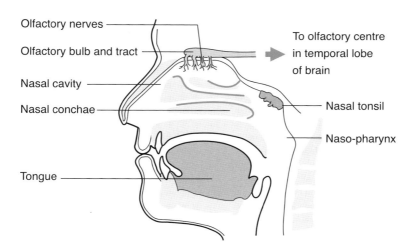

Olfactory nerves

Olfactory bulb and tract

Nasal cavity

Nasal conchae

Tongue

To olfactory centre in temporal lobe of brain

Nasal tonsil

Naso-pharynx

**Figure 66:** The nose

## The tongue

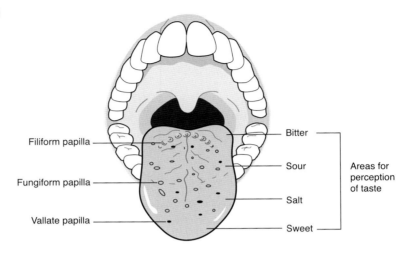

Filiform papilla

Fungiform papilla

Vallate papilla

Bitter

Sour

Salt

Sweet

Areas for perception of taste

**Figure 67:** The tongue

## The tongue

This muscular organ, attached to the **hyoid bone**, contains the **taste buds** and special **receptor cells** which convey the sense of taste (salt, bitter, sweet and sour) to the brain for interpretation. These are found within specialised structures known as **papillae** (*see Figure 67*).

Other flavours are appreciated in conjunction with the sense of smell. It is for this reason that the sense of taste is affected when the person is suffering from a cold. For the perception of these sensations, the membranes in which the special cells are situated, must be moist.

Taste buds are also present in the mucous membrane of the **palate** and **pharynx**.

## Abbreviations

| | |
|---|---|
| **ABR** | auditory brainstem response |
| **Acc** | accommodation |
| **AD** | right ear (auris dextra) |
| **AMD** | age-related macular degeneration |
| **AS** | left ear (auris sinister) |
| **Ast** | astigmatism |
| **AU** | both ears (aures unitas) or each ear |
| **D** | diopter (lens strength) |
| **db** | decibel (measurement of sound) |
| **ENT** | ear, nose and throat |
| **EOM** | extraocular movement |
| **HM** | hand movement |
| **IOFB** | intraocular foreign body |
| **IOP** | intraocular pressure |
| **L&D** | light and dark perceived |
| **LASIK** | laser *in situ* keratomileusia |
| **LCS** | left convergent squint (eye turns inwards) |
| **LDS** | left divergent squint (eye turns outwards) |
| **OD** | oculus dexter (right eye) |
| **OS** | oculus sinister (left eye) |
| **OU** | oculus uterque (each eye) |
| **PERLA (PERRLA)** | pupils equal (round), react to light and accommodation |

| | | | | |
|---|---|---|---|---|
| **PDT** | photodynamic therapy | | | optic disc area where there are no sensory visual receptors |
| **PND** | post-nasal drip (catarrh dripping down the back of the throat from the nasal passages and sinuses) | | **Fovea** | see Macula |
| | | | **Fundus of eye** | the whole of area at the back of the eye opposite the pupil |
| **PRK** | photo-refractive keratotomy | | **Macula (fovea)** | area on the retina with the greatest number of receptors for sight (central vision) |
| **RCS** | right convergent squint (eye turns outwards) | | | |
| **RDS** | right divergent squint (eye turns inwards) | | **Ophthalmic optician** | person qualified to examine eyes, and prescribe and dispense spectacles |
| **REM** | rapid eye movement | | | |
| **SC** | without correction (spectacles) | | **Ophthalmologist** | specialist in the diseases of the eye |
| **Ts & As** | tonsillectomy and adenoidectomy | | **Ophthalmology** | scientific study of the eye |
| **T+** | increased intraocular pressure | | **Optician** | person who makes and fits spectacles |
| **T−** | decreased intraocular pressure | | **Optometrist** | person who measures/tests eyes and fits spectacles |
| **VA** | visual acuity (clarity or accuracy of vision) | | **Orthoptist** | therapist who treats squints |
| | | | **Otologist** | medical specialist in treating ear disease |
| **VF** | visual field | | **Otology** | study of ear disease |

## Terminology

| | |
|---|---|
| **Blephar/o** and **Tars/o** | stem for eyelid |
| **Cor, core/o** | stem for pupil |
| **Irid/o** | stem for iris (of eye) |
| **Kerat/o** | stem for cornea |
| **Dacry/o** **Lachrym/o** **Lacrim/o** **Lacrym/o** | stems for tear |
| **Ocul/o** and **Ophthalm/o** | stems for eye |
| **Opt/o** | stem for vision |
| **Ot/o** and **Aur/i** | stems for ear |
| **Phak/o** | stem for eye lens |
| **Retin/o** | stem for retina |
| **Tars/o** | stem for eyelid |
| **Tympan/o** and **Myring/o** | stems for ear drum |
| **Uve/o** | stem for uveal tract |
| **Blind spot** | area of no vision due to |

| | |
|---|---|
| **Otorhino-laryngologist** | medical specialist in ear, nose and throat disease |
| **Otorhino-laryngology** | study of the ear, nose and throat |
| **Refraction** | bending of light rays to measure the focusing of the eye mechanisms |

## Diseases and disorders

| | |
|---|---|
| **6/6 vision** | the normal ability to be able to read line six of the Snellen chart at six metres |
| **Amblyopia** | dimness of vision |
| **Aphakia** | condition where there is no lens present, e.g. after removal of cataract |
| **Astigmatism** | eye defect usually of shape of cornea which is irregular in curvature, causing blurring of vision |
| **Aural polyp** | pedunculated (stalk-like) tumour in the ear – not malignant |

| | |
|---|---|
| **Blepharitis** | inflammation of the eyelids |
| **Cataract** | an opacity of the lens or its capsule causing blurring of sight |
| **Cauliflower ear** | enlargement/deformity of the external ear due to haematoma formation after injury |
| **Choroiditis** | inflammation of the choroid layer of eyeball |
| **Conduction deafness** | loss of hearing due to the failure of the vibrations caused by sound waves to be conducted to specialised nerve cells of the inner ear |
| **Conjunctivitis** | inflammation of the conjunctiva membrane covering eyeball and lining eyelids |
| **Corneal ulcer** | open sore on cornea |
| **Dacryo-cystectomy** | surgical removal of a tear sac |
| **Dacryocystitis** | inflammation of the tear sacs |
| **Dacryolith** | stone in the tear duct |
| **Dacryostenosis** | narrowing of tear duct |
| **Dendritic ulcer** | corneal ulcer that has tree-like branches in shape (caused by the herpes simplex virus – cold sore) |
| **Ectropion** | eversion of eyelid (outward) |
| **Entropion** | inversion of the eyelid (inward) |
| **Exophthalmos** | abnormal protrusion of the eye |
| **Glaucoma** | a condition where intraocular pressure is raised, which in turn causes damage to the retina leading to blindness if not controlled |
| **Glue ear/serous otitis media** | presence of catarrh (fluid/pus) in middle ear |
| **Hemianopia** | partial blindness – ability to see only half the visual field |

| | |
|---|---|
| **Hordeolum** | 'stye' – infection of the eyelash follicle |
| **Hypermetropia** | long-sightedness |
| **Intraocular pressure** | pressure within the eyeball |
| **Iridocyclitis** | inflammation of the iris and ciliary body (from where the lens is suspended) |
| **Iritis** | inflammation of the muscular iris of the eye |
| **Keratitis** | inflammation of the cornea |
| **Labyrinthitis** | inflammation of the inner ear |
| **Macular degeneration** | a degeneration of vision due to changes to the macular area of the eye (*see Figure 63*) which is responsible for maximum vision – at present there is little effective treatment |
| **Mastoiditis** | inflammation of the mastoid antrum (cavity containing porous sieve-like bone) of the temporal bone of the skull |
| **Meibomian cyst** | blockage of ducts of specialised sebaceous glands of the eyelid known as meibomian glands |
| **Ménières disease** | a syndrome causing vertigo (dizziness), tinnitus and deafness |
| **Myopia** | short-sightedness |
| **Myringitis** | inflammation of the eardrum |
| **Nerve deafness** | loss of hearing due to damage or disease of the nerve fibres |
| **Optic disc** | area at the back of the eyeball where there are no rods or cones, and where the optic nerve enters the eyeball – examined with an ophthalmoscope to detect swelling or abnormality to blood vessels or nervous system |

| | |
|---|---|
| **Otalgia** | earache |
| **Otitis externa** | inflammation of the external ear |
| **Otitis media** | inflammation of the middle ear |
| **Otorrhoea** | discharge from the ear |
| **Otosclerosis** | progressive hardening of the membranous bony labyrinth (lining of inner ear); hereditary in females – otoliths in middle ear also become fixed so cannot vibrate |
| **Papilloedema** | oedema (free fluid present) of the optic disc |
| **Presbyopia** | (old sight) long-sightedness due to failure of the lens capsule to accommodate, i.e. change shape of lens in order to focus close up objects – lens capsule becomes less elastic with the process of ageing |
| **Proptosis** | eyeballs protrude outwards/forwards |
| **Ptosis** | drooping of the eyelid |
| **Retinal detachment** | detachment of the retinal layer of eyeball from the choroid |
| **Retinitis** | inflammation of the retina (nerve layer of the eyeball) |
| **Retinopathy** | disease of the retina |
| **Rodent ulcer** | slow growing malignant tumour of the top layer of skin causing destruction of tissue |
| **Scleritis** | inflammation of the sclera (tough outer coat of eyeball) |
| **Scotoma** | normal and abnormal 'blind spots' in the visual fields |
| **Strabismus** | squint, i.e. failure of eyes to work evenly together |
| **Uveitis** | inflammation of the uveal tract (iris, choroid and ciliary body) |

## Procedures and equipment

| | |
|---|---|
| **Audiogram** | the recorded measurement of hearing |
| **Audiometer** | instrument used to measure hearing |
| **Audiometry** | measurement of hearing |
| **Auriscope (otoscope)** | lighted instrument used to examine ear canal and eardrum |
| **Corneal graft** | grafting a donor cornea into place |
| **Cryosurgery** | cooling or freezing the area which is being operated upon |
| **Decibels** | a unit of hearing (measurement of sound) |
| **Ear syringing** | removal of excessive wax by syringing external auditory canal with warm water |
| **Enucleation** | removal of an organ from its place, e.g. eyeball from socket |
| **Grommets** | special valves fitted into eardrum to release pressure in middle ear and drain fluid |
| **Iridectomy** | surgical removal of portion of iris, forming an artificial 'hole' |
| **Laser *in situ* keratomileusia (LASIK)** | a procedure in which the cornea is moulded surgically to correct short sight |
| **Laser surgery** | surgery using a laser beam instead of scalpel or stitching |
| **Miotics** | drops which constrict the pupil of the eye |
| **Mydriatics** | drops used to dilate the pupil of the eye |
| **Myringotomy** | cutting into the eardrum |
| **Ophthalmoscope** | a lighted instrument used to examine the interior of the eyeball |
| **Otoscope** | instrument for examining the ear (see Auriscope) |

**Otoscopy** — examination of the ear with a lighted instrument

**Paracentesis tympani** — drawing off of fluid within the middle ear

**Perimetry** — plotting of the visual fields

**Photodynamic therapy (PDT)** — used to treat macular degeneration. A light-sensitive substance is injected via the blood stream. It reaches the eye and a light is directed to the area, which activates the chemical causing it to stick to leaking blood vessels. This prevents formation of scar tissue on the retina

**Photo-refractive keratotomy (PRK)** — an older method of correcting short sight by surgery

**Radical mastoidectomy** — removal of large area of mastoid bone area to prevent further infection and drain area of pus (common before advent of antibiotics), a complication of otitis media

**Removal of cataract** — operation to remove the opaque lens

**Rinne's Test** — test for deafness using a tuning fork placed on the auditory opening of the ear. When the patient ceases to hear the ringing tone it is placed on the bony area below, known as the mastoid process. In normal hearing it will not be heard at this point, but in conditions of middle ear deafness a tone will still be heard by the patient

**Slit lamp** — special machine used to examine the eyes

**Snellen chart** — chart used to test visual acuity, i.e. sight

**Stapedectomy** — surgical removal of the stapes (stirrup bone) of the middle ear

**Tarsoplasty** — reshaping of the eyelid

**Tonometer** — an instrument used to measure intra-ocular pressure (within the eyeball)

**Trephine** — instrument used for cutting away a circle of tissue

**Tympanoplasty** — reshaping the eardrum

**Visual acuity** — the acuteness of sight

**Visual fields** — measurement or plotting of the area of vision (perimetry) to establish any damage (blind spot will be normal area)

**Weber's test** — test for comparison of the bone conduction of hearing in both ears. A tuning fork is struck and placed on the vertex of the skull. The patient indicates in which ear it is heard the loudest. In conditions of middle ear deafness it is louder in the affected ear.

Chapter **15**

# The endocrine system

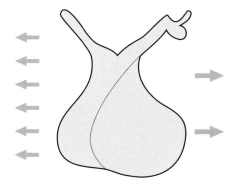

## Function

This is the system concerned with the production of chemical messengers (**hormones**) which are secreted from a ductless gland (**endocrine gland**) directly into the blood stream to activate a target organ (*see Figure 68*).

## Structure

The endocrine system consists of the following:

- **Pituitary gland**
- **Adrenal glands**
- **Thyroid gland**
- **Parathyroid glands**
- **Pancreas**
- **Ovaries**
- **Testes**
- **Thymus**
- **Pineal body**

### Pituitary gland

This is situated at the base of the brain and is the size of a pea. It is known as the master gland or 'leader of the endocrine orchestra' because it controls many of the other endocrine glands. It has an **anterior** and **posterior** lobe which produce many hormones (*see Figure 69*). It is controlled by the **hypothalamus** of the brain, situated immediately above.

## The endocrine system

1. Pineal gland
2. Parathyroid glands
3. Adrenal glands
   (Suprarenal)
4. Testes (male)
   Ovaries (female)
5. Pancreas
6. Thymus gland
7. Thyroid gland
8. Pituitary gland

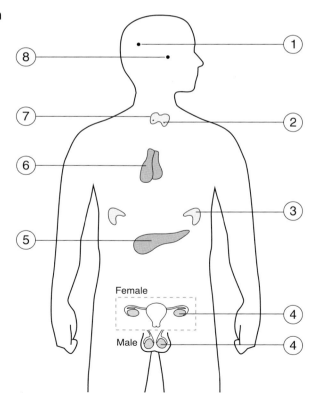

**Figure 68:** The endocrine system

*Anterior lobe*

This produces the following hormones:

**Adrenocorticotrophic hormone (ACTH)**
stimulates adrenal gland cortex to produce corticosteroids and sex hormones

**Growth hormone (GH)**
stimulates growth of bone especially long bones

**Thyroid stimulating hormone (TSH)**
stimulates thyroid gland to produce thyroxin

**Melanin stimulating hormone (MSH)**
produces pigmentation of skin but is normally inhibited by action of adrenal cortex hormones

**Gonadotrophic hormones (FSH & LH)**
follicle stimulating hormone (FSH) stimulates the follicles of ovaries causing egg (ovum) to ripen ready for release. In males it stimulates the testes

**Prolactin or luteotrophic hormone (LTH)**
stimulates production of milk

Growth hormone (GH) affects the growth of long bones. A deficiency will cause stunted growth or **dwarfism** in children. Excess will cause **gigantism**, while in adults, whose long bones can no longer grow, it will cause enlargement of flat bones of the face, hands and feet (**acromegaly**).

The other hormones mentioned act upon target organs, which are influenced in the production of their own hormones. These include the **ovaries, testes, thyroid** and **adrenal** function. The production of **milk** by the breast is stimulated by **prolactin**.

*Posterior lobe*

This produces:

- **Oxytocin**

- **Pitressin** or **vasopressin**

Oxytocin affects the contraction of the **smooth muscle** of the **uterus** in pregnancy and childbirth, and the ejection of milk from the breast in **suckling**.

**Pitressin**, also known as **antidiuretic hormone (ADH)**, stimulates the tubules of the kidney to reabsorb water and mineral salts, keeping the correct balance in the body. Absence of ADH produces a disease known as **diabetes insipidus**, where copious dilute urine is produced.

# Pituitary gland

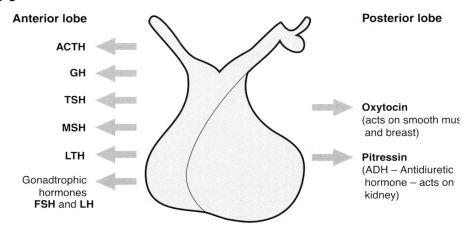

**Anterior lobe**

ACTH

GH

TSH

MSH

LTH

Gonadtrophic hormones **FSH** and **LH**

**Posterior lobe**

Oxytocin
(acts on smooth mus
and breast)

Pitressin
(ADH – Antidiuretic
hormone – acts on
kidney)

**Figure 69:** The pituitary gland

## Adrenal glands

The adrenal glands (**suprarenal glands**), situated on the top of each **kidney**, are composed of two parts – an outside portion (**cortex**) and a middle (**medulla**) which produce different secretions and are stimulated by the pituitary gland.

### Cortex

The cortex produces **steroids** which affect salt balance, protein and glucose metabolism, growth and muscle tone. Sex hormones are also produced.

In deficiency of these hormones, the patient suffers from **Addison's disease** and is administered **cortisone**. Excess produces **Cushing's syndrome**.

### Medulla

The medulla produces **adrenaline**, the stress hormone concerned with preparation of the body for the **'fight or flight'** mechanism, whereby heart rate and respirations quicken, energy is released by the liver and muscles, and the body can respond to fear and excitement.

## Thyroid gland

This gland is stimulated by the pituitary gland. It is situated in the neck, in front of the larynx and is concerned with the basic metabolism of the body. It produces a hormone called **thyroxine** which requires **iodine** in the diet for its production. Iodine is added to salt used for cooking purposes for this reason.

Excessive secretion causes **hyperthyroidism** or **thyrotoxicosis** with increased heart rate, excessive energy, nervousness, protruding eyeballs, etc. Treatment is usually surgical and a **partial thyroidectomy** is performed.

Under-secretion, or **hyposecretion**, causes a disease known as **myxoedema** where the patient is mentally and physically slow and all body functions are sluggish as metabolism is at a minimal rate. Treatment is with **thyroxine** and the effect can be miraculous as the patient returns to normal.

In childhood, deficiency produces **cretinism** and this is routinely tested (**screened**) for at birth.

## Parathyroid glands

Deep within the thyroid gland lie the parathyroids. These produce **parathyroid hormone (PTH)**, which is involved in the control of **calcium metabolism** and the level of calcium in the bloodstream and in the bone.

## Pancreas

The endocrine function of the pancreas, situated in the abdominal cavity close to the stomach, is the control of **carbohydrate** metabolism in the body.

**Insulin** is produced directly into the bloodstream from special cells known as the **'islets of Langerhans'**. These regulate the levels of **glucose** in the blood and allow conversion of sugars to glucose for storage in the liver and muscles, ready for release when required.

Deficiency of insulin causes a condition known as **diabetes mellitus**, which may be treated with insulin injections. Insulin cannot be taken by mouth as it is destroyed by the gastric secretions of the stomach.

## Ovaries and testes

These are the **gonads** (and produce the sex cells). Their role in hormone secretion is to produce **oestrogens** and **progesterone** in the female and **androgens** in the male, the main one being **testosterone**. They are stimulated by the pituitary gland.

## Thymus

This is situated in the chest (thoracic) cavity near the trachea upon the major blood vessels. It is important in childhood and puberty for growth and development. It is concerned with the production of **lymphoid tissue**, **lymphocytes** and **immunity**.

## Pineal body

This is a structure within the **cerebrum** of the brain which was probably a vestigial third eye (remains from animal development). Its endocrine function is not clear, but it may have effects upon '**diurnal rhythm**' ('body clock') and production of sex hormones.

## Abbreviations

| | |
|---|---|
| **ACTH** | adrenocorticotrophic hormone |
| **ADH** | antidiuretic hormone (pitressin) |
| **FBS** | fasting blood sugar |
| **FSH** | follicle stimulating hormone |
| **GH** | growth hormone |
| **IDDM** | insulin-dependent diabetes mellitus |
| **LH** | luteinising hormone |
| **LTH** | luteotrophic hormone (prolactin) |
| **MSH** | melanin stimulating hormone |
| **NIDDM** | non-insulin-dependent diabetes mellitus |
| **PBI** | protein-bound iodine |
| **PTH** | parathyroid hormone |
| **RAI** | radioactive iodine |
| **RAIU** | radioactive iodine uptake |
| **T3** | triiodothyronine (thyroid hormone) |
| **T4** | thyroxine (thyroid hormone) |
| **TSH** | thyroid stimulating hormone |

## Terminology

| | |
|---|---|
| **Aden/o** | stem for gland |
| **Adren/o** | stem for adrenal gland |
| **Basal metabolic rate (BMR)** | the rate at which the body cells work in using food substances and oxygen to create energy and waste products of carbon dioxide ($CO_2$) and water ($H_2O$) – measured at complete rest |
| **Cortic/o** | stem referring to the cortex (outer portion) of an organ |
| **Endocrin/o** | endocrine (concerning hormones) |
| **Hypophys/o** | pituitary gland |
| **Medull/o** | medulla (middle/inside portion) |
| **Parathyr/o** | stem for parathyroid gland |
| **Pitressin (vasopressin)** | antidiuretic hormone (ADH) increases reabsorption by the kidney tubules to prevent dehydration (water loss by the body) |
| **Thym/o** | thymus gland |
| **Thyr/o** | stem for thyroid gland. |

## Diseases and disorders

| | |
|---|---|
| **Acromegaly** | overgrowth of flat bones of face, hands and feet caused by excessive growth hormone in adults |
| **Addison's disease** | insufficient adrenal cortex hormones produced causing weakness, pigmentation of skin, wasting etc |
| **Cretinism** | under-secretion of thyroxine hormone in babies – present at birth (congenital) causing mental and physical retardation |
| **Cushing's syndrome** | excessive adrenal cortex hormones (steroids) causing abnormal distribution of hair, fat and shrinking (atrophy) of genitals |
| **Diabetes insipidus** | deficiency of pitressin hormone resulting in copious amounts of urine being produced |
| **Diabetes mellitus** | deficiency of pancreatic hormone, insulin – or development of insensitivity to insulin, leading to failure to metabolise carbohydrates |
| *type 1 (IDDM)* | early onset |
| *type 2 (NIDDM)* | late onset or very high levels of insulin leading to insensitivity to insulin |
| **Dwarfism** | insufficient growth hormone produced causing lack of growth of long bones in children |

**Exophthalmos**    abnormal protrusion of the eyeball

**Gigantism**    excessive growth hormone in children, causes excessive growth of long bones

**Goitre**

   *Simple goitre*    enlargement of the thyroid gland in the neck – can cause pressure upon the trachea embarrassing breathing. Enlargement of the thyroid gland due to lack of iodine in the diet, also known as 'Derbyshire neck' as there is no iodine in Derbyshire water

   *Malignant goitre*    enlargement of thyroid gland due to hyperthyroidism causing severe toxic symptoms which are dangerous to health

**Hyperparathyroidism**    excessive production of parathyroid hormone (PTH) from parathyroid glands – causes excessive calcium in the blood and can cause deposits of calcium salts (stones) in the kidneys

**Hypersecretion**    oversecretion

**Hypoparathyroidism**    insufficient production of hormone PTH from parathyroid glands causing insufficient calcium in the blood

**Hyposecretion**    undersecretion

**Myxoedema**    undersecretion of thyroxine hormone in adults causing slowed metabolism, mental and physical dullness, loss of eyebrows and hair, oedema (free fluid) of the face, etc.

**Osteitis fibrosis cystica**    formation of cysts in the bone due to excess parathyroid hormone production, calcium salts are removed from the bones into the blood

**Tetany**    involuntary spasms of the muscles, particularly of the hands and feet, caused by low levels of calcium in the blood

**Thyrotoxicosis**    hyperthyroidism – oversecretion of the hormone thyroxine, causing raised pulse, tremor, bulging eyes (exophthalmos), loss of weight, enlargement of thyroid gland etc

## Procedures and equipment

**Hypophysectomy**    surgical removal of the pituitary gland (or partial removal)

**Thyroidectomy**    partial or complete surgical removal of the thyroid gland

# Chapter 16

# Clinical imaging

The X-ray department and its services

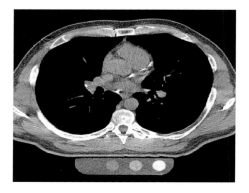

This hospital department is primarily concerned with the diagnosis and investigation of disease using **X-rays (ionising rays)**. It is also involved with newer types of investigations such as **ultrasound**, and **magnetic resonance imaging (MRI)**.

In hospitals which do not have a separate **nuclear medicine department**, diagnostic techniques which use radioactive isotopes are performed in the X-ray department. Therapy involving the use of **radioactive isotopes**, and **radiotherapy** used in the treatment of cancer, may also form part of the work of this department.

The diagnostic **radiologist** is the medical doctor who specialises in this field, while diagnostic **radiographers** are the professional staff involved in the many procedures. Where such staff are involved in treatment of disease they are known as therapeutic radiologists and ragiographers.

## X-rays

X-rays, also known as **Röentgen** rays, are short waves which are potentially very harmful, unless carefully controlled, and extreme precautions are enforced to ensure safety to both patients and staff. Scatter of the rays from the X-ray table will occur as the pictures are taken.

Careful technical design, regular testing of machines and stringent training of all staff are employed to this effect. Monitoring of **exposure to the radiation** by staff, is measured by a special type of counter (usually a **'film badge'**) attached to the person's clothing.

The wearing, by the radiographers and other personnel involved in procedures, of **lead aprons**, through which X-rays will not penetrate, is essential for their protection. Children and pregnant women are given a shield of lead material to prevent the ovaries or testes, containing immature ova and sperm, becoming affected by the radiation. X-rays of pregnant women are only performed when absolutely essential, to avoid potential damage to the fetus.

### Genetic damage

While all cells are sensitive to radiation, dividing or immature cells are even more vulnerable and damage to the genetic material can occur.

Whenever possible, routine X-ray investigations are avoided during the latter part of the menstrual cycle, when a woman of childbearing age could have conceived. It is for this reason that a section for lmp (last menstrual period) is to be found on X-ray request forms.

## Diagnostic radiology

This is the term used when X-rays are used for diagnosis. The term, diagnostic radiology, is also sometimes used to refer to other imaging processes which do not use X-rays but are carried out in the clinical imaging/X-ray department.

### Medical imaging

X-rays are able to pass through skin and soft tissue. They can then act upon certain photographic chemicals to produce a permanent record known as a **radiograph**. They also have the property of being able to 'light up' a **fluorescent screen**, so producing a visible image of body organs on the screen, which can then be transferred to a TV monitor.

### Preparation of the patient

Some X-ray investigations require special preparation of the patient by fasting, giving of laxatives or other special requirements.

### Simple straight X-rays

X-rays will penetrate different types of tissue at different intensities, according to the thickness and density of the body structures through which they are passing. They are reflected by bone tissue containing calcium salts, i.e. the latter are **opaque** to X-rays. Soft tissues will appear more transparent than bone, which will appear as dense opaque structures; air present in the lungs and abdomen will give a completely transparent appearance on an X-ray film or **radiograph**. In

**simple straight X-rays**, only a certain amount of information will be obtained from the varying degree of shadow produced. These pictures are taken on a special film and developed by the dark room technician for later reading and report by the radiologist.

**Examples:**
Investigations for:

■ **fractured bones**

■ **pneumonia**

■ swallowed **foreign bodies** (e.g. safety pins).

## Image enhancement

However, with the use of modern techniques, the scope of investigation of the body by X-ray has been transformed. The investigation of soft tissues requires lower radiation doses which will travel more slowly through the differing densities of tissues producing varying degrees of shadow. This differentiation of soft tissue to a higher resolution is also enhanced by implementation of techniques such as the application of the photographic process (**xeroradiography**), by use of specially sensitised film (as in the process of **mammography**) and computer-enhanced imaging techniques such as in **CAT (CT) scanning**, allowing the clear demonstration of **lesions** (abnormal changes). These techniques are now widely used in diagnostic procedures.

## Fluoroscopy

This procedure is used for live visual examination of the patient by the radiologist; the image appears upon a fluorescent screen or monitor. This technique is particularly useful for examining movements such as **swallowing** and the propulsion of food along the alimentary canal by **peristalsis**. Pictures are also taken for later inspection by the radiologist. **Contrast medium** is usually used in these investigations, which include those of the urinary tract, gastrointestinal tract and blood vessels.

### Contrast medium

The introduction of a **'contrast medium'** or **radio-opaque substance** (a substance which

will absorbs X-rays) allows blood vessels and hollow organs to be clearly demonstrated. Substances, such as **barium sulphate** and radio-opaque **iodine dyes**, are used either by swallowing (ingestion) or via injection.

**Examples:**
■ Investigation for gastric ulcer etc. by **barium meal, barium enema** for tumours of the bowel.

■ **Intravenous pyelogram (IVP)** for introduction of radio-opaque iodine to show kidneys and bladder.

Air may also be used as a contrast medium when injected into a structure which normally absorbs X-rays. As the air will absorb considerably less X-radiation, it is said to be **radio-translucent** and will give a transparent effect on the screen or film.

**Example:**
■ Introduction of air in a **ventriculogram** for investigation of the brain.

## Examples of organ imaging

The following are examples of special procedures performed in organ imaging investigations:

### Mammography

This special X-ray procedure involves the compression of the breast tissue between plastic plates which, together with low density X-rays, allows enhanced imaging of the soft tissues. Special film plate and processing are also used. It is now widely used in the detection of cancerous lesions before any clinical signs or symptoms are apparent (see Chapter 20).

### Thermography

This is a method which records the emission of infrared radiation or heat rays from the body. Actively dividing cells produce more heat than other less active cells and show 'hot' spots in a picture. Inflammation of tissue will also have this effect.

**Example:**
■ Investigation and monitoring of arthritis.

### CAT or CT scan (computerised axial tomography or computerised tomography)

This is a method whereby the tissue density of any part of the head and trunk is examined by X-rays in minute layered sections (see Figure 70). The whole process is computerised to produce numerous pictures which are used to detect any abnormality. A **radio-opaque** substance may also be injected during the procedure to give further information to aid diagnosis.

**Example:**
- Investigation for tumours of the central nervous system etc.

### MRI (magnetic resonance imaging)

This is a procedure which is mainly used to investigate the **central nervous system** (*see Figure 71*). Powerful **magnets** are used to activate the **hydrogen** component of body cells. Sensitive detectors reflect this activity, which is then translated into high resolution images by a computerised system.

As this procedure does not involve the use of X-rays, there is less risk to the patient than with CAT (CT) scanning. It will also detect smaller abnormalities. **Radioactive dye** is injected intravenously during the scanning process to give a better demonstration of any abnormality.

**Example:**
- Investigation of neurological conditions, e.g. multiple sclerosis.

### Functional MRI scanning (FMRI)

This new type of MRI scanning, demonstrates the **functioning** of specific areas of the brain. Colourful pictures of the brain can be obtained performing complicated tasks, such as working out complicated mathematical problems. It has enabled scientists to understand differences in normal brain activity and that in those patients with certain disorders such as **schizophrenia** and **Alzheimer's disease**.

As it does not expose the patient to radioactivity, it can be used in **serial scans** which follow up

## CAT scan

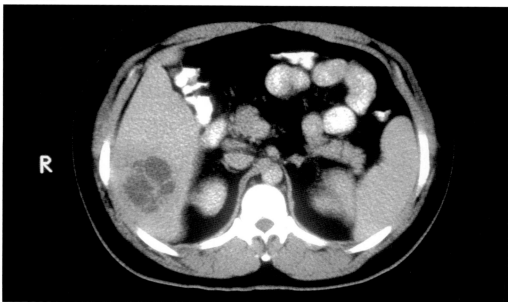

**Figure 70:** A CT scan showing an amoebic liver abscess
*(Photograph courtesy of Lanarkshire Infectious Unit/Wellcome Photo Library)*

the effects of treatment in psychiatric diseases and the use of newer drugs which actively change the way in which the brain works. Removal of much of the stigma of mental illness may hopefully follow, the demonstration that mental illness results from definable organic disease and not from the failure of personality.

### PET – Positron emission tomography

This type of scan demonstrates the **functioning** of cells. With the use of an isotope it shows visually oxygen uptake, blood flow and glucose metabolism of specific areas of the body.

### Nuclear medicine

This method of investigation uses **radio-isotopes**, i.e. unstable compounds which give off radiation. These substances are introduced into the body, usually orally or by injection.

Because different tissues absorb chemicals at different rates, specific organs can be investigated using this method. A special detector picks up

the radiation being given off from the area where it has been absorbed and converts it into a coloured picture.

### Bone scan or scintigram

This is used to detect bone cancer at a very early stage; cancerous bone cells absorb more of the isotope than normal bone cells and so a brighter, or 'hotter', area is produced on the picture.

### Ultrasonic scan

The ultrasound department is found within the X-ray department of many hospitals, although sometimes it is part of the obstetric department.

Ultrasound is a term used to describe high frequency vibration beyond the audible range, known as **ultrasonic waves**. 'Echoes' are reflected backwards when a beam of ultrasonic sounds is made to travel through the body tissues. Images are produced on a television-type screen which give information concerning

## MRI scan

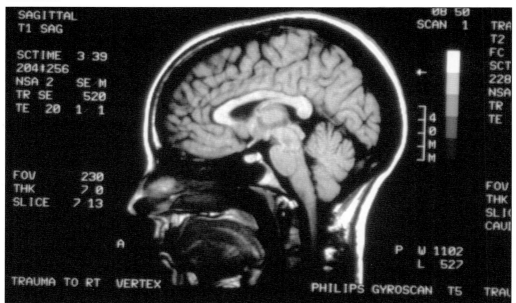

**Figure 71:** An MRI scan of the sagittal section of the brain
*(Photograph courtesy of Wellcome Photo Library)*

position, size and shape of the body structures. There are two types of scanning, type A and type B, each of which gives a different range of imaging. As ultrasound does not involve the use of X-rays, it is a safer procedure for the patient.

**Examples:**

- Investigation of fetal development (*see Figure 72*)

- Investigation of prostatic enlargement etc.

### Doppler system

This is a type of ultrasonic scanning which produces audible signals and records movement within the body.

**Examples:**

- Investigation of blood flow in blood vessels, e.g. for diagnosis of **DVT (deep vein thrombosis)** or heart movements.

### Electron beam tomography (EBT) scan

A new, non-invasive technique, which produces an improvement on conventional, CT scanning, is now available in the private sector. It produces a better quality picture with no discomfort to the patient. It is especially useful in determining those patients **at risk of developing heart disease**, who require invasive tests and possible treatments (*see Figure 73*).

The scanner works on the **gantry** principle, in that it slowly moves over the patient, who lies fully clothed on a couch. It is silent and does not require the patient to disappear into a cigar like tube, as in some scanning techniques, (a daunting and panic producing procedure for many!).

Radiation doses are at least 25% less than in CT and the speed and angle of the scanning produces clearer images. The procedure takes only 15 minutes in all. Both stills and video

## Ultrasound scan

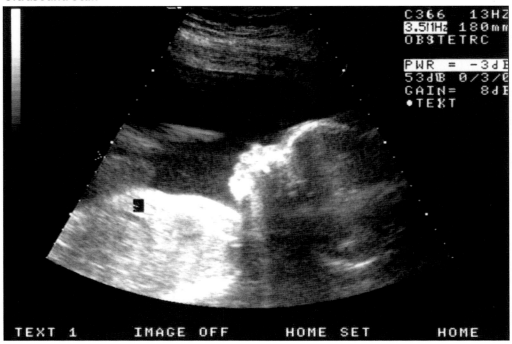

**Figure 72:** An ultrasound image of a normal 24 week fetus
*(Photograph courtesy of Wellcome Photo Library)*

recordings are made of the heart, main artery (aorta), lungs, ribs and spine.

### Terahertz scanning

Research on a so far hidden spectrum of light known as 'terahertz', has been recently tested at Addenbrooke's Hospital, Cambridge and a trial on humans is commencing at St Thomas Hospital, London. Images of tumours are being produced using terahertz radiation. The light is absorbed differently by healthy and cancerous tissue. The difference is then measured, giving surgeons a clear picture of the tumour's location. This method would appear to enable cancers to be discovered earlier and with more precision than is achievable with MRI, ultrasound or X-Ray scans, which use different types of light and sound. 85% of all cancers are not visible with the conventional techniques. Terahertz scanning is said to be as big a break through as the discovery of X-Rays.

## Use of X-rays as therapy

This is usually part of the department of nuclear medicine. The doctor in charge of this department is a **radiotherapist**.

Radio-isotopes, usually of **radium** or **cobalt**, are used to treat conditions such as cancerous tumours. Cancerous cells are, by their nature, immature, rapidly dividing cells and are more susceptible to exposure by radiation than normal cells. This is the principle of radiation treatment.

Normal dividing cells, such as blood cells, are also damaged by the treatment, which is why anaemia and lowered immunity can be side-effects of the treatment.

Carefully controlled dosages are given, measured for each individual patient. Great care must be taken of the skin surrounding the

## EBT scan

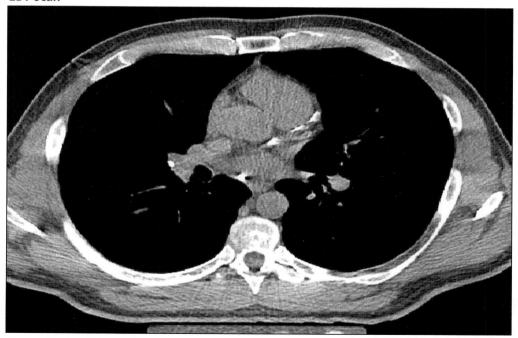

**Figure 73:** An EBT scan showing calcium deposits in the coronary arteries – and indication of coronary heart disease
*(Courtesy of Nathan D. Wong, PhD, Univ of California, Irvine, USA)*

target area, which must be kept dry throughout and after treatment to avoid breakdown of the tissue.

## X-ray requests

Special request forms for X-ray procedures are completed with the details of the patient and the type of X-ray required. *It is important that all details are correct, including the information concerning the LMP (last menstrual period).*

After the radiologist at the hospital has reported on the results of the investigation, copies are despatched to the doctor/GP who requested the procedure.

Costing for X-rays is divided into various categories, according to the complexity of the procedures.

## Abbreviations

| | |
|---|---|
| **AP&L** | anterior, posterior and lateral |
| **DEXA** | dual energy x-ray absorptometry (for osteoporosis) |
| **EBT** | electron beam tomography |
| **ERCP** | endoscopic retrograde cholangio-pancreatography |
| **FMRI** | functional magnetic resonance imaging |
| **IVP** | intravenous pyelogram |
| **IVU** | intravenous urogram |
| **PET** | positron emission tomography |
| **RP** | retrograde pyelogram |

(See also abbreviations in other specialities)

## Terminology

**Angiogram (-ography)**
X-ray investigation of blood vessels using an opaque medium

**Aortogram (-ography)**
1. recording of pulse in graph form
2. demonstration of aorta using opaque medium

**Barium X-ray**
X-ray using barium sulphate as contrast medium to demonstrate any abnormality in the digestive tract

| | |
|---|---|
| **Meal** | the stomach and small intestine. |
| **Swallow** | the oesophagus |
| **Enema** | the large intestine |
| **Follow through** | the whole tract |

**Bronchogram (-ography)**
X-ray examination of bronchi and bronchioles using an opaque medium

**Cephalopelvimetry**
measurement of fetal head in relation to maternal pelvis

**Cholangiogram (-ography)**
X-ray examination of the ducts of the gallbladder using an opaque medium

**Cholecystogram (-ography)**
X-ray examination of the gallbladder using an opaque medium given by mouth

**Encephalogram (-ography)**
X-ray of the brain by insertion of air

**Endoscopic retrograde cholangio-pancreatography (ERCP)**
special X-ray examination of the bile and pancreatic ducts by insertion of a radio-opaque dye via an endoscope

**Hysterosalpingogram (-ography)**
X-ray of uterus and fallopian tubes using an opaque medium to detect blockage or abnormality

**Intravenous pyelogram (-ography)**
X-ray of the kidney and its pelvis after injection of an opaque medium

**Intravenous urogram (-ography)**
X-ray of urinary tract highlighting bladder after injecting opaque medium

**Mammogram (-ography)**
special X-ray of the breast to detect early cancer

**Micturating cystogram**
X-ray of the bladder for investigation of stress incontinence etc.

**Myelogram**
X-ray of spinal cord using
a radio-opaque dye

**Nuclear medicine**
the use of radio-active isotopes in diagnosis
and treatment of disease

**Radiculogram**
X-ray of spinal cord using radio-opaque
dye which highlights the roots of the
lumbar-sacral spinal nerves

**Radiographer**
a professional person qualified in:

**1.** technical use of X-rays (diagnostic)

**2.** applying treatment with radiation
    (therapeutic)

**Radiologist**
medical specialist concerned with radiation
and X-rays

**Radiology**
scientific study of radiation and its effects

**Radiotherapy**
the use of radiation to treat disease

**Retrograde pyelogram (-ography)**
X-ray of ureters, bladder and pelvis of kidney
by insertion of an opaque dye via catheters in
the ureters from the urethra below

**Sialogram (-ography)**
X-ray of salivary glands using an
opaque medium

**Ventriculogram**
X-ray of the ventricles of brain by insertion
of air

**N.B. for other types of investigations see
various specialities.**

Chapter **17** | The pathology department and its services

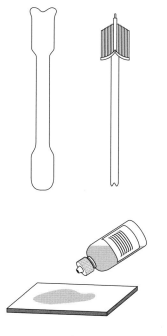

This hospital department is involved in special tests concerning various samples from the living body used to assist in the diagnosis and prognosis of disease. The **mortuary** is also part of the pathology department and **post-mortems** are performed by the **pathologist**, who is also the specialist doctor in charge of the whole department. Recently, private laboratories have been involved with providing services.

## Organisation

As previously mentioned, apart from the chief pathologist, there will be the following personnel employed in the department:

- **Pathologists**
  (doctors) dependent on size of hospital
- **Scientific officers**
- **Trainees**
- **Laboratory assistants**
- **Phlebotomists**
  (staff who take blood from patients)
- **Administrative and clerical staff**
- **Morticians**
- **Porters**

## Safety

Stringent health and safety precautions must be observed in this department as in any other hospital area. The risk is immense, as the specimens handled are hazardous due to their disease-producing potential.

### Recent requirements for transport and packaging of diagnostic specimens

**International agreements** under the auspices of the **United Nations** have recently been introduced, in order to prevent cross-infection caused by the transporting of diagnostic specimens including those used in medicine. This involves numerous statutory regulations, which cover strict requirements for transport by road, rail, air and sea. In the UK, various legislation including the present **Carriage of**

**Dangerous Goods by Road Regulations 1996 (amended 1999)** is to be replaces in early **2004** with the **'ADR'** known as **'The European Agreement'**. There are also other regulations, covering transport by rail and air, in force.

**All postal specimens must comply with road, rail and air regulations.**

The following strict requirements for diagnostic specimens (complying with UN650) are all considered on the basis of the level of safety required:

- **Classification of risk**
- **Quality of packaging**
- **Marking of diagnostic specimens**
- **Mode of transport used**
- **Volume of specimen** (50ml maximum).

*NB: there is a list of infectious substances forbidden as diagnostic specimens, as well as a stated emergency response procedure, to be followed in the event of spillage or exposure.*

## Sections

The following sections are part of the pathology laboratory:

- **Haematology** (including **serology**)
- **Biochemistry** or **clinical chemistry**
- **Cytology**
- **Histology** or **histopathology**
  (including oncology)
- **Microbiology**
- **Virology**
- **Epidemiology**

**The Public Health Laboratory** is also usually part of the pathology department, sharing facilities. This is involved in routine checking of food, milk and water samples, as well as being involved in the control of infectious diseases. Suspected carriers of infection are screened and samples from them are tested in this laboratory.

## Haematology

This is one of the largest sections of the laboratory and is sometimes connected with the work of the **Regional Blood Transfusion Centre** where blood for donation is stored. Any blood ready for transfusion will be kept here in a special refrigerated unit. Dried **plasma** ready for use will also be available for emergencies.

The areas within the department will include those investigating blood cells, and the **serology section** involved with investigations on the **serum** of blood.

### Tests

Various tests will be performed on cells and serum sent from the hospital and general practice in the various containers required, e.g. **haemoglobin estimation**. The department's phlebotomists also collect blood from patients attending for this purpose.

## Biochemistry

This section is involved in investigation of the chemical content of the blood, urine or other body fluid.

### Tests

As well as routine tests for **electrolytes**, **hormones** etc, samples from patients suffering from **drug overdose** are analysed here.

### Tumour markers

The appearance or increase of certain substances in the blood, appear to indicate the likelihood of developing **cancers** and other processes occurring in the body. More is being understood about this in recent years. However, many can give **false positive results**, so care is needed in their interpretation. **Genetic markers** are also indicative of a person's tendency to develop certain diseases.

Tumour markers which indicate the likelihood of developing cancer include:

| | |
|---|---|
| **AFP (alpha-fetoprotein)** | liver, ovary, testicle cancer |
| **BRCA1** and **BRCA2** | genetic markers for breast cancer and ovarian cancer |
| **CA 15-3** | breast cancer |
| **CA 19-9** | colorectal cancer, stomach, bile duct |

| | |
|---|---|
| **CA 72-4** | stomach cancer |
| **CA 125** | ovarian cancer |
| **CEA** | colorectal, pancreas, lung, breast, stomach, thyroid, female genital cancers |
| **BHCG** | testicular, ovarian, liver, pancreas, stomach cancer |
| **B2M** | blood forming (haematopoietic system) |
| **NSE** | lung cancer |
| **SCLC** | pancreas, brain cancer |
| **CYFRA 21-1** | lung cancer |
| **NSCLC** | uterus, breast cancer |
| **PSA** | prostate cancer |
| **HCG** | human chorionic gonadotrophic hormone found in pregnancy but also a marker for testicular cancer |

(*See Table 5 for further information*).

A number of tumour markers are already very commonly used by doctors and specialists everywhere. However the combination of improvements in biochemistry (and its 'tools' such as **computerized analysis equipment**) *and* available statistics of cases (showing which markers have actually shown up in which quantities and in what combination in actual cases), have increased the specificity and reliability of tumour marker screening dramatically.

### Examples:

- **Prostate cancer:** the use of the FPSA/TPSA relationship improves our ability to distinguish between cancer and non-cancer, avoiding invasive examination procedures;

- **Lung cancer** (a very complex cancer): the use of the CYFRA 21-1/NSE associated with CEA and CA-125 allows:

  - the determination of the type of cancer we are dealing with;

  - the detection of the appearance, during the course of the treatment, of cell-clones different from the initial clone, which would bring about the immediate modification of the current treatment (having become ineffective).

**Table 5:** Known tumour markers – and their normal and abnormal values.

| CEA | | |
|---|---|---|
| Levels | Normal: <5 ng/ml | Moderate: 5 – 10 ng/ml | High: 10 – 100,000 ng/ml |

| Cancers that may be indicated by high levels | **Colon:** colorectaladenocarcinoma<br>**Pancreas:** adenocarcinoma and endocrine<br>**Lung:** adenocarcinoma<br>**Breast**<br>**Stomach:** adenocarcinoma<br>**Thyroid**<br>**Ovary:** mucoid adenocarcinoma<br>**Uterus:** mucoid tumours<br>**Liver:** hepatocarcinoma<br>**Oesophagus:** adenocarcinoma<br>**Thyroid:** medullar |
|---|---|

| AFP | | |
|---|---|---|
| **Levels** | Normal: <15 ng/ml | Moderate: 15 – 200 ng/ml | High: 200 – 10,000 ng/ml |

| Cancers that may be indicated by high levels | **Ovary:** germinating<br>**Testicle:** germinating; non-seminomatous tumours<br>**Liver:** hepatocarcinoma |
|---|---|

| PSA and Free PSA (FPSA) | | |
|---|---|---|
| **Levels** | Normal: <4 ng/ml | Moderate: 4 – 10 ng/ml | High: 10 – 1,000 ng/ml |

| Cancers that may be indicated by high levels | **Prostate:** adenocarcinoma (The FPSA/PSA ratio improves the diagnostic differential between prostate cancer and benign prostate hypertrophy) |
|---|---|

| CA 15-3 | | |
|---|---|---|
| **Levels** | Normal: <40 U/ml | Moderate: 40 – 60 U/ml | High: 60 – 30,000 U/ml |

| Cancers that may be indicated by high levels | **Breast:** epithelial tumours<br>**NB:** High rates of CA 15-3 *can* also apply to other cancers: colon, stomach, kidney, lung, ovary, uterus, pancreas, liver |
|---|---|

| CA 19-9 | | |
|---|---|---|
| **Levels** | Normal: <35 U/ml | Moderate: 35 – 100 U/ml | High: 100 – 1 million U/ml |

| Cancers that may be indicated by high levels | **Colon:** colorectal adenocarcinoma<br>**Pancreas:** adenocarcinoma and endocrine<br>**Stomach:** adenocarcinoma<br>**Bile duct**<br>**Ovary:** mucoid adenocarcinoma<br>**Uterus:** mucoid tumour<br>**Lung:** adenocarcinoma |
|---|---|

**Table 5:** Known tumour markers – and their normal and abnormal values (continued).

| CA 125 | | | |
| --- | --- | --- | --- |
| **Levels** | Normal: <35 U/ml | Moderate: 35 – 50 U/ml | High: 50 – 50,000 U/ml |

| | |
| --- | --- |
| Cancers that may be indicated by high levels | **Ovary:** adenocarcinoma<br>**Uterus:** adenocarcinoma (5%) and corpus adenocarcinoma (95%)<br>**Fallopian tubes**<br>**Colon:** Colorectal adenocarcinoma<br>**Lung:** adenocarcinoma and small cell carcinoma |

| CA 72-4 | | | |
| --- | --- | --- | --- |
| Levels | Normal: <5.2 U/ml | Moderate: 6 – 30 U/ml | High: 30 – 10,000 U/ml |

| | |
| --- | --- |
| Cancers that may be indicated by high levels | **Stomach:** adenocarcinoma<br>**NB:** Diagnosing gastric carcinoma is often complicated and can be extremely difficult due to presentation with vague, nonspecific symptoms which are sometimes associated with non-malignant disease. Although endoscopy, coupled with histological evalua-tion of biopsy specimens, is most often used to make definitive diagnosis, the search for additional non-invasive diagnostic procedures has continued: strong new clinical evidence has recently emphasized the clinical value of the CA 72-4 serum tumour marker assay in the diagnosis and monitoring of gastric cancer |

| HCG and Beta HCG (BHCG) | | |
| --- | --- | --- |
| Levels | Normal: <5 mUI/ml | Moderate/High: 5 – 100,000 mUI/ml |

| | |
| --- | --- |
| Cancers that may be indicated by high levels | **Ovary**<br>**Liver**<br>**Stomach**<br>**Pancreas**<br>**Lung**<br>**Testicle:** seminoma and non-seminomatous tumours |

| B2M | | |
| --- | --- | --- |
| Levels | Normal: <2 mg/l | Moderate/High: 2 – 10 mg/l |

| | |
| --- | --- |
| Cancers that may be indicated by high levels | **Haematopoietic system:**<br>**NB:** B2M, the beta2microglobulin, is used as a tumour-marker in various illnesses of the haematopoietic system, mainly where B lymphs cells are concerned |

**Table 5:** Known tumour markers – and their normal and abnormal values (continued).

### NSE

| Levels | Normal: <15 ng/ml | Moderate: 15 – 40 ng/ml | High: 40 – 4,000 ng/ml |
|---|---|---|---|

| Cancers that may be indicated by high levels | **Lung:** small cell lung carcinomas (SCLC) |
|---|---|
| | **Pancreas:** endocrine |
| | **Nervous system:** neuroblastomas |
| | **Thyroid:** medullar |

### CYFRA 21-1

| Levels | Normal: <3.5 ng/ml | Moderate/High: 3.5 – 1,000 ng/ml |
|---|---|---|

| Cancers that may be indicated by high levels | **Lung:** non-small cell lung carcinomas (NSCLC) |
|---|---|
| | **Uterus** |
| | **Breast:** epithelial tumours |
| | **Oesophagus:** epidermoid |

## Cytology

This section of the pathology department examines cells to detect any abnormality.

### Tests

These include cervical cells present in **cervical smears**, as well as cells from the respiratory tract and other areas under investigation. The aim, in many cases, is to detect early abnormalities (**precancerous conditions**) in order to prevent the development of a cancerous condition.

## Histology or histopathology

This section is involved in preparing sections of tissue which have been removed from the living patient at a **biopsy**.

### Tests

These tissue sections are then examined under the microscope to diagnose and classify any abnormality, such as cancer.

## Oncology

This section, often part of the histology department, examines cells from tumours.

### Tests

These involve microscopic examination of sections of suspected malignant tumours from any area of the body.

## Microbiology

This section is involved in investigation of samples taken from wounds and other areas to detect microscopic organisms which are causing disease.

### Classification of micro-organisms

The main ones are:

- **bacteria**    e.g. staphylococcus
- **viruses**    e.g. measles virus (Morbilli)
- **fungi**    e.g. thrush
      (Candida albicans)
- **protozoa**    e.g. amoeba

Although not a micro-organism **'Prions'**, rogue proteins, are capable of causing diseases such as **BSE (bovine spongiform encephalopathy)** and **CJD (Creudzfeldt Jacob Disease)**. The mechanism of their actions is not fully understood.

### Tests

These include those on urine, sputum and blood samples etc, from which the organisms are **cultured**, i.e. put into or onto a **medium** which allows the organism to grow.

### Culture

The **culture plate**, or other medium, impregnated with the specimen, is placed in an **incubator** at body temperature and left for any organisms present to multiply. The resulting culture is then removed and stained with special dye. This is taken up by the cells, which enables them to be viewed under the microscope. In this way the organism can be recognised and named.

**Agar** (from seaweed) is commonly used as culture medium and blood can be added as a nutrient. Not all micro-organisms will grow outside the body. Viruses require living tissue, such as blood or eggs, for culture.

### Sensitivity

Bacteria respond to antibiotic treatment, but it is important that the most effective one is used to fight the infection in the patient. The culture plate used contains various areas of specific antibiotics to determine to which of them the organism is **sensitive**. The bacteria will grow around and over those antibiotics to which they have become **resistant**. A space will be left around those to which the organism is sensitive.

## Virology

This section is concerned with the isolation and culture of viruses. As with all areas in the laboratory, stringent safety precautions must be taken, but here special **fume cupboards** are used to prevent the spread of any viruses present.

### Tests

These are for the isolation and classification of any viruses in the specimens. Only viruses large enough to be filtered can be detected.

## Epidemiology

This department, which is concerned with the study of the causes of disease (including social factors), may be attached to the pathology department or be a separate unit. Recently, some epidemiology departments have been involved in the monitoring of extra-contractual referrals of patients (patients referred to a hospital with which the health authority has no contract for services).

## Collection of specimens

### Types of specimen

The following are some of the common specimens sent for investigation:

| | |
|---|---|
| **Wound swabs** | plain swabs usually placed |
| **Nasal swabs** | in nutrient broth |
| **Throat swabs** | after collection |
| **Urine** | |
|   **MSU** | midstream specimen of urine usually for C&S (culture and sensitivity) |
|   **EMU** | early morning urine usually for pregnancy test |
|   **CSU** | catheter specimen of urine, if patient has an indwelling catheter; not usually a routine specimen |
| **Blood** | there are different containers for differing tests. Anti-clotting agents are included in some containers from laboratories. Tops and labels of bottles are colour-coded. |
| **Cervical smears** | on special named slides. Fixative must be added immediately after collection and allowed to dry, before placing in container (*see Figure 74*) |
| **Faeces** | for culture or content, e.g. fat, usually a series of three specimens |
| **High vaginal swab (HVS)** | charcoal swab often used for culture |
| **Histology** | tissue placed in pot with preservative (prevents drying out of cells) |
| **Sputum** | for culture or oncology, single or three specimens |
| **Vomit** | this may be sent in cases of overdose or poisoning, together with any urine passed. |

In hospital, specimens of **pleural fluid**, **cerebrospinal fluid** etc. are also taken.

## Cervical smear equipment

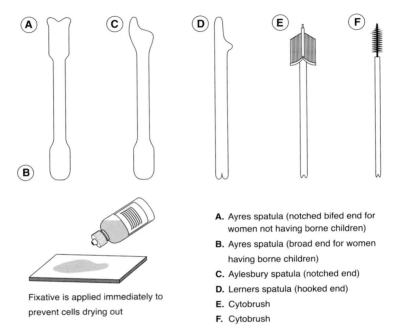

Fixative is applied immediately to
prevent cells drying out

**A.** Ayres spatula (notched bifed end for
women not having borne children)

**B.** Ayres spatula (broad end for women
having borne children)

**C.** Aylesbury spatula (notched end)

**D.** Lerners spatula (hooked end)

**E.** Cytobrush

**F.** Cytobrush

**Figure 74:** Cervical smear equipment

### Rules for collection and dispatch of specimens

It is most important that all rules are followed concerning pathology specimens. They are classed as a hazard within the **COSHH (Control of Substances Hazardous to Health) Regulations** in health and safety requirements. If five or more people are employed, general practices and hospitals should have written health and safety policies to protect the safety of their staff, and the handling of specimens should be included in those policies.

- Specimens must be clearly identifiable as to the patient and the source; laboratory personnel will not accept specimens which do not comply.

- Gloves should be worn when handling specimens – if a rigid container is kept in the reception area, patients can be requested to place their specimens in it themselves when bringing them to the surgery. In this way the box can be collected by the practice nurse and the receptionist does not normally need to handle the specimen.

- All forms and labels must be correctly completed and legible; clinical details **must** be included.

- All tops **must** be firmly fixed.

- Specimens (except smears) should remain upright.

- The request form must be placed in the plastic envelope provided and **must not** be in contact with the specimen itself.

- **High-risk specimens** must be labelled with the warning label as well as the form.

## Royal Mail Safebox

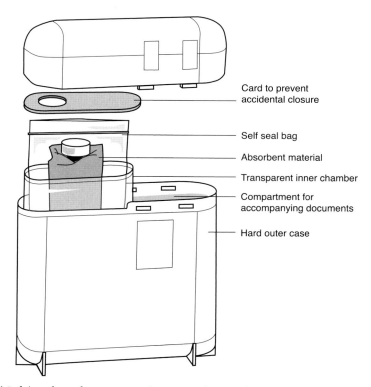

Card to prevent accidental closure

Self seal bag

Absorbent material

Transparent inner chamber

Compartment for accompanying documents

Hard outer case

**Figure 75:** The Royal Mail Safebox for safe transportation or posting specimens
*(Courtesy of The Royal Mail)*

- Special care must be taken with common names, e.g. John Smith, and any middle names included.

- Posted specimens **must** comply with **United Nations requirements** (see above). The Royal Mail provides special specimen containers, known as **'Royal Mail Safebox'**, (*see Figure 75*) which comply with all transport requirements.

- These specimens should be sent by **first class post** (or similar such as 'Special Delivery' or 'Recorded Delivery'), in order to avoid delay which would increase the risk factor. If sent by 'Royal Mail Safebox' this may be simply placed in the post box in the usual way. ('Safeboxes' are prepaid at time of purchase).

- **High-risk specimens must not be posted.**

Patients should be given the following instructions:

- How to collect their own specimen (a leaflet is preferable);

- Where it must be taken and the opening times of the laboratory;

- How to obtain the results and that an appointment should be made accordingly.

- All specimens should be stored in a cool place and not left on window ledges in the sun or near radiators etc.

### Delay

If there is any delay in the dispatch of specimens to the laboratory (apart from cervical smears and histology specimens) they should be placed in the ordinary part of the refrigerator. A separate refrigerator should be provided for this purpose and must not be the one used for food. **Never place specimens of blood etc. on a radiator**. Stale specimens can give false results.

## Prevention of cross-infection

It is important that hands are washed after handling any specimen. Waterproof plasters should always be placed on any broken skin surfaces when working at the surgery.

Blood and body fluids may contain the viruses of **hepatitis B**, **HIV** or other **pathogens**. **Needles** and other **sharps**, such as scalpel blades, must be placed in the **sharp** boxes provided, together with used syringes. These are collected and effectively disposed of by incineration to prevent spread of disease. They should never be more than two-thirds full.

There have been incidents of **'needle-stick injuries'** occurring where needles have been placed in the ordinary waste bin and unsuspecting staff have been injured in this way when handling the bag involved. This can only occur with bad practice by other members of staff.

### Needle-stick injuries

In the event of a 'needle-stick' injury, there are certain rules which must be followed. The wound should be immediately washed under cold water and encouraged to bleed as a first measure. These events must be **reported immediately** to the named person in the health and safety policy and to the doctor responsible. Details of the relevant patient whose used needle has caused the injury (if possible), should be traced together with their relevant history. Blood should be taken as a precaution from the person injured and kept as a control specimen.

### Clinical waste

This is also a hazard and includes dressings and linen soiled with body fluid. Special colour-coded bags are used to prevent ordinary disposal or accidental mishandling.

## Immunisation

It is recommended that those staff exposed to the risk of hepatitis B infection are offered protection with immunisation. This is given to practice nurses and personnel regularly coming into contact with blood and body fluids. Some GPs offer it to all surgery staff.

## Reports

Results of tests will be returned to the doctor requesting the investigation. Urgent results may be sent by telephone from the laboratory, but would only usually be given to the doctor directly. The growing use of modems on computers will probably result in direct transmission of results, but the important requirement of **confidentiality** must be ensured. Similarly, this must be maintained in the use of fax machines, where mistakes can so easily be made.

## Abbreviations

NB: Many of the terms relating to pathology have already been included in the terminology of the blood (Chapter 4), but a further explanation is included here for some of the common tests performed in the laboratory.

| | |
|---|---|
| **AHF** | antihaemophilic factor VIII |
| **APTT** | activated partial thromboplastin time |
| **AST\*** | aspartate transaminase (cardiac enzyme) |
| **BUN** | blood urea nitrogen |
| **C&S** | culture and sensitivity |
| **CPK\*** | creatinine phosphokinase (cardiac enzyme) |
| **CRP** | C-reactive protein indicates the presence of inflammation within the body. It may be a truer indication of those at risk of an acute heart attack (coronary thrombosis, myocardial infarction) as inflammation of the fatty plaques in the lining of the |

| | |
|---|---|
| | arteries cause them to break away and block blood vessels |
| **ESR** | erythrocyte sedimentation rate (rate at which red cells drop to the bottom of the tube) – it is read after one hour, raised in cases of tuberculosis, rheumatic fever and other inflammatory diseases – shows the progress of a disease |
| **FBC** | full blood count – gives the total numbers of all the different blood cells for a comparison with the normal ranges. White cells increase in the presence of infection: |
| **Erythrocytes** | red cells |
| **Leucocytes** | white cells: **polymorphonuclear leucocytes:** neutrophils basophils eosinophils **non-granular leucocytes:** lymphocytes mononocytes |
| **Platelets or thrombocytes** | clotting cells |
| **FBS** | fasting blood sugar to determine diabetes mellitus or low blood sugars, performed in early morning before any intake of food |
| **GFR** | glomerular filtration rate (estimation of kidney function) |
| **GOT**∗ | glutamicoxalo-acetic transaminase (cardiac enzyme) |
| **GTT** | glucose tolerance test to diagnose diabetes mellitus |
| **HAI** | hospital acquired infection |
| **Hb** | haemoglobin is the iron compound carrying oxygen Normal levels are: **women -** 12.5 - 16.0 g/dl (grams per decilitre). **men -** 14.0 - 18.0 g/dl. *The variation in the female is caused by blood loss at menstruation.* |

| | |
|---|---|
| **HbA1c** | blood test for diabetes which shows the amount of glucose that has bound to the haemoglobin of the red cell |
| **HDL** | high-density lipoprotein |
| **HUS** | haemolytic uraemic syndrome |
| **LBC** | liquid based cytology |
| **LD**∗ | lactate dehydrogenase (cardiac enzyme) |
| **LDL** | low-density lipoprotein |
| **LFT** | liver function test, to diagnose liver disease |
| **MC&S** | microscopy culture and sensitivity |
| **MCV** | mean corpuscular volume (size of cell) |
| **MRSA** | multiple resistant staphylococcus aureus, a resistant strain of bacteria |
| **RBC** | red blood cells |
| **T$_4$** | serum thyroxine test for thyroid disease |
| **TPHA** | treponema pallidum haemagglutination assay (blood test for syphilis) |
| **U&Es** | urea and electrolytes; urea is the part of protein broken down by the liver for excretion by the kidneys – raised in kidney damage and dehydration; electrolytes in body fluid include sodium, potassium, calcium, magnesium, bicarbonates, chlorides and phosphates |
| **VDRL** | veneral disease research laboratory (for syphilis) |
| **WBC** | white blood count – this is raised in infection, inflammation and leukaemia, different types according to the type of cause |

∗ These enzymes also show changes in metabolism of other tissues

## Units used in biochemistry

| | |
|---|---|
| **IU or U** | international unit |
| **mmol** | millimole |
| **mmol/l** | millimole per litre |
| **nmol** | nanomole |
| **µmol** | micromole |

## Common abbreviations used in laboratory results

| | |
|---|---|
| **d, deci** | $10^{-1}$ (divided by 10) |
| **f, femto** | $10^{-15}$ (divided by 1 000 000 000 000 000) |
| **g/dl** | grams per decilitre |
| **g/l** | grams per litre |
| **IU/l** | international units per litre |
| **m, milli** | $10^{-3}$ (divided by 1 000) |
| **mg/ml** | milligrams per millilitre |
| **mm3** | cubic millimetre |
| **mU/l** | milliunits per litre |
| **ng/ml** | nannograms per millilitre |
| **n, nano** | $10^{-9}$ (divided by 1 000 000 000) |
| **p, pico** | $10^{-12}$ (divided by 1 000 000 000 000) |
| **µ, micro** | $10^{-6}$ (divided by 1 000 000) |

## Terminology

| | |
|---|---|
| **Abscess** | collection of pus in a cavity |
| **Acid-fast bacteria** | takes up the acid stain |
| **Adenovirus** | virus which affects the glands, e.g. mumps |
| **Aerobic bacteria** | type of bacteria which requires $O_2$ to maintain its life |
| **Airborne or droplet infection** | transmission of infection via the air as tiny droplets |
| **Anaerobic bacteria** | type of bacteria that thrives in the absence of $O_2$ |
| **Anaplasia** | abnormal cell formation (malignant) |
| **Animal vectors** | infection transmitted from animals, e.g. rabies from cats, foxes etc. |

| | |
|---|---|
| **Arbovirus** | virus that is transmitted from types of insect vectors such as mosquitos, e.g. Yellow fever/Colarado Fever |
| **Bacillus** | rod-shaped bacteria |
| *Campylobacter* | type of bacteria which causes food poisoning |
| **Carbuncle** | a boil discharging through many openings |
| **Communicable** | transmissible from one person to another by either direct or indirect contact |
| **Contact** | direct or indirect (see Contagious and Fomites) |
| **Contagious** | transmitted by direct contact with a person or fomites |
| **Coombs' test** | test for Rhesus incompatibility |
| **Coronavirus** | virus which appears to have a crown-like halo around it, e.g. SARS |
| **Diplococcus** | bacteria which are like berries and are found in pairs |
| **Dysplasia** | formation of abnormal cells |
| **Endemic** | a disease always present in an area |
| **Enterovirus** | virus which affects the gut (intestine), e.g. Norwalk virus, polio virus |
| **Epidemic** | a disease attacking a large number of people at one time in an area |
| *Escherichia coli* | type of bacillus bacteria responsible for some types of food poisoning, normally found in the bowel; can cause illness when present elsewhere in the body. Type E0157:H7 is responsible for virulent illness |
| **Exudation** | oozing of fluid into, and out of, capillaries |
| **Fibrosis** | excessive formation of fibrous tissue |

| | |
|---|---|
| **Fomites** | objects which are contaminated with organisms of disease, e.g. a toy from a child with chicken-pox |
| **Fulminating** | sudden onset of an infection which is rapid in its course |
| **Gangrene** | death of a piece of body tissue |
| *Dry* | tissue is dry and shrivelled/mummified |
| *Wet* | bacterial infection is present causing cellulitis of the affected area |
| **Gram-negative bacteria** | do not take up Gram stain |
| **Gram-positive bacteria** | take the Gram stain into their cell |
| **Granulation** | healing of a wound where capillaries and other tissues renew from the surface |
| *Haemolytic streptococcus* | type of bacteria which causes sore throats and wound infections |
| **Healing by first intention** | edges of clean wound heal together side by side - little scarring |
| **by second intention** | edges of a wound not held together; gap between forms granular tissue before upper skin can grow across the wound |
| **Herpes zoster** | shingles |
| **Immunoglobulins** | antibodies of various types, i.e. Igm, IgG, IgA, IgD and IgE |
| **Infection** | the successful invasion, establishment and growth of micro-organisms in the body |
| **Infectious** | disease transmissible from one host to another |
| **Infectious parotitis** | mumps |
| **Infestation** | the presence of animal parasites in, or on, a living body |

| | |
|---|---|
| **Inflammation** | reaction of living tissues to injury, infection or irritation (a body defence) |
| **Insect vectors** | transmission of infection via insects, e.g. flies, lice |
| **Keloid scar** | overgrowth of scar tissue forming an elevated ridge |
| **Koplik's spots** | small white spots found on the mucous membranes of the mouth – indicative of measles (morbilli) |
| **Legionella** | organism which causes legionnaire's disease |
| **Liquid-based cytology (LBC)** | a relatively new cervical cytology test now approved by NICE as routine testing |
| **Lymphadenitis** | inflamed lymph gland |
| **Lymphangitis** | inflammation of lymph vessel as infection spreads |
| **Metaplasia** | a type of cell that grows beyond where it is usually found |
| **Morbilli** | measles |
| **Necrosis** | death of tissue |
| **Neurotropic virus** | virus with an affinity for nerve tissue, e.g. rabies |
| **Nosocomial** | hospital acquired infection, e.g. MRSA |
| **Oncovirus** | virus which can cause cancer, e.g. herpes virus |
| **Pandemic** | as epidemic, but worldwide |
| **Parotitis (infectious)** | mumps |
| **Paul-Bunnell test** | serology test for glandular fever |
| **Pertussis** | whooping cough |
| **Phagocytosis** | the action of the white blood cells which engulf foreign particles of bacteria etc |
| **Pus** | yellowish liquid composed of bacteria and dead leucocytes – the result of infection. |
| **Putrefaction** | breaking down of tissue by bacteria accompanied |

| | |
|---|---|
| | by offensive odour, due to gases produced |
| **Pyaemia** | pus in the blood stream |
| **Resolution** | subsidence of an infection (recovery) |
| **Rose-Waaler** or **Waaler-Rose test** | blood test for rheumatoid arthritis |
| **Retrovirus** | virus which has the ability to alter genetic material; often slow-growing, e.g. leukaemia, HIV. (Retroviruses are also used in gene transfer therapy) |
| **Rubella** | German measles |
| *Salmonella* | type of bacillus bacteria which causes food poisoning, including typhoid fever |
| **Septicaemia** | bacteria multiply in the blood stream |
| **Slough** | dead tissue which separates from healthy tissue in a wound |
| **Sporadic** | disease occurring in isolated cases |
| *Staphylococcus* | bacteria which are shaped like berries and are found in clusters |
| *Staphylococcus aureus* | type of bacteria which causes food poisoning, skin and wound infections and sore throats |
| *Streptococcus* | bacteria which are shaped like berries and are found in chains |
| **Suppuration** | formation of pus |
| **Toxaemia** | generalised spread of toxins (poisons) in the body – products from |

| | |
|---|---|
| | bacteria or other invasive micro- organisms |
| **Varicella** | chicken-pox |
| **Viraemia** | viruses circulating and multiplying in the blood stream |
| **Waterborne** or **faecal infection** | transmission of infection via contaminated water usually taken in by eating or drinking |
| **WR** and **Kahn tests** | blood tests for syphilis |

## Classification of bacteria

| | |
|---|---|
| **-bacillus** | bacteria which are rod-shaped |
| **-coccus** | types of bacteria which are round-shaped (like berries) |
| **Spirochaete** | shaped like a corkscrew |
| **Vibrio** | bacterium shaped like a comma |

Bacteria are also classified by the stains which they absorb and which show under the microscope, e.g:

| | |
|---|---|
| **Acid fast bacillus** | takes up the acid stain |
| **Gram-negative (-ve) bacteria** | does not take the gram stain |
| **Gram-positive (+ve) bacteria** | takes the gram stain |

*Some bacteria causing gastro-enteritis:*

- *Campylobacter*
- *E. Coli* (and haemolytic uraemic syndrome)
- *Giardiasis*
- *Salmonella*
- *Shigella* (bacillary dysentery)

Chapter **18**

# Drugs

# and

# prescribing

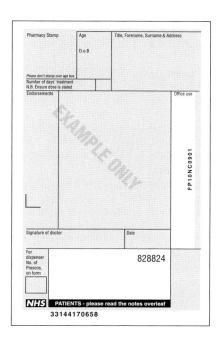

| Pharmacy Stamp | Age | Title, Forename, Surname & Address |
| | D.o.B | |

Please don't stamp over age box

Number of days' treatment
N.B. Ensure dose is stated

Endorsements                                                    Office use

EXAMPLE ONLY

FP10NC0901

Signature of doctor                          Date

For
dispenser
No. of
Prescns.
on form                                    828824

**NHS**   PATIENTS - please read the notes overleaf

33144170658

A drug is any substance which, when taken into the body or onto its surface, alters the body's structure or function.

Drugs or medicines are powerful chemicals and the greatest care must be taken to avoid **abuse** or **misuse** of these substances. Dependency or addiction may be physical or psychological. Prevention of abuse is an important responsibility of the doctor and his/her staff.

Misuse or abuse of drugs within medicine refers to any drug that is used in any other way than that for which it is intended.

## Legal responsibility

Drugs used in medicine are subject to legislation, introduced to prevent harmful or illegal use of these substances. Various regulations have been drawn up and **must** be followed. The doctor is legally responsible for that which he or she prescribes, and also for the storage and disposal of any drugs within his/her control. In the case of a hospital consultant advising a GP which drugs to prescribe for a patient, it is the doctor signing the prescription who is held responsible.

The main legislation involved is:

- The *Medicines Act* 1968
- The *Misuse of Drugs Act* 1971 and its subsequent MODA regulations.

### The Medicines Act 1968

This includes **all** drugs used in medicine and is concerned with their manufacture, supply, use and storage. It divides medicines into three categories:

1. **General Sales List (GSL)** – those which can be sold over the counter at retail stores, no pharmacist needed. Small quantities only and must be in childproof containers (foil packs accepted), e.g. up to 16 aspirin or paracetamol. There is a list of drugs.

2. **Pharmacy Only Drugs (P)** – all other medicinal products which are not on the GSL and are marked with a P. Pharmacist must be present for sale (on premises). Includes small quantities (up to 32 tablets of aspirin 300 mg and paracetamol), some antihistamines etc. **NB**: Tablets aspirin 75 mg are exempt from these quantity restrictions.

3. **Prescription Only Medicines (POM)** – lists products which may only be supplied with a prescription and are marked POM. Includes antidepressants, antibiotics, ampoules etc. Large quantities of paracetamol and aspirin are now included in this category. Controlled drugs are also included, but these have added requirements under MODA.

## The Misuse of Drugs Act (MODA) 1971 (and subsequent regulations)

This Act controls the manufacture, supply, storage and prescribing of so-called controlled drugs, i.e. drugs of addiction. They are classified into various schedules according to their potential for addiction. There are five schedules, the most important in medicine being schedules two and three.

| | |
|---|---|
| **Schedule one (S1)** | is concerned with drugs not used in medicine, e.g. LSD, marijuana etc. **It is an offence to possess them without a special licence from the Home Office.** |
| **Schedule two (S2)** | includes derivatives of opium, such as morphine and heroin (diamorphine), as well as cocaine and amphetamines. |
| **Schedule three (S3)** | includes most barbiturates, minor stimulants, and the tranquilliser Temazepam. |

Drugs in schedules two and three are known as **controlled drugs**.

Stringent rules must be observed for these prescriptions and for **storage** of the drugs within Schedule two and for some in three. **No 'repeat' prescribing of these drugs is allowed.**

| | |
|---|---|
| **Schedule four (S4)** | includes anabolic steroids and tranquillisers, e.g. diazepam. There are no special prescribing requirements at present for these drugs (other than POM requirements). |

**Schedule five (S5)** contains drugs which have a very small amount of schedule two or three in their formula, e.g. codeine compound tablets. There are no special requirements at present for these drugs within these regulations, although a pharmacist must be present for their sale.

## Controlled drugs

Controlled drugs are those referred to in schedules 2 and 3 of the *Misuse of Drugs Act (MODA), 1971* (see page 184).

The abbreviations **CD** or **cd** or the symbol CD refer to controlled drugs.

Controlled drugs also have very strict requirements concerning both supply and disposal. A special **register** is required for supply of schedule 2 drugs. Invoices for controlled drugs (S2 & S3) and S5 should be kept for 2 years. It is unwise for staff to accept any return of controlled drugs from a patient and they should be referred to the dispensing pharmacist or GP.

## Prescriptions for controlled drugs

Controlled drugs for schedule 2 and schedule 3 (see The *Misuse of Drugs Act 1971*, Section 18) have very stringent requirements for prescriptions. These must be prepared by the doctor who is prescribing.

The following requirements are in addition to those for ordinary prescriptions (see later):

- It must be written throughout in the **doctor's own handwriting**.

- **Name and address** of patient.

- The **form and strength** of preparation.

- **Total quantity** of preparation or number of dose units in words and figures.

- The date on the script must be the **date that the prescription is signed**. A date stamp may be used but not a computer generated date.

The prescribing doctor must be known to the dispensing pharmacist so that his/her writing and signature are recognised. **It is an offence for a doctor to issue an incomplete prescription**

**for these drugs and the pharmacist must not dispense it.** No repeats are allowed on the same prescription.

There are other rules concerning **instalments** of the drug being issued, and the issuing of quantities to travellers going abroad is limited to 14 days' supply.

A prescription for a controlled drug is valid for only 13 weeks, whereas an ordinary prescription is valid for six months.

### Phenobarbitone

*Although barbiturates are controlled drugs, phenobarbitone is **exempt** from the strict rules of handwriting by the doctor. It can be placed on a computer and printed, **but** the date must be handwritten at the time of signing. This drug is extensively used to control epilepsy.*

*N.B. Any prescription for a controlled drug should be placed in a sealed envelope and locked in a drawer or other safe place while awaiting collection.*

### Temazepam

***Temazepam** is exempt from **all** special writing requirements for prescription **but** special storage requirements are applicable.*

## Rules for prescriptions

The following details must be included on all prescription forms (FP10) which must be written in ink or be otherwise indelible:

- Full name and address of patient (to include surname, one forename and initials).

- **Age and date of birth** of the patient should preferably be stated. It is a **legal requirement**, in the case of prescription only medicines (POM), to **state the age for children under 12 years**. It is also recommended to print the age of adults over 60 years, and to incluse years and months for children under 5 years.

- **Name of drug**.

- **Form of drug**.

- **Strength of drug**.

- **Dosage of drug** with instructions to patient on administration.

- **Quantity of drug** to be dispensed or number of days' treatment in box provided.
- **Signature** in ink by the prescriber.
- **Date** of signing.

The directions to the patient **should never** say simply 'as directed' as this can lead to mistakes being made e.g. it is not acceptable to say 'one as directed'. Similarly prn should also state the time interval, e.g. 4 hourly prn.

The name, address and telephone number of the doctor prescribing, together with his PCT number, will be printed or stamped on the prescriptions supplied by the PCT. **Private prescriptions**, often written on the doctor's headed notepaper, **must always** contain the doctor's name, qualifications, address and telephone number.

## Supply of NHS prescription pads FP10

These are supplied to GPs directly by the Prescribing and Pricing Authority (PPA) paid for by PCTs. Each prescription (*see Figure 76*) is already printed with the name, address and

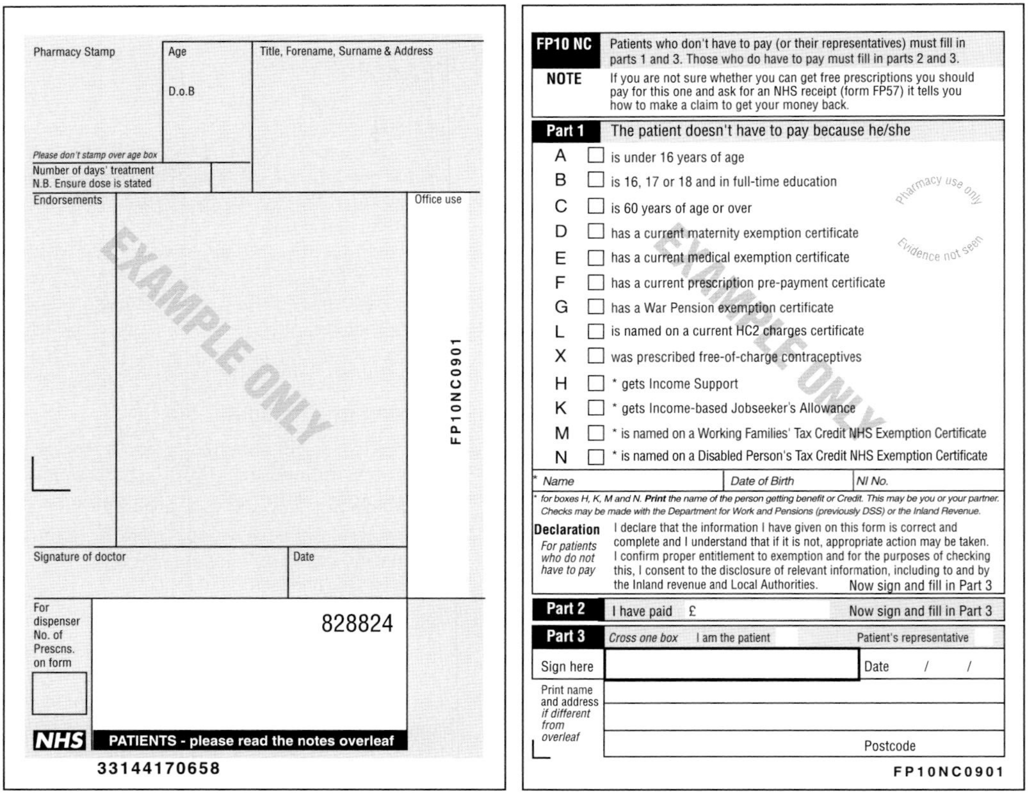

Pharmacy Stamp | Age | D.o.B | Title, Forename, Surname & Address

Please don't stamp over age box

Number of days' treatment
N.B. Ensure dose is stated

Endorsements | Office use

EXAMPLE ONLY

FP10NC0901

Signature of doctor | Date

For dispenser No. of Prescns. on form

828824

NHS PATIENTS - please read the notes overleaf

33144170658

**FP10 NC** Patients who don't have to pay (or their representatives) must fill in parts 1 and 3. Those who do have to pay must fill in parts 2 and 3.

**NOTE** If you are not sure whether you can get free prescriptions you should pay for this one and ask for an NHS receipt (form FP57) it tells you how to make a claim to get your money back.

**Part 1** The patient doesn't have to pay because he/she

- A ☐ is under 16 years of age
- B ☐ is 16, 17 or 18 and in full-time education
- C ☐ is 60 years of age or over
- D ☐ has a current maternity exemption certificate
- E ☐ has a current medical exemption certificate
- F ☐ has a current prescription pre-payment certificate
- G ☐ has a War Pension exemption certificate
- L ☐ is named on a current HC2 charges certificate
- X ☐ was prescribed free-of-charge contraceptives
- H ☐ * gets Income Support
- K ☐ * gets Income-based Jobseeker's Allowance
- M ☐ * is named on a Working Families' Tax Credit NHS Exemption Certificate
- N ☐ * is named on a Disabled Person's Tax Credit NHS Exemption Certificate

Pharmacy use only
Evidence not seen

* Name | Date of Birth | NI No.

* for boxes H, K, M and N. **Print** the name of the person getting benefit or Credit. This may be you or your partner. Checks may be made with the Department for Work and Pensions (previously DSS) or the Inland Revenue.

**Declaration** *For patients who do not have to pay* I declare that the information I have given on this form is correct and complete and I understand that if it is not, appropriate action may be taken. I confirm proper entitlement to exemption and for the purposes of checking this, I consent to the disclosure of relevant information, including to and by the Inland revenue and Local Authorities. Now sign and fill in Part 3

**Part 2** I have paid £ Now sign and fill in Part 3

**Part 3** *Cross one box* I am the patient | Patient's representative

Sign here | Date / /

Print name and address *if different from overleaf*

Postcode

FP10NC0901

**Figure 76:** Example of a prescription Form FP10 NC

**Form FP 57:** a receipt of prescription charge, issued to patient to claim a refund

**Form FP 95:** Prepayment Certificate for patients requiring multiple items each month – available from GP practices, Post Offices and Benefit Agencies – completed form is sent to the PCT

**Form HCII:** explains eligibility for free prescriptions and information on prepayment certificates and refunds. This should be displayed prominently at the surgery.

telephone number of the doctor. Also included is the doctor's PCT number. All now carry a serial number and have a coloured background to deter photocopying. A message, which is visible under ultraviolet light, also aids in the detection of forged prescriptions by addicts.

## Repeat prescriptions

Patients on long-term medication form a large part of the GP's prescribing requirement. It is essential that certain rules are followed to prevent dependency occurring and also to monitor compliance by the patient, i.e. taking the required amount of medication at the correct intervals.

Regular review of prescribing and examination of the patient by the doctor will also highlight any side-effects produced by the treatment being given. Requests to see the patient before the next prescription is supplied may be placed on the computerised slip accompanying the prescription.

### Procedures for repeat prescriptions

In many general practices the receptionist will be involved in the process of the provision of 'repeat prescriptions'. Prescriptions must **never** be signed by the doctor before all details have been entered.

**It is essential that a recognised procedure for repeat prescriptions is adopted by every GP and that the staff involved are aware of the part they must play in its implementation.**

The procedures for repeat prescriptions may be divided into the following stages:

- **Requests**
- **Preparation**
- **Storage and collection.**

## Requests for repeat prescriptions

### Minimum period of notice

Most surgeries require a minimum period of notice for these prescriptions but it must always be flexible. There are always circumstances where it is imperative that a patient does not miss dosages of their prescribed drugs, e.g. conditions of epilepsy, asthma etc.

### Methods of request

These may be by the provision of a computerised 'tear-off' sheet from the prescription or a special card provided to the patient by the doctor, listing all repeat medications to be provided. The patient may bring it in person or post it, stating which drugs are required. A stamped addressed envelope may also be provided for return of the new prescription.

Alternatively, patients may telephone a request. This should then be written in a special book or in the general message book according to the practice policy. Writing messages on scraps of paper should be avoided. If telephones are involved, a special number should be used especially for this purpose. This should never be listed in the telephone book, as addicts can easily use this method to try to obtain illegal supplies.

Telephone requests are prone to errors and for this reason many GPs do not encourage this method. Although nowadays most prescriptions are computer-generated, handwritten ones are required if the computer fails, or in emergencies.

## Preparation of repeat prescriptions

### Methods of preparing repeat prescriptions (manual) on FP10 NC green

The following procedures should be followed:

- Check the **notes are correct** for the patient requesting repeat prescription.

- Check that the drug requested **is to be repeated** by checking the patient's request card and notes for the 'rep' instruction.

- Check the **date of the last prescription** and the **amount of drug** given. **Any discrepancy must be reported to the doctor before any script is written.**

- Check if the **review date is due**. If so a note must be attached to the prescription requesting the patient to make an appointment to see the doctor **before** requesting the next prescription.

- Write the prescription following the entry on the **notes and request card** – ensure spelling of drug, dosages and total quantity are all correct; **nothing that the doctor has written on the card or notes should be altered in any way**.

- **Quantity** to be supplied may be stated indicating the number of days of treatment required in the box provided. In most cases the exact amount will be supplied. This does **not** apply to items directed to be used 'as required' – if the dose and frequency are **not** given, the quantity to be supplied needs to be stated.

- Ideally, instructions should not be abbreviated, but should be **written in full**, e.g. twice a day. Care should be taken with decimal points, e.g. '.5' should be written as '0.5' but only when the dosage cannot be expressed as milligrams or micrograms (e.g.'0.5 g' will become '500 mg').

- The use of a capital 'L' in mL is a printing convention throughout the BNF: both 'mL' and 'ml' are recognised standard abbreviations in medicine and pharmacy. The terms cc or cubic centimetre must not be used.

- Directions should preferably be **in English without abbreviation**; it is recognised that some Latin abbreviations are used (details are given in the British National Formulary. See also page 195 of this book.)

- The strengths microgram and nanogram, **should never be abbreviated** (death of patients has resulted with errors made because these have been mistaken for milligram). Similarly, the word 'units' must **not** be abbreviated.

- A maximum of **three items** is recommended to be placed on one prescription form. Any space underneath the written instructions should be cancelled with a **diagonal line or Z pattern** to fill the space. This prevents unauthorised addition at a later date

- The request card and the notes should all have entries made with the **date, drug** and **amount** as a record of prescribing

- A prescription for a preparation that has been withdrawn or needs to be specially imported for a named patient should be handwritten. The name of the preparation should be endorsed with the prescriber's signature and the letters **'WD'** (withdrawn or specially imported drug). There may be considerable delay in obtaining the drug.

- It is permissible to issue carbon copies of NHS prescriptions as long as they are individually signed in ink (**apart** from for controlled drugs).

- Computer-generated facsimile signatures **do not** meet the legal requirement.

**If there are any queries or discrepancies, the doctor must be informed before any prescription is issued.**

The prepared prescription should now be placed, together with the patient's notes, ready for signing by the appropriate doctor.

## Preparing computerised repeat prescriptions (on FP10 C green)

The drugs required by individual patients will have already been entered into the particular system used by the practice, usually by the doctor. A procedure for these computerised prescriptions should have been agreed with the doctor, and it should ensure safety and prevention of drug abuse similar to the process for manual repeat prescriptions.

- **Care must be taken to ensure that it is the correct patient's computer file that is accessed.**

- It is also important that a routine check is made each time a prescription is processed to ensure that the drug is **authorised** and that it is **due** by date etc.

- The number of items on the script can be entered on the prescription at the bottom of the completed items section, or the space can be cancelled by other printed signs, so preventing **unauthorised additions**.

- The number of items per form need be limited only by the ability of the printer to produce **clear and well demarkated instructions** with sufficient space for each item. A space line **must** be placed before each fresh item.

- Entries should also be made in the **patient's notes** (or other permanent record) stating dates and quantities of the drug concerned for recording purposes.

- The accompanying sheet with the computerised prescription may be used for many purposes and can be given to the patient as a future request slip. However, no code must appear on this sheet although the name of the patient is allowed but the word 'CONFIDENTIAL' should be inserted before it.

- Alterations are best avoided and only made in exceptional circumstances. **It is preferable to print out a new prescription.** However, if any alterations are made, they should be clear and unambiguous; strike through incorrect items and **add prescriber's initials against altered items. Any alteration must be made in the doctor's own writing.**

- Names of medicines **must come from a dictionary held in the computer's memory**, to provide a check on spelling and to ensure that the name is written in full. Programming of the computer, to recognise the generic and proprietary names and to print out the preferred choice is recommended. It must **not print out BOTH names.**

- For **medicines NOT in the dictionary, separate checks are required** and the user should be warned that no dictionary check was possible.

- **Names of controlled drugs must not be printed from computers in any form (see exceptions for phenobarbitone and Temazepam on page 185).**

The requirements for the doctor's own name, address etc. are the same as with ordinary prescriptions:

## Reference books

The main reference books used in prescribing are the *British National Formulary*, the recognised authorative publication on prescribing (now also available for use with computers) and *MIMS (Monthly Index of Medical Specialities)* a book of proprietary preparations published on behalf of drug companies.

The *BPC* or *British Pharmaceutical Codex* is the official publication on drugs. The *ABPI Compendium of Data Sheets and Summaries of Product Characteristics*, supplied by the pharmaceutical companies in the UK, contains information on storage, legal requirements, drug categories and overdose etc.

*The Drug Tariff* from the Prescription Pricing Authority for the Department of Health, contains information on the costing of drugs and appliances on the NHS and information on the 'blacklist', i.e. drugs not available on the NHS, 'endorsement' requirements, prescribable appliances and prescription charges, and is updated each month and supplied free to GPs.

## Food substances – borderline substances

Prescriptions for these substances, which are foods and not drugs, e.g. soya milk, must have **'ACBS'** (Advisory Committee on Borderline Substances) marked on the prescription or they will not be dispensed.

## Dressings and appliances

Prescriptions for these must be precise and include substances such as **oxygen cylinders, surgical hosiery** and **urine testing equipment.** They must always be written on a separate FP10 from drugs.

## SLS prescribing for specific conditions

There is a list of specific conditions for which individual patients may receive NHS prescriptions (further information is found in the Drug Tariff list). These prescriptions must be endorsed with SLS (**i.e. selected list scheme**), e.g. "Viagra".

## Generic names

This is the official name for the drug, e.g. salbutamol, and the one that doctors are requested to use in prescribing. Many manufacturers produce the substance and so costs are lower. However, the base of the preparation may not be the same as the proprietary brand and it may have different effects on some individuals.

## Proprietary names

This is the individual brand or 'trade name' of the drug, e.g. Ventolin, and is usually more expensive than the generic name drugs. However, in a proprietary drug, a standard preparation will be produced to acceptable standards, with which the prescribing doctor will be familiar.

## EU directives on information

**Bubble packs in containers with written information and warnings have been introduced for all tablets and capsules. This will ensure compliance with the EU directive** which requires information to be provided for the person being dispensed or purchasing medicines.

Pharmacists can provide the bubble pack quantity nearest to the amount stated on the prescription. In order to ensure accuracy, care will have to be taken to adjust the patient's repeat prescription records.

## Oral syringes

When liquid medicines for the oral route, (i.e. by mouth) are prescribed in doses other than multiples of 5 ml, an oral syringe (marked in divisions of 0.5 ml from 1 to 5 ml) is provided. This helps to ensure that doses of less than 5 ml are accurately measured. It is provided with an adaptor and instruction leaflet. The 5 ml spoon is used for doses of 5 ml or multiples of 5 ml.

## Limited list NHS

Since 1985, regulations have been introduced which name a list of preparations which are not allowed to be prescribed on the NHS as they were considered too expensive and many had cheaper generic equivalents. It is known as the limited list and also as the **blacklist**. This includes preparations such as proprietary pain-killers (analgesics), e.g. Disprin, as well as other types of drugs. Should these be accidentally prescribed, the doctor will be charged for the preparation him/herself.

## PACT (prescribing analysis and cost) and PPA

Information is issued to each general practice at regular intervals from the Prescription Pricing Authority (PPA), comparing the prescribing habits of the doctor with the average for the area.

## Practice formulary

Many practices will have a practice formulary. This is a standard list of drugs in different categories, produced by the practice. The list will be the first choice of drugs to be prescribed by the doctors for various conditions from which patients may be suffering. Partners will all have agreed to the choice of drugs within it. All practices will have a practice formulary as part of their budgeting process.

## National Institute for Clinical Excellence (NICE)

This is an agency, which examines clinical treatments and drugs for their efficacy and cost benefit, advising which new drugs may be prescribed on the NHS

# Storage and collection of repeat prescriptions

The following rules apply:

- The signed prescriptions should be placed in an appropriate box away from the reach of anyone coming to the reception desk. They must **never** be left for patients to help themselves.

- The identity of the person collecting the prescription must be **verified**, e.g. request for a date of birth or a middle name etc. of the patient for whom it is written.

- Ensure two pages are **not** stuck together.

- Take care that it is the **correct** prescription for the correct patient – verify address, spelling etc.

- Repeat prescriptions should **not** be handed to children unless the doctor or parent has made special provision.

- All uncollected prescriptions should be **locked away at night** and when the desk is unattended.

## Prescriptions directed to outside pharmacies

Some general practices have arrangements with local pharmacists for prescriptions to be sent directly to the pharmacist ready for dispensing. If this procedure is in force it is essential that individual patients have signed that they consent to this arrangement.

## Exemptions from prescription charges

Certain categories of patients are exempt from prescription charges, these include those aged under-16, students aged 17 and 18 years in full-time education, the over-60s, pregnant women and those patients suffering from some named chronic conditions:

- **Colostomy, tracheostomy** or **ileostomy** patients.

- **Epilepsy**, on continuous anticonvulsant treatment.

- **Diabetes mellitus**, unless the treatment is by diet alone.

- Patients requiring supplemental **thyroxine**.

- **Hypoparathyroidism**.

- **Diabetes insipidus** or **hypopituitarism**.

- **Hypoadrenalism** including **Addison's disease**.

- **Myasthenia gravis**.

The details of other exemptions are to be found on the back of an FP10 form. Many patients may require assistance from the receptionist with the completion of this form.

## Measures taken to recognise drug addicts

The previous requirement for GPs to report the name of anyone whom they suspect of being a drug addict to the Home Office has been removed, except for in Northern Ireland.

There is a new special centre, **'The National Drugs Treatment Monitoring System'** whom GPs should notify when commencing treatment of a patient for drug addiction. This is an anonymised, database system. There are various regional offices in England, Scotland and Wales which may be contacted by telephone.

**NB:** Only doctors with a special licence issued by the Home Secretary, are allowed to treat drug addiction to diamorphine, dipipanone or cocaine; other practitioners must refer any addict requiring these drugs, to a special treatment centre.

Special FP10 (MDA) prescription forms are used by GPs for prescribing controlled drugs to addicts in installments. There are 10 light blue double-sided, numbered forms in each pad.

However, a GP or other doctor may prescribe these drugs in the usual way, for any patient requiring them for the relief of pain, due to organic disease or injury.

Letters are sent from each PCT, warning GPs of suspicious people in the area. This is in order that the doctor may be aware of a particular ruse used to obtain drugs by that person. If the receptionist has any suspicions about someone visiting the premises, s/he should immediately inform the practice manager or doctor.

The regular review of repeat prescribing for all patients plus the alertness of the receptionist involved in writing repeat prescriptions, helps in the prevention and awareness of any abuse of drugs.

## Security of the premises

A good burglar alarm system is vital and the surgery window curtains are usually drawn back at night and lights left on so that policemen are able to inspect premises more easily.

## Further requirements to prevent drug abuse

FP10 prescription pads are now designed to prevent unauthorised alteration and photocopying. Special print and coloured paper are used for various categories of prescription. Special inscriptions, visible only in UV light, also aid detection of forgeries. All prescriptions now include serial numbers.

Batches of prescription pads, delivered to the surgery from the PCT, should be checked to ensure that all are present. Any discrepancy must be reported to the PCT and the police. All unused prescription pads must be stored in a safe place and should be locked away at night and when the doctor's room is unattended. Should any prescriptions be stolen there is a procedure for writing all future prescriptions in red. This is for a stated period of time. It alerts the pharmacist to the possibility of an illegal script.

Drugs should not be stored in cupboards where patients have access, e.g. in the waiting room. Clear directions must be given to patients concerning the dosage and mode of administration. Drug storage cupboards should be locked and should not be marked. The controlled drugs (CD) cupboard keys should be kept on the person of a suitable member of staff, usually the doctor and the practice nurse.

If the doctor's bag contains drugs (as is usual) it must be kept locked and in a safe place. If controlled drugs are contained in the bag, a locked car is not recognised as being a sufficiently secure place. **It must be locked in the case in the locked boot of the car.** Prescription pads should **never** be left in a car where the public may see them.

Any drugs left in the doctor's room, e.g. by drug firm representatives, should be collected and locked away in the appropriate place (usually by the practice nurse).

## Disposal of drugs

Drugs are sometimes returned to the surgery by patients. These should be returned to the pharmacist or placed in the special collection service provided by some PCTs. This complies with the requirements of the *Environmental Protection Act*. Controlled drugs have stringent requirements and should only be handled by appropriate designated staff. Returned drugs must never be reused. **Expired drugs should be disposed of in the same way. Expired drugs must never be mixed with other batches of drugs already in the surgery, for re-use.**

## Supply and disposal of controlled drugs in general practice

There are stringent requirements under The *Misuse of Drugs Act*, covering Schedules 2 and 3 (drugs of addiction used in medicine).

The requirements cover:

- Supply
- Prescription writing (see previous section)
- Safe custody
- **The Controlled Drugs Register**
- Destruction/disposal.

### The Controlled Drugs Register

Supply of and dispensing of Schedule 2 controlled drugs is required to be recorded and signed for in the Controlled Drugs Register.

**Entries must include:**

- **Drugs received**
- **Date received**
- **Name and address of GP authorised to hold and supply the drugs or the supplying person/firm**
- **Amount received**
- **Form in which supplied**, e.g. ampoule/tablet.

**The Register itself must:**

- Be **bound** with ruled and headed columns
- Entries written in **ink** or indelible form
- Have separate sections for **each class** and **form** of drug
- Have transactions entered **on the day of occurrence** or, at latest, the following day
- Have **no cancellations or alterations** (any corrections **must** be made in the margin provided **or** as a footnote and must be signed and dated)
- Be **kept on the premises** to which the register relates
- Be **kept for two years** from the date of the last entry
- Be **available for inspection** at any time (by

medical officer or a Home Office drugs inspector).

**The following are also recommended:**

- A separate column to record **the balance of stock** remaining (this allows the actual stock to be checked easily, enabling any stock discrepancies to be immediately reported and investigated)

- A separate Controlled Drug Register for *each* **GP's bag**.

## Disposal/destruction of controlled drugs

Normally, controlled drugs in Schedule 2, must be destroyed, only, in the presence of **an authorised person**, such as a police officer or Home Office drugs inspector. The name of the drug, the amount and date of destruction is entered in the Controlled Drugs Register and signed by the person in whose presence the drugs were destroyed.

There is an **audit trail** (from importation) at every stage, ending at the supply to the patient. However, there is no requirement within The *Misuse of Drugs Act*, of any recording to be made of any drugs returned to the GP by the patient or patient's relatives, or of their destruction.

Following the terrible revelations of the **Shipman murders**, interim proposals by Professor Richard Baker are being considered for implementation.

### Professor Richard Baker's report

The main proposals of Professor Richard Baker's report are:

- Systems for **monitoring GPs** should be reviewed and include routine monitoring of **death rates** and improved methods for overseeing the prescribing of controlled drugs and quality of medical records.

- A system for collecting information about the number of deaths of GPs' patients, and **death certificates** issued by them, should be investigated and a practical system introduced as soon as possible.

- Information about the circumstances of death and the patient's clinical history should be recorded both in the case of **cremations** and **burials**.

- The procedure for **revalidating GPs** should include an assessment of appropriate samples of a GP's records.

- The policy of offering to return **records** to GPs after the expiry of the period of storage by PCTs should be reviewed. If GPs are allowed to retain records, arrangements for their **secure storage** should be established.

- An effective system for the **inspection of GPs' Controlled Drugs Registers** should be introduced.

- GPs should record **batch numbers** in clinical records when they personally administer controlled drugs, and batch numbers should be included in the Controlled Drugs Registers of GPs and pharmacists.

The need to ensure that there are more effective controls on controlled drugs is abundantly clear. The loop-hole of returned Schedule 2 drugs, such as heroin, (diamorphine), and morphine, to doctors from the relatives of deceased patients, who have received palliative (terminal care), has illustrated enormous potential for their misuse. The lack of any requirement for GPs to record possession or destruction of these controlled drugs, enabled the means for Dr Shipman to enact his evil crimes with relative ease.

### PCT controls

Primary Care Trusts are trying to ensure that steps are being taken to ensure that all controlled drugs are witnessed as they are being destroyed. The list of persons to be present as witnesses, has been extended to include :

- Primary Care Trust Chief Pharmacists

- Registered medical practitioner appointed with responsibility for Clinical Governance or Risk Management

- Medical Director of a Primary Care Trust.

## Further information

### CSM reporting of adverse reactions

Reporting on the 'yellow card' to the CSM (Committee on the Safety of Medicines) via the

Medicines and Health Care Products Regulatory Agency (MHRA) is an important part of research in general practice and can help to avoid another thalidomide disaster, i.e. the deformities produced in children born to mothers who had been prescribed this drug during pregnancy in the late 1950s and early 60s. reporting may also be made at the website: www.medicines.mhra.gov.uk

**New drugs are always monitored in this way and are marked with a *black triangle* for at least the first *two years* following the release to the public on prescription, in order to alert the doctor to the necessity of reporting any untoward side-effects.**

## Prescription event monitoring

In addition to the CSM's Yellow Card scheme, an independent scheme monitors the safety of new medicines using a different approach. The **Drug Safety Unit** identifies patients who have been prescribed selected new medicines and collects data on clinical events in these patients. This is a voluntary scheme and the data is submitted by general practitioners using green forms.

## Adverse Reactions to Medical Devices

Suspected adverse reactions to medical devices, including dental or surgical materials, intra-uterine devices and contact lens fluid, should also be reported to the MHRA.

## Nurse practitioners and community nurses

Some of these personnel have been given the legal right to prescribe certain drugs directly to patients. The nurse's NMC (Nurses and Midwives' Council) PIN number must be included on the prescription as well as the practice identification number and address.

Practice nurses qualified as District Nurses or Health Visitors who have attended an approved nurse prescribers' course may prescribe from a limited list of drugs (see BNF, NPF [Nurses' Prescribing Formulary] or Drug Tariff). The FP10 PN used is coloured lilac. Community Nurses and Health Visitors who have also attended the required course may prescribe from the same list on FP10 CN which is coloured grey.

There is also an extended list for those first level nurses and registered midwives nurses who have completed the, 'Extended Formulary Nurse Prescriber' Course, which allows approximately 140 prescription only medicines, (POMs), to be prescribed for therapeutic areas of:

- **Minor illness**
- **Minor injury**
- **Health promotion**
- **Palliative care**

## Private prescriptions

These may be required when substances are not available on the NHS. All requirements for prescriptions are as for the Medicines Act. Private headed notepaper is normally used and the name and qualifications are required, as well as all other details as already stated for other medicines. Charges are suggested in the BMA list.

## Complimentary medicine

It is important to remember that a number of herbal medicine have been found to interfere with conventional therapy, e.g. St John's Wort. Information on this subject can be found at www.mhra.gov.uk

## Abbreviations

| | |
|---|---|
| **BNF** | British National Formulary |
| **CD** or **cd** or CD | controlled drug (schedule 2 or 3 of MODA, 1971) |
| **HRT** | hormone replacement therapy |
| ~~**NHS**~~ | not available on the NHS |
| **NIDDM** | non-insulin dependent diabetes mellitus |
| **IDDM** | insulin dependent diabetes mellitus |
| **NSAID** | nonsteroidal anti-inflammatory drug |
| **OP** | original pack (manufacturer's own pack) |

| | |
|---|---|
| **P** or P | pharmacy only drugs |
| **PGD** | patient group direction/directive – a written direction on the supply and/or administration of medicines by a healthcare professional (not a doctor) for a stated type of patient, e.g. "morning after pill" |
| **POM** or POM | prescription only medicine |
| **PPI** | proton pump inhibitor (reduces amount of acid stomach produces) |
| **SLS** | selected list scheme |
| **SSRI** | selective serotonin reuptake inhibitor (antidepressant) |
| **TTA** | to take away |
| ▲ | special reporting requirements |

## Prescriptions

| Abbreviation | Meaning [Latin] |
|---|---|
| **a.a.** | of each – equal amount [ana] |
| **a.c.** | before food [ante cibum] |
| **alt die** | alternate days [alt die] |
| **alt noct.** | alternate nights [alt nocte] |
| **b.d.** | twice daily [bis die] |
| **c.** | with [cum] |
| **ex. aq.** | water [ex aquain] |
| **h.n.** | tonight [hac nocte] |
| **mane** | in the morning [mane] |
| **nocte** | at night [nocte] |
| **NP** | proper name [nomen proprium] |
| **o.d.** | every day/daily [omni die] |

| | |
|---|---|
| **o.m.** | every morning [omni mane] |
| **o.n.** | every night [omni nocte] |
| **p.a.** | to the affected part [parti affectae] |
| **p.c.** | after food [post cibum] |
| **p.r.n.** | whenever necessary [pro re nata] |
| **q.d.s.** | four times daily [quater die sumendum] |
| **q.i.d.** | four times daily [quater in die] |
| **q.q.h.** | every four hours [quarta quaque hora] |
| **R$_x$** | take [recipe] |
| **rep.** | let it be repeated [repetitur] |
| **s.o.s.** | if necessary (one dose only) [si opus sit] |
| **stat.** | at once [statim] |
| **t.d.s.** | three times daily [ter die sumendum] |
| **t.i.d.** | three times daily [ter in die] |

*BNF approved abbreviations for directions*

The following are **approved** for use by the BNF:

| | |
|---|---|
| **a.c.** | before food |
| **b.d.** | twice daily |
| **o.d.** | every day / daily |
| **o.m.** | every morning |
| **o.n.** | every night |
| **p.c.** | after food |
| **p.r.n.** | whenever necessary |
| **q.d.s.** | four times daily |
| **q.q.h.** | every four hours |
| **stat.** | at once |
| **t.d.s.** | three times daily |

## Preparations

| Abbreviation | Meaning [Latin] |
|---|---|
| **caps.** | capsules |
| **neb.** | nebulizer |
| **occ.** or **oc.** | for the eyes [occulentae] |
| **p.o.c.** | for the eyes |
| **p.r.** | via the rectum [per rectum] |
| **p.v.** | via the vagina [per vaginam] |
| **pessary** | for the vagina |
| **suppos.** | suppository |
| **tabs.** | tablets |

| Abbreviation | Meaning [Latin] |
|---|---|
| **tinct.** | tincture [tincture] |
| **troch.** | lozenge [trochisci] |
| **ung.** | ointment [unguentum] |
| **vap.** | vapour [vapore] |

## Measurements

| | |
|---|---|
| **g** | gram |
| **mcg** | microgram |
| **mg** | milligram |
| **ml** | millilitre |
| **ng\*** | nanogram |
| **S.I.** | International System |
| **µg\*** | microgram |

*must not be used on prescriptions according to British National Formulary recommendations*

## Terminology

### Classification of drugs etc.

| | |
|---|---|
| **Continuous subcutaneous infusion** | drugs given into the layer under the dermis via a syringe driver or 'pump' |
| **Intradermal (ID)** | into the skin |
| **Intramuscular (IM)** | into the muscle |
| **Intravenous (IV)** | via the vein |
| ***Materia medica*** | drugs used in medicine |
| **Oral** | by mouth |
| **Parenteral** | drugs administered, other than by the oral route |
| **Pharmacologist** | specialist in drugs |
| **Pharmacology** | study of drugs |
| **Systemic** | by injection – affects whole body. |

### Types of preparation

| | |
|---|---|
| **Elixir** | a sweetened aromatic substance containing alcohol |
| **Enema** | a liquid substance inserted into the rectum |
| **Lavage** | a washout – fluid inserted through a tube usually into the stomach to remove contents |
| **Linctus** | sweet syrupy liquid for coughs |
| **Pessary** | solid form of drug inserted in the vagina (pv) |
| **Suppository** | solid form of drug inserted in the rectum (pr) |
| **Tincture** | solution of a drug in alcohol |

## Drug types (classification)

| | |
|---|---|
| **ACE inhibitor** | (ACE: angiotensin-converting enzyme) drug which is used for treatment of hypertension or heart failure |
| **Anaesthetic** | drug for removal of feeling |
| *General* | to the whole body – produces unconsciousness. |
| *Local* | to a part – produces numbness |
| **Angiotensin-II receptor antagonists** | drug used to treat hypertension |
| **Analgesic** | drug for relief of pain |
| **Antacid** | a substance which neutralises stomach acid |
| **Anti-arrhythmic** | drug which controls abnormal rhythm of the heart |
| **Antibiotic** | drug which kills bacteria |
| **Anticoagulant** | drug which reduces clotting |
| **Antidepressant** | drug which lifts the patient's mood |
| **Anti-emetic** | drug which reduces nausea |
| **Antifungal** | drug which kills fungi |
| **Antihistamine** | drug which reduces production of histamine – for allergies |
| **Antihypertensive** | drug which reduces blood pressure |
| **Anti-inflammatory** | drug which reduces inflammation |
| **Anti-obesity** | drug which helps reduce weight |
| **Antipyretic** | drug which reduces fever |
| **Antipsychotic** | also known as 'neuroleptics', drug which quietens disturbed patients suffering from mania, hallucinations etc. used as a short term measure |
| **Antispasmodic** | drug which reduces spasms of muscle, e.g. colic |
| **Antitussic** | drug which reduces coughing |
| **Anxiolytic** | drug which reduces anxiety |
| **Beta-blocker** | drug which lowers blood pressure etc. – by affecting specific beta-nerve receptors |
| **Bronchodilator** | drug which dilates the bronchial tubes as in treatment for asthma |
| **Calcium channel blockers** | drugs which depress cardiac function |
| **Carminative** | drug which reduces flatulence (wind) |
| **Chemotherapy** | toxic drugs which are given to kill malignant cells |
| **Contraceptive** | drug which prevents conception |
| **Cox 2 inhibitor** | drug to reduce inflammation in arthritis better tolerated by the gastro-intestinal system than NSAIDs |
| **Cytotoxic** | drugs which kill cells – used to treat malignant disease by killing cancerous cells |
| **Decongestant** | drug which relieves congestion of mucous membranes |
| **Depressant** | a drug which depresses function of the central nervous system |
| **Diuretic** | drug which increases the production of urine |
| **Expectorant** | liquid form of drug which encourages coughing up of secretions from the respiratory tract |
| **Hypnotic** | drug which induces sleep |
| **Miotic** | for the eyes – to constrict the pupil |

**Mydriatic**  for the eyes – to dilate
the pupil

**Narcotic**  drug derived from opium
which will induce deep
sleep

**Prophylactic**  a substance used to prevent
disease

**Proton pump**  drugs which inhibit the
production of hydrochloric
acid in the stomach

**Sedative**  a drug which lowers
function

**Statins**  drug which lowers
cholesterol blood levels

**Steroids**  drugs containing hormones –
usually of the adrenal cortex

**Corticosteroids**  drugs from the cortex
of the adrenal glands or
synthetic preparations,
which reduce inflammation
etc., e.g. prednisolone

**Stimulant**  a drug which increases
function of the central
nervous system

**Tranquilliser**  a drug which reduces
anxiety

**Vaccine**  a substance prepared
specially to stimulate the
body to produce its own
antibodies or antitoxins

# Chapter **19** | Preventive medicine

# Health

### The World Health Organisation's definition of health states:

*"Health is a state of complete physical, mental and social well-being and not merely the absence of disease or infirmity . . . Good Health is held to be fundamental to all peace and security."*

This is the ideal state and is very difficult to achieve.

Each one of the three factors (**physical, mental,** or **social**) will affect the other two, e.g. problems with physical health will cause mental and social problems for the patient; similarly, problems with social factors will affect mental and physical well-being.

**Preventive medicine** is concerned with the prevention of disease in all forms. It is aimed at all people worldwide of all age ranges, *not just* the developing countries. Based on the concept 'prevention is better than cure', it is intended to provide a better span and quality of life for human beings wherever possible. It is also considered cheaper to prevent disease than cure it.

Prevention can be divided into three main categories:

1. **Primary prevention**
2. **Secondary prevention**
3. **Tertiary prevention.**

## Primary prevention

This is the complete **avoidance** of the disease, e.g. by **immunisation** and **lifestyle modifications**.

## Secondary prevention

This is concerned with the **early detection** of disease in patients who have **no symptoms**, e.g. **screening of babies, cervical cytology,** routine **mammography**. All screening processes are secondary prevention.

## Tertiary prevention

This is concerned with the **limitation of chronic disease** by the discovery and management of the disease before complications have produced disability or handicap; e.g. **careful management** of diabetes mellitus, hyperten-

sion and asthma, as well as care of those with the effects of diagnosed coronary heart disease

# Data

The setting up of **age-sex registers** and use of **Read Codes** on computers are essential tools for the implementation of preventive medicine in general practice. The New GP Contract 2003 requirements for setting up of specific disease registers will provide a useful tool in complying with clinical governance.

Read codes provide a clinical coding system on the data of patients, concerning disease, drugs, etc. These systems enable easy recall of information which can be used for research, statistics and regular recall of patients.

# Primary Health Care Team (PHCT)

The Primary Health Care Team is a group of professional health care workers within the community, each contributing their own special skills to the benefit of patients' well-being (*see Figure 77*). They are normally the first professionals involved in the care of the patient.

In general practice, it is the PHCT who is at the front line of preventive medicine. This aspect was given a definite emphasis in the 1990 GP Contract and continues to be regarded as of vital importance in the **2003 GP Contract** as a part of the quality requirements.

The PHCT requires:

- Clear **goals**
- Clear **roles** and **responsibilities** ensuring best use of different expertise
- Good **relationships**
- Good **communication.**

## Goals

It is important that the PHCT work together as a team towards a common goal. Each member should be aware of the specialist skills provided by each of the other members, thus providing support to each other and the best care for the patient. It is always important to remember what the overall achievement should be, i.e. the best care of the patient.

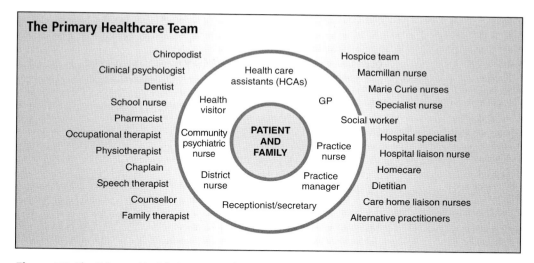

**Figure 77:** The Primary Health Care Team (PHCT) *(Reproduced from The Primary Care Nurses' Companion, edited by Sue Hinchliff. In press: Magister Consulting)*

Among the common goals is that of preventive medicine. The new **'Primary Care Organisations' (PCOs)**, include all disciplines and (together with the **National Plan** and the continuing expansion and implementation of the **National Service Framework**) should help to achieve the overall targets for 2010, of the 1999 White Paper, *'Saving Lives: Our Healthier Nation'*.

## Members

The basic PHCT is composed of:

- **GP**
- **Health visitor**
- **Community nurse/midwife**
- **Nurse practitioner**
- **Practice nurse**
- **Health care assistants**
- **District nurse**
- **Social worker**
- **Practice manager**
- **Receptionist/secretary**
- **Community psychiatric nurse**

The administrative support from the practice manager, receptionists and secretaries is absolutely vital and ensures the smooth running of the team. Good communication is vital and it is here that the receptionist can bring invaluable support by ensuring accuracy in conveying messages.

The other specialist members of the primary team include (*see Figure 77*):

- **Counsellors**
- **Clinical Nurse Specialist in Palliative Care (CNS) – Macmillan nurse**
- **School nurses**
- **Continence advisors**
- **Chiropodists**
- **Dietitians**
- **Domiciliary physiotherapists**
- **Occupational therapists**
- **Speech therapists**
- **Orthoptists**
- **Pharmacists**
- **Dental officers.**

Nurses at **'NHS Direct'** and **'Walk in Centres'** can be described as part of the PHCT as they are often the first contact the patient has with a health professional.

*The patient and his/her carer (voluntary or a Home Care Assistant), are the basis of the team, allowing the patient to remain in the community.*

## Areas of primary preventive medicine

These include:

- **Immunisation**
- **Public health and housing controls**
- **Health education**
- **Dental fluoridation.**

### Immunisation

This is one of the main areas of prevention (*see Chapter 22*). Before the advent of immunisation of children against infectious diseases (such as **diphtheria**), many children died before reaching puberty.

### Public health and housing controls

Without the sweeping changes in these areas, which came about in the late 19th century ensuring better **housing**, clean **water** supplies and **disposal of sewage**, the general standard of health would be very poor. These controls should never be under-estimated as control of the **environment** is paramount in the battle for health. Increasing **pollution** of the atmosphere is producing health hazards for many of the population at the present time.

### Health education/promotion

Health education and promotion is aimed at persuading people to live **healthy lifestyles** and adopt a positive view towards taking responsibility for their own, and their children's, health.

The greatest problem is the 'it won't happen to me' attitude. Anti-smoking, anti-drugs and AIDS campaigns, together with all the other areas in which the **Health Development Agency** is involved, play a major part in these fields.

The provision of the many available health education leaflets is of great help to the GP practice and to the health visitor in their relationship with the patient. Leaflets can be obtained from the **'Health Promotion and Resources'** department within Primary Care Organisations.

Health education begins with **preconceptual advice** and continues through to, and includes, old age. Parents and teachers play a major role in childhood: **'example'** is the greatest teacher of all.

## Important areas of preventive medicine

There are many different areas of health promotion in different sectors of the community. Some examples of the wide range of preventive medicine are described below:

### Maternal care (antenatal and postnatal)

- Screening for defects in the **fetus**
- Screening for diseases in the **mother**
- Early detection or prevention of **toxaemia** of pregnancy.

### Child care

- Detection of abnormalities by **screening** tests – physical, mental and social
- **Developmental surveillance** – hearing, speech and visual defects etc
- **Immunisation**
- **Prevention of accidents** – avoidance of poisoning, burns etc
- **Prevention of child abuse** – **non-accidental injury** and **sexual abuse**
- **Prevention of dental caries**
- **Prevention of drug abuse.**

### Adolescents

- **Smoking** prevention/cessation
- **Contraception** and dealing with unwanted pregnancy

- **Accident prevention** at work and home.
- **Alcohol** and **drug abuse**
- **Sexually transmitted disease** including AIDS
- **Suicide/self-harm.**

## Adults: 16 to 64 years

- Complications of **pregnancy**
- **Smoking**
- **Chronic Obstructive Airway/ Pulmonary Disease (COAD** or **COPD)**
- **Sexually transmitted disease** including HIV and AIDS
- **Rubella** (German measles)
- **Motor accidents**
- **Alcohol and drug abuse**
- **Cancer of the breast and cervix**
- **Testicular and prostate cancer**
- **Hypertension**
- **Coronary heart disease**
- **Suicide/self-harm**
- **Cancer of the oesophagus and colon.**

## Elderly: 65 years and over

- **Hypertension**
- **Loss of autonomy**
- **Dementia**
- **Hearing defects**
- **Feet problems**
- **Visual defects**
- **Influenza,** with emphasis on those at risk due to other diseases
- **Hypothermia**
- **Accidents** and loss of **balance**
- **'Granny bashing'** – abuse of the elderly by carer/relative.

## All age ranges

- **Diet** and **obesity**
- **Asthma**
- **Diabetes mellitus type 2**
- **Exercise.**

The range of preventive medicine is a vast one and these are only examples of the many areas where the individual may benefit from the prevention of disease, health education or screening processes.

## Opportunistic screening

Instead of special health promotion clinics, it is now accepted and recognised that **opportunistic screening** is more effective in primary and secondary preventive medicine.

The GP and his/her staff have always been involved in the routine testing of **urine** and recording of **blood pressure**, and hidden cases of **diabetes mellitus** and **hypertension** have been regularly detected. Hypertension is a 'silent killer' as no symptoms occur until there has already been extensive damage to the body.

## The role of the receptionist in preventive medicine

The receptionist in general practice will be involved in the collection and programming of **statistics** and also the maintenance of the **age/sex register** or **morbidity register**. Various letters and questionnaires will need to be given or sent to patients. Efficient recording and filing of notes are essential.

Ensuring there is always a good supply of **health education leaflets** available for patients, is a valuable contribution to the work of the PHCT. Local Health Promotion Departments will readily supply these on request as well as assist in the setting up of specialist displays on many aspects of preventive medicine.

**Immunisation** and **cervical smear** targets will also be a priority. An understanding of the reasons for these important requirements will enable the receptionist to assist the PHCT with an even greater motivation.

## Saving Lives: Our Healthier Nation

A white paper issued by the government in 1999 entitled *'Saving Lives: Our Healthier Nation'* stated their intentions for the planned improvement of the nation's health up to the year **2010**.

The paper states that good health is a top priority for the government. The aim is to prevent people falling ill in the first place by **'tackling the root causes of the avoidable illnesses'**. In recent years emphasis has been placed on the individual's responsibility to live healthy lives via **lifestyle** changes. This has been beneficial but has also led to an attitude which blames the individual for his/her poor health. The plan now is for more attention and government action to be placed on controlling those factors which damage health and are beyond the individual's control.

## Inequality

Poor health has complex causes, some of which are fixed, such as **genetic factors** and **ageing**. However, many other factors which may cause bad health can be changed, e.g. lifestyle, diet, physical exercise, sexual behaviour, smoking, alcohol and drugs.

**Social and economic factors** also play a part, for instance **poverty, unemployment** and **social exclusion**. Our environment, including air and water quality, housing, as well as access to good services such as education, transport, social services provision and the NHS, all affect our health. It is a fact that poor people are ill more often and die sooner.

There is now an emphasis on fundamental inequalities and attention and resources are being given to the areas most affected by: air pollution, low wages, unemployment, poor housing, and crime and disorder, all of which can make people both mentally and physically ill.

## Linked programmes

A series of programmes linked to improving factors affecting health are to be implemented by the government, including measures on:

- **'Welfare to work'** (tackling unemployment)
- **Crime**
- **Housing**
- **Education**
- **Health.**

## Key aims

There are two key aims for improving the health of the population:

1. **'To improve the health of the population as a whole by increasing the length of people's lives and the number of years people spend free from illness.'**

2. **'To improve the health of the worst off in society and to narrow the health gap.'**

The government has set out a new way to achieve this goal 'between the old extremes of individual victim blaming' and 'nanny state social engineering on the other' by introducing the **National Contract for Better Health**.

### Partnerships

To achieve the main aims, the following groups work together:

- **Government**
- **Health care trusts**
- **Local authorities**
- **Businesses**
- **Voluntary bodies.**

**Individuals** also play a part in taking decisions about their own health

## Targets of
*Saving Lives: Our Healthier Nation*

Based on health statistics from 1996, four priority areas are targeted for 2010. The new goals are as follows:

**1. Cancer**

to reduce the death rate in people under 75 by at least a fifth (20%)

**2. Coronary heart disease and stroke**

to reduce the death rate in people under 75 by at least two fifths (40%)

**3. Accidents**

to reduce the death rate by at least a fifth (20%) and to reduce the incidence of serious injury by at least a tenth (10%)

**4. Mental Illness**

to reduce the death rate from suicide and undetermined injury by at least a fifth (20%)

**Additionally wider action has been taken on the following:**

- **Smoking**

- **Sexual health**

- **Drugs**

- **Alcohol**

- **Food** safety (Food Standards Agency established)

- **Fluoride** and **oral health**

- **Communicable diseases**

- **Genetic factors** (Genetics Task Force)

- The health of **black and minority ethnic groups.**

## Local targets

Other health problems, particular to each locality in the country, are also targeted, according to the local needs – e.g. problems of the elderly in localities with high levels of retired residents and their associated health problems. The relevant areas targeted, will be decided by the Local Primary Care Trusts and Local Authorities. Auditing and monitoring will be performed by the **Strategic Health Authority (SHA)**

The Department of Health issued the following advice:

## Ten Tips - your guide to better health

1. Don't smoke. If you can, stop. If you can't, cut down.

2. Follow a balanced diet with plenty of fruit and vegetables.

3. Keep physically active.

4. Manage stress by, for example, talking things through and making time to relax.

5. If you drink alcohol, do so in moderation.

6. Cover up in the sun, and protect children from sunburn.

7. Practise safer sex.

8. Take up cancer screening opportunities.

9. Be safe on the roads: follow the Highway Code.

10. Learn the First Aid ABC - airways, breathing and circulation.

issued by Liam Donaldson, Chief Medical Officer

## National Service Framework (NSF)

Following the white paper 'A First Class Service: quality in the new NHS' (Department of Health, 1998), the National Institute for Clinical Excellence (**NICE**) has established the 'National Service Framework' for specific named conditions. This has been introduced with the aim of ensuring all patients are treated in the same clinical way, regardless of their post code, so that health is not a lottery according to the area in which you live. Each framework lays down the ways in which risk assessment is made as well as the recommended treatment which should be given to the patient.

Each National Service Framework covers:

- **Prevention**
- **Diagnosis**
- **Management**
- **Rehabilitation**

for each specific condition.

These frameworks are intended for use in:

- **Public health**
- **Primary care**
- **Secondary care**

Their aim is to ensure that the main targets of *'Saving Lives: Our Healthier Nation'*, will be achieved by 2010.

To date there are **National Service Frameworks** established for:

- **Coronary heart disease**
- **Diabetes mellitus**
- **Mental health**
- **Older people**
- **Renal health**
- **Children**

and

- a National Health Service Plan has also been introduced for **cancer.**

(A summary of the current NSFs and the NHS Cancer Plan are given below).

They are delivered by means of clinical governance, underpinned by professional self-regulation and lifelong personal development plans

They are monitored by the:

- **Commission for Health Improvement (CHI)**
- **NHS Performance Assessment Framework**
- **National Survey of NHS Patients.**

**Strategic Health Authorities** are responsible for the auditing of compliance with these standards and the new **2003 GP Contract** is heavily orientated to the provision of these quality requirements. GPs' remuneration will reflect their performance in these fields.

## Summary of NSF standards and the NHS Cancer Plan

### Coronary Heart Disease (CHD)
- Reducing heart disease in the population
- Preventing CHD in high risk patients
- Heart attack and other acute coronary syndromes
- Stable angina
- Revascularisation
- Heart failure
- Cardiac rehabilitation.

### Diabetes mellitus
- Prevention of type 2 diabetes
- Identification of people with diabetes
- Empowering people with diabetes
- Clinical care of adults with diabetes
- Clinical care of children and young people with diabetes
- Management of diabetic emergencies
- Care of people with diabetes during admission to hospital
- Diabetes and pregnancy
- Detection and management of long-term complications.

### Mental Health Services for Working Age Adults
- Promoting Social Inclusion
- Service User and Carer Empowerment
- Promotion of opportunities for fulfilling and socially inclusive patterns of daily life
- Equitable, accessible services
- Commissioning effective, comprehensive and responsive services
- Delivering effective, comprehensive and responsive services
- Effective client assessment and core pathways
- Ensuring a well-staffed, skilled and supportive workforce.

**Older People**

- Rooting out age discrimination

- Person centred care

- Intermediate care

- General hospital care

- Stroke

- Falls

- Mental health in older people

- Promoting an active healthy life in older age.

**Renal**

- Primary prevention, pre-dialysis and acute renal failure

- Effective delivery of dialysis

- Transplantation

- Alternative models of care.

**Children, young people and maternity services**

This framework is still being developed as a partnership between health and social care with links to education, housing, leisure, the voluntary sector and other stakeholders including parents/ carers, children and young people. The aim of the Children's NSF is that *"all children and young people achieve optimum health and well being and are supported in achieving their potential"*. The scope of the Children's NSF includes all children and young people from pre-conception to 18th birthday (and beyond for young people with special needs).

The standards for children, young people and maternity services will cover nine specific groups:

- Children and young people with acute and chronic illness or injury

- Disabled children and young people

- Improving health and well-being of all children and young people

- Children and young people in special circumstances

- Mental health and psychological well-being of children and young people

- Maternity

- Medicines

- Workforce development

- Performance development.

**NHS Cancer Plan**

More than one in three people in England will develop cancer at some stage in their lives. One in four will die of cancer. This means that, every year, over 200,000 people are diagnosed with cancer, and around 120,000 people die from cancer. So better prevention of cancer, better detection of cancer, and better treatment and care, matter to us all.

The Cancer Plan has four aims:

- to save more lives

- to ensure people with cancer get the right professional support and care as well as the best treatments

- to tackle the inequalities in health that mean unskilled workers are twice as likely to die from cancer as professionals

- to build for the future through investment in the cancer workforce, through strong research and through preparation for the genetics revolution, so that the NHS never falls behind in cancer care again.

For the first time this plan provides a comprehensive strategy for bringing together prevention, screening, diagnosis, treatment and care for cancer and the investment needed to deliver these services in terms of improved staffing, equipment, drugs, treatments and information systems.

At the heart of the Plan are **three new commitments**. These will be:

- In addition to the existing *Smoking Kills* target of reducing smoking in adults from 28% to 24% by 2010, new national and local targets to address the gap between socio-economic groups in smoking rates and the resulting risks of cancer and heart disease

- New goals and targets to reduce waiting times for diagnosis and treatment

- Additional NHS investment in hospices and specialist palliative care, to improve access to these services across the country.

## General lifestyle advice

**Opportunistic screening** for lifestyle risks is probably most effective as the patient is more receptive to advice when attending the surgery for a visit for some other condition, or prescription review, than actually having to make a separate appointment to attend a well-person clinic.

Opportunistic screening includes assessment of:

- **Smoking**
- **Diet**
- **Alcohol consumption**
- **Exercise**
- **Stress** levels with a view to increasing an awareness of the concept of good mental health
- Awareness of the benefits of regular **breast self-examination** for women or **testicular self-examination** for men (*see Chapter 20: Screening tests*).

## Health risks of cigarette smoking

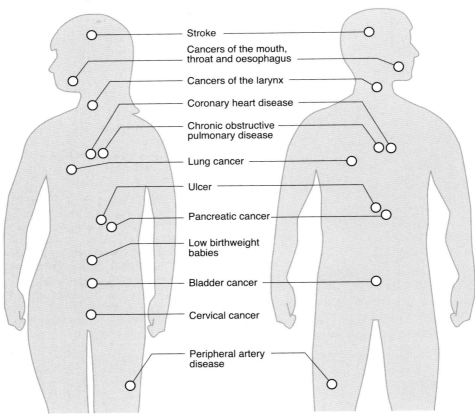

Stroke

Cancers of the mouth, throat and oesophagus

Cancers of the larynx

Coronary heart disease

Chronic obstructive pulmonary disease

Lung cancer

Ulcer

Pancreatic cancer

Low birthweight babies

Bladder cancer

Cervical cancer

Peripheral artery disease

**Figure 78:** The health risks of cigarette smoking *(based on "Smoke-free for Health" [Department of Health, 1994] and the US Office on Smoking and Health, Centres for Disease Control and Prevention Report [1990])*

## Smoking

Complete cessation should be the overall aim. Smoking is a very large factor in both the development of cancers and coronary heart disease (*see Figure 78*). Helpful advice, as well as medication, in the form of patches and oral tablets (on NHS prescription), are available.

### Benefits of stopping smoking

The benefits of cessation of smoking are:

- A decrease in the ease of blood clotting within two weeks, **lowering the risk of thrombosis**
- A **lowering of blood cholesterol** to normal for the individual within one month
- A **reduction in the complications associated with chronic heart disease** within one year
- A restoration of the **risk of stroke to 'normal' range** within five years
- A **reduction** of the chances of **atheroma** (furring up of arteries with fatty deposits).

### Passive smoking

The damage suffered through passive smoking is now an accepted fact and parents should be advised on the effect it has on their children.

## Diet

The following is recommended:

- Regular intake of five portions of **fruit** or **vegetables** per day (80g each)
- Eat *less* **fat, salt** and **sugar**
- Eat *more* **fibre**
- Drink at least **3 litres of fluid** per day

The British Heart Foundation produced a newsletter for children and adolescents called *"Intake"*. It provides advice on diet and, while it is aimed at children, the advice is sound for people of all ages (*see Figure 79*).

The **Food Standards Agency** monitors food and farming methods, acting as a watch dog following the **BSE (bovine spongiform encephalopathy)** disaster. Recently it has prevented a chocolate manufacturer's planned competition in schools, which would have encouraged large amounts of chocolate consumption by children.

## Alcohol

The government's recommended sensible drinking advice is **2 to 3 units of alcohol maximum per day for women** and **3 to 4 units maximum per day for men** (*see Figure 80*).

However, overall and as the guidelines from the British Hypertension Society state, people should be advised to limit their **weekly** alcohol intake to < 21 units (men) <14 units (women).

It is not intended that these daily unit totals are to be drunk **every** day, 7 days a week! There should be days of abstinence or lesser consumption. A maximum daily total has been advised in order to prevent "binge drinking", because it has been found that individuals have drunk a whole week's recommended total intake in one session!

For **pregnant women**: when planning conception or when pregnant, women are advised to consume fewer units (or abstain from alcohol completely). The potential damage to the fetus from alcohol – especially in the first weeks of pregnancy– can be devastating.

### Damage to health

Alcohol travels to every cell in the body, every tissue, and every organ. It is a **poison** and has to be broken down by the **liver**. Over time, using too much alcohol can damage the heart, raise the blood pressure, and cause cancer, liver disease, and brain damage; it can cause ulcers, weaken the muscles, and even lead to death. In pregnancy it can severely damage the fetus causing a condition of deformities, known as **'fetal alcohol syndrome'** in which there is extensive damage to the brain and major organs.

## Physical exercise

The Health Development Agency (2001) recommended that individuals should take 30 minutes exercise of moderate intensity on five days a week. Brisk walking, swimming, dancing and gardening are all recommended. Two 15-minute sessions is acceptable, providing they are both performed on the same day. The aim of increasing the rate of breathing is an important factor (i.e. **aerobic exercise**). As well

## Food "rools!"

How we look and feel has a lot to do with what we eat.
If you want less spots, great hair and bags of energy just follow these simple tips:

### We're only human!

Don't make drastic changes to your diet. The "naughty" things
we like (cakes, chocolate, chips, fizzy drinks, crisps) are okay every
now and then – but just not everyday!

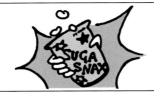

### Variety is the spice of life!

Eat a variety of foods everyday so that you don't get bored
with eating the same things all the time.

### Don't skip breakfast!

Breakfast gives your body the energy you need to kick-start the day.
Try high fibre cereals instead of sugary ones; or baked beans on
wholemeal toast; or fresh fruit and low fat yoghurt – and if you're
running really late, grab a couple of pieces of fresh fruit.

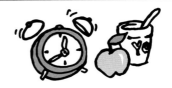

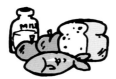

### Be wary of adverts!

Don't just believe what they say in the adverts. Work out for
yourself which foods are the healthiest to eat – and which
advertisers are trying to get you to eat unhealthy stuff.

### Be radiant!

Eat five portions of fruit or veg every day. Not only are they good
for your insides but it makes your hair and skin healthier too
– a difference that shows on the outside!

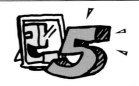

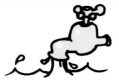

### Drink lots of water!

Water is good for your looks and it's important for your health.
Our bodies are about two-thirds water. We need plenty of water
– especially after exercise and in hot weather.

**Figure 79:** Dietary advice for children and young people but applicable to all age groups
*(adapted from the British Heart Foundation newsletter "Intake")*

## Sensible drinking

**If you drink 3 or more units a day there is an increased risk to your health!**

**Women**
2 or 3 units per day

- Most women can drink up to 2 or 3 units of alcohol a day without significant risks to their health

- Women who are trying to conceive or who are pregnant should avoid getting drunk and are advised to consume no more than 1 or 2 units of alcohol once or twice a week

- After the menopause there is evidence that drinking one to two units a day, **but no more**, can result in positive health benefits

**Men**
3 or 4 units per day

- Most men can drink up to 3 or 4 units of alcohol a day without significant risks to their health

- For men aged 40 and over there is evidence that drinking 1 or 2 units a day, **but no more**, can result in positive health benefits

**NB. These 'benchmarks' are not targets to drink up to. There are times and circumstances when it makes sense not to drink at all**

 **Don't**

- Drink and drive

- Operate machinery, use electrical equipment or work at heights after drinking

- Drink before playing sport or swimming

- Drink while on certain medications – check labels and ask a doctor if unsure

- Drink when it would affect the quality of your work

- Drink if your doctor advised you not to

- Binge drink – it can lead to health and other problems

 **Remember**

- Drinks poured at home are often more generous than pub measures

- If you drink heavily in the evening you may still be over the drink/drive limit the following morning

 **Do**

- Abstain for 48 hours, if you have an episode of heavy drinking, to let your body recover

- Remember drinks poured at home are often bigger than pub measures

- Work out how much you drink and try to stick to the guidelines – which are daily benchmarks not weekly targets

- Get help from a doctor or a specialist agency if worried about your drinking

- Remember that drinking responsibly can be enjoyable and is compatible with a healthy lifestyle

**Figure 80:** Government guidelines on sensible drinking *(adapted from "It all adds up: the sensible drinking guidelines explained" published by The Portman Group: www.portmangroup.org.uk and "Think about drink" a leaflet published by the Health Education Authority)*

# What is 1 unit of alcohol?

**1 unit of alcohol =**
- about half a pint (284ml) of ordinary strength lager, beer or cider, typically 3.5% alcohol by volume (ABV)
- a 25ml pub measure of spirit, typically 40% ABV
- a small glass of 9% ABV wine.

# What does this mean in terms of drinks?

### Beer, lager and cider
- 330ml bottle at 4% or 5% ABV = 1.5 units
- 440ml can at 4% or 5% ABV = 2 units
- 440ml can at 8% or 9% ABV = 3.5 to 4 units
- 500ml can at 8% or 9% ABV = 4 to 4.5 units

### Low alcohol beer and lager
- 440ml can at 1.2% ABV = 0.5 units

### Wine
- 125 ml glass of wine at 11% or 12% ABV = 1.5 units
- 175ml glass of wine at 11% or 12% ABV = 2 units

### Spirits
- 25ml measure of spirit at 40% ABV = 1 unit

### Sherry, port, madeira and vermouth
- 50ml measure at 20% ABV = 1 unit

### Alcopops
- 330ml bottle at 4% to 6% ABV = between 1.3 and 2 units
- 200ml bottle at 13.5% ABV = 2.7 units

### A word of caution
Some drinks are stronger than others. For example, a pint of premium lager has more units of alcohol in it than a standard strength beer. Most bottles of wine at 11% or 12% ABV. You can work out the number of units in a drink by multiplying the volume in ml by the percentage ABV and dividing the total by 1000. The figures listed here are rounded to the nearest half unit.

---

**If you drink heavily you have an increased risk of:**

- **Hepatitis** (inflammation of the liver)

- **Cirrhosis** (scarring of the liver) – up to 3 in every 10 long-term heavy drinkers develop cirrhosis

- **Stomach disorders**

- **Pancreatitis** (severe inflammation of the pancreas)

- **Mental health problems** including **depression, anxiety** and various other problems

- **Sexual difficulties**, such as **impotence**

- **Muscle** and **heart muscle disease**

- **Hypertension** (high blood pressure)

- **Damage to nervous tissue**

- **Accidents** – drinking alcohol is associated with a much increased risk of accidents, in particular injury and death from fire and car crashes (about 1 in 7 road deaths are caused by drinking alcohol)

- **Some cancers** – mouth, gullet, liver, colon and breast

- **Obesity** – alcohol has many calories

- **Damage to an unborn baby** in pregnant women

- **Alcohol dependence (addiction)**.

In the UK about 33,000 deaths a year are related to drinking alcohol – about one quarter of these are due to accidents.

---

as other benefits, exercise brings a feeling of 'well-being', because the body produces chemicals known as **'endorphins'**. (These are similar to the effects of morphine which produces a feeling of euphoria.)

## Obesity

According to the National Audit Office (NAO, 2001), obesity predisposes the individual to a higher risk of associated diseases. The increase in incidence of obesity is a worrying factor for the overall health of the population at the present time. A useful tool for measuring this is to calculate the **Body Mass Index (BMI)** of people.

### Body Mass Index (BMI) recordings

The body mass index (BMI) of an individual can be used to calculate the obesity risk to health of that individual (*see Tables 6, 7 and 8*).

The BMI is calculated with the following formula:

$$\frac{\text{Weight (kg)}}{\text{Height (m) squared}} = \text{BMI}$$

**Classification for adults is as follows:**

| | |
|---|---|
| Underweight | **BMI <18.5** |
| Normal | **BMI 18.5 – 25** |
| Overweight | **BMI 25 – 30** |
| Obese | **BMI 30 – 40** |
| Extreme obesity | **BMI > 40** |

### Girth

Waist circumference is another useful measure for 'at risk patients', as it may indicate **intra-abdominal fat mass**, which is linked to various diseases such as **coronary heart disease** (CHD), **insulin resistance, type 2 diabetes mellitus, hyperlipidaemia** (raised blood fats) and **hypertension** (high blood pressure).

The typical **'apple shaped'** figure, where extra weight is carried on the waist area is a warning sign as opposed to the **'pear shaped'** figure

**Table 6:** Body mass Index as an indicator of health weight

weight in kilograms

| height | 124 | 122 | 120 | 118 | 116 | 114 | 112 | 110 | 108 | 106 | 104 | 102 | 100 | 98 | 96 | 94 | 92 | 90 | 88 | 86 | 84 |
|---|---|---|---|---|---|---|---|---|---|---|---|---|---|---|---|---|---|---|---|---|---|
| 2.00 m | 31 | 30 | 30 | 29 | 29 | 28 | 28 | 27 | 27 | 26 | 26 | 25 | 25 | 24 | 24 | 23 | 23 | 22 | 22 | 21 | 21 |
|  | 32 | 32 | 31 | 31 | 30 | 30 | 29 | 29 | 28 | 28 | 27 | 27 | 26 | 26 | 25 | 24 | 24 | 23 | 23 | 22 | 22 |
| 1.92 m | 34 | 33 | 33 | 32 | 31 | 31 | 30 | 30 | 29 | 29 | 28 | 28 | 27 | 27 | 26 | 25 | 25 | 24 | 24 | 23 | 23 |
|  | 35 | 35 | 34 | 33 | 33 | 32 | 32 | 31 | 31 | 30 | 29 | 29 | 28 | 28 | 27 | 27 | 26 | 25 | 25 | 24 | 24 |
| 1.84 m | 37 | 36 | 35 | 35 | 34 | 34 | 33 | 32 | 32 | 31 | 31 | 30 | 30 | 29 | 28 | 28 | 27 | 27 | 26 | 25 | 25 |
|  | 38 | 38 | 37 | 36 | 36 | 35 | 35 | 34 | 33 | 33 | 32 | 31 | 31 | 30 | 30 | 29 | 28 | 28 | 27 | 27 | 26 |
| 1.76 m | 40 | 39 | 39 | 38 | 37 | 37 | 36 | 36 | 35 | 34 | 34 | 33 | 32 | 32 | 31 | 30 | 30 | 29 | 28 | 28 | 27 |
|  | 42 | 41 | 41 | 40 | 39 | 39 | 38 | 37 | 37 | 36 | 35 | 34 | 34 | 33 | 32 | 32 | 31 | 30 | 30 | 29 | 28 |
| 1.68 m | 44 | 43 | 43 | 42 | 41 | 40 | 40 | 39 | 38 | 38 | 37 | 36 | 35 | 35 | 34 | 33 | 33 | 32 | 31 | 30 | 30 |
|  | 46 | 45 | 45 | 44 | 43 | 42 | 42 | 41 | 40 | 39 | 39 | 38 | 37 | 36 | 36 | 35 | 34 | 33 | 33 | 32 | 31 |
| 1.60 m | 48 | 48 | 47 | 46 | 45 | 45 | 44 | 43 | 42 | 41 | 41 | 40 | 39 | 38 | 37 | 37 | 36 | 35 | 34 | 34 | 33 |
|  | 51 | 50 | 49 | 48 | 48 | 47 | 46 | 45 | 44 | 44 | 43 | 42 | 41 | 40 | 39 | 39 | 38 | 37 | 36 | 35 | 35 |
| 1.52 m | 54 | 53 | 52 | 51 | 50 | 49 | 48 | 48 | 47 | 46 | 45 | 44 | 43 | 42 | 42 | 41 | 40 | 39 | 38 | 37 | 36 |
|  | 57 | 56 | 55 | 54 | 53 | 52 | 51 | 50 | 49 | 48 | 47 | 47 | 46 | 45 | 44 | 43 | 42 | 41 | 40 | 39 | 38 |
| 1.44 m | 60 | 59 | 58 | 57 | 56 | 55 | 54 | 53 | 52 | 51 | 50 | 49 | 48 | 47 | 46 | 45 | 44 | 43 | 42 | 41 | 41 |
|  | 63 | 62 | 61 | 60 | 59 | 58 | 57 | 56 | 55 | 54 | 53 | 52 | 51 | 50 | 49 | 48 | 47 | 46 | 45 | 44 | 43 |
| 1.36 m | 67 | 66 | 65 | 64 | 63 | 62 | 61 | 59 | 58 | 57 | 56 | 55 | 54 | 53 | 52 | 51 | 49 | 49 | 48 | 46 | 45 |

|   | 19 st | | 18 st | | 17 st | | 16 st | | 15 st | | 14 st | |

Extreme obesity > 40   Obese 30 – 40   Overweight 25 – 30

where the excess weight is carried on the hips and thighs. Present recommendations are that waists should be less than 40 inches (preferably 37 inches) for men and less than 35 inches, (preferably under 32 inches) for women.

## Sexual health/diversity and mental well-being

More recent developments in treatments for impotence (**erectile dysfunction**) and **frigidity**, as well as the addressing of such areas as **'gender identity'**, **sexual orientation** and other areas, together with changing attitudes to diversity of lifestyle, will hopefully assist in more fulfilled lives for the individual. In this context, this should help in the prevention of mental illness such as depression with its ultimate risk of suicide.

## School bullying and child health

More recognition and prevention of this distressing problem in our society will hopefully continue and cases of subsequent suicide, be reduced.

## Environment

Government efforts to reduce **pollution**, reduce **speed limits**, cut **crime**, improve **social attitudes** and opportunities for all members of society etc. are all geared to produce better health in its widest sense.

## Skin cancer and sun

Skin cancer is increasing and warnings of risk exposure are now included in weather

weight in kilograms

| 82 | 80 | 78 | 76 | 74 | 72 | 70 | 68 | 66 | 64 | 62 | 60 | 58 | 56 | 54 | 52 | 50 | 48 | 46 | 44 | 42 | |
|----|----|----|----|----|----|----|----|----|----|----|----|----|----|----|----|----|----|----|----|----|---|
| 20 | 20 | 19 | 19 | 18 | 18 | 17 | 17 | 16 | 16 | 15 | 15 | 14 | 14 | 13 | 13 | 12 | 12 | 11 | 11 | 10 | height |
| 21 | 21 | 20 | 20 | 19 | 19 | 18 | 18 | 17 | 17 | 16 | 16 | 15 | 15 | 14 | 14 | 13 | 12 | 12 | 11 | 11 | 6 ft 6 in |
| 22 | 22 | 21 | 21 | 20 | 20 | 19 | 18 | 18 | 17 | 17 | 16 | 16 | 15 | 15 | 14 | 14 | 13 | 12 | 12 | 11 | |
| 23 | 23 | 22 | 22 | 21 | 20 | 20 | 19 | 19 | 18 | 18 | 17 | 16 | 16 | 15 | 15 | 14 | 14 | 13 | 12 | 12 | 6 ft 3 in |
| 24 | 24 | 23 | 22 | 22 | 21 | 21 | 20 | 19 | 19 | 18 | 18 | 17 | 17 | 16 | 15 | 15 | 14 | 14 | 13 | 12 | |
| 25 | 25 | 24 | 23 | 23 | 23 | 22 | 21 | 20 | 20 | 19 | 19 | 18 | 17 | 17 | 16 | 15 | 15 | 14 | 14 | 13 | 6 ft 0 in |
| 26 | 26 | 25 | 25 | 24 | 23 | 23 | 22 | 21 | 21 | 20 | 19 | 19 | 18 | 17 | 17 | 16 | 15 | 15 | 14 | 14 | 5 ft 9 in |
| 28 | 27 | 26 | 26 | 25 | 24 | 24 | 23 | 22 | 22 | 21 | 20 | 20 | 19 | 18 | 18 | 17 | 16 | 16 | 15 | 14 | |
| 29 | 28 | 28 | 27 | 26 | 26 | 25 | 24 | 23 | 23 | 22 | 21 | 21 | 20 | 19 | 18 | 18 | 17 | 16 | 16 | 15 | 5 ft 6 in |
| 30 | 30 | 29 | 28 | 28 | 27 | 26 | 25 | 25 | 24 | 23 | 22 | 22 | 21 | 20 | 19 | 19 | 18 | 17 | 16 | 16 | |
| 32 | 31 | 30 | 30 | 29 | 28 | 27 | 27 | 26 | 25 | 24 | 23 | 23 | 22 | 21 | 20 | 20 | 19 | 18 | 17 | 16 | 5 ft 3 in |
| 34 | 33 | 32 | 31 | 30 | 30 | 29 | 28 | 27 | 26 | 25 | 25 | 24 | 23 | 22 | 21 | 21 | 20 | 19 | 18 | 17 | |
| 35 | 35 | 34 | 33 | 32 | 31 | 30 | 29 | 29 | 28 | 27 | 26 | 25 | 24 | 23 | 23 | 22 | 21 | 20 | 19 | 18 | 5 ft 0 in |
| 37 | 37 | 36 | 35 | 34 | 33 | 32 | 31 | 30 | 29 | 28 | 27 | 26 | 26 | 25 | 24 | 23 | 22 | 21 | 20 | 19 | 4 ft 9in |
| 40 | 39 | 38 | 37 | 36 | 35 | 34 | 33 | 32 | 31 | 30 | 29 | 28 | 27 | 26 | 25 | 24 | 23 | 22 | 21 | 20 | |
| 42 | 41 | 40 | 39 | 38 | 37 | 36 | 35 | 34 | 33 | 32 | 31 | 30 | 29 | 28 | 27 | 26 | 24 | 23 | 22 | 21 | 4 ft 6 in |
| 44 | 43 | 42 | 41 | 40 | 39 | 38 | 37 | 36 | 35 | 34 | 32 | 31 | 30 | 29 | 28 | 27 | 26 | 25 | 24 | 23 | |

13 st | 12 st | 11 st | 10 st | 9 st | 8 st | 7 st |

Normal 18.5 – 25 [ ]    Underweight < 18.5 [ ]

forecasts. A high **barrier cream** should always be applied, especially to children. The less time spent in direct sunshine, especially during peak times the better. **Malignant melanoma** is the most serious type of skin cancer and is the most frequently occurring although incidents of squamous cell carcinoma are increasing and can be equally invasive if not treated at an early stage.

**Warning signs of skin cancer:**

- An existing mole becomes larger
- A new mole is growing
- A mole has a ragged, irregular outline
- A mole has a mixture of different shades of brown or black
- A new growth or sore does not heal within 4 weeks

- A spot or sore continues to itch, hurt, scab or bleed
- Skin ulcers persist which are not explained by other causes.

## Stress

Teaching people the nature of stress, its benefits and dangers and how to recognise and cope with it, plays an important part in prevention of wider ill health. Recent research indicates that prolonged stress lowers the body's immunity, thus allowing many medical problems to arise

**Signs of stress include:**

- Feeling guilty when relaxing – uneasy if not always busy
- Lying awake at night worrying about tomorrow

**Table 7:** Interpretation of height/weight ratios for adults

**MEN**

| Mean weight for medium build (kg) | | | | | Mean weight for medium build (st lb) | | | | |
|---|---|---|---|---|---|---|---|---|---|
| Height (cm) | Mean -10% | Mean | Mean +10% | Mean +20% | Height (ft in) | Mean -10% | Mean | Mean +10% | Mean +20% |
| 155 | 49 | 54 | 59 | 64 | 5. 1 | 7. 9 | 8. 7 | 9. 4 | 10. 2 |
| 157 | 50 | 55 | 61 | 66 | 5. 2 | 7.12 | 8.10 | 9. 8 | 10. 6 |
| 160 | 51 | 57 | 63 | 68 | 5. 3 | 8. 1 | 8.13 | 9.11 | 10.10 |
| 162 | 52 | 58 | 64 | 69 | 5. 4 | 8. 3 | 9. 2 | 10. 1 | 10.13 |
| 165 | 54 | 60 | 66 | 71 | 5. 5 | 8. 7 | 9. 6 | 10. 4 | 11. 3 |
| 167 | 55 | 62 | 68 | 74 | 5. 6 | 8.10 | 9. 10 | 10. 9 | 11. 8 |
| 170 | 57 | 64 | 70 | 76 | 5. 7 | 9. 0 | 10. 0 | 11. 0 | 12. 0 |
| 172 | 59 | 65 | 72 | 78 | 5. 8 | 9. 4 | 10. 4 | 11. 4 | 12. 4 |
| 175 | 60 | 67 | 74 | 80 | 5. 9 | 9. 7 | 10. 8 | 11. 9 | 12. 9 |
| 177 | 63 | 69 | 76 | 83 | 5.10 | 9.11 | 10.13 | 12. 0 | 13. 1 |
| 180 | 64 | 71 | 79 | 85 | 5.11 | 10. 2 | 11. 3 | 12. 5 | 13. 6 |
| 183 | 66 | 74 | 80 | 88 | 6. 0 | 10. 6 | 11. 8 | 12. 9 | 13.11 |
| 186 | 68 | 75 | 83 | 90 | 6. 1 | 10.10 | 11.12 | 13. 0 | 14. 3 |
| 188 | 70 | 78 | 85 | 93 | 6. 2 | 10.14 | 12. 3 | 13. 6 | 14. 9 |
| 191 | 72 | 80 | 88 | 96 | 6. 3 | 11. 5 | 12. 8 | 13.11 | 15. 0 |

**WOMEN**

| Height (cm) | Mean -10% | Mean | Mean +10% | Mean +20% | Height (ft in) | Mean -10% | Mean | Mean +10% | Mean +20% |
|---|---|---|---|---|---|---|---|---|---|
| 142 | 40 | 45 | 49 | 54 | 4. 8 | 6. 5 | 7. 0 | 7.10 | 8. 6 |
| 145 | 41 | 46 | 51 | 55 | 4. 9 | 6. 7 | 7. 3 | 7.13 | 8. 9 |
| 147 | 43 | 47 | 52 | 56 | 4. 10 | 6.10 | 7. 6 | 8. 2 | 8.12 |
| 150 | 44 | 49 | 54 | 58 | 4. 11 | 6.12 | 7. 9 | 8. 6 | 9. 2 |
| 152 | 45 | 50 | 55 | 60 | 5. 0 | 7. 1 | 7.12 | 8. 9 | 9. 6 |
| 155 | 46 | 51 | 56 | 61 | 5. 1 | 7. 4 | 8. 1 | 8.12 | 9. 9 |
| 157 | 48 | 53 | 58 | 63 | 5. 2 | 7. 7 | 8. 5 | 9. 2 | 9.13 |
| 160 | 49 | 55 | 60 | 65 | 5. 3 | 7.10 | 8. 8 | 9. 6 | 10. 4 |
| 162 | 51 | 57 | 63 | 68 | 5. 4 | 8. 0 | 8.13 | 9.11 | 10. 9 |
| 165 | 52 | 59 | 64 | 70 | 5. 5 | 8. 4 | 9. 3 | 10. 1 | 11. 0 |
| 167 | 54 | 61 | 66 | 72 | 5. 6 | 8. 7 | 9. 7 | 10. 6 | 11. 5 |
| 170 | 57 | 63 | 68 | 74 | 5. 7 | 8.11 | 9.11 | 10. 10 | 11. 9 |
| 172 | 58 | 64 | 70 | 76 | 5. 8 | 9. 1 | 10. 1 | 11. 0 | 12. 0 |
| 175 | 59 | 66 | 72 | 79 | 5. 9 | 9. 4 | 10. 5 | 11. 5 | 12. 5 |
| 177 | 61 | 68 | 74 | 81 | 5.10 | 9. 8 | 10. 9 | 11. 9 | 12. 10 |

- Feeling tense – neck feels 'knotted up'
- Being impatient or irritable – interrupting others when they are talking
- Feeling you have a lot on your mind – finding it difficult to concentrate
- Smoking more and/or drinking more alcohol – eating in a hurry

- Life seems full of crises – and a tendency to have more rows
- Difficulty in make decisions
- Feeling frustrated when people do not do what you want
- Frequently experiencing 'butterflies in the stomach', a dry mouth, sweaty palms or a 'thumping heart'.

**Table 8:** The increased relative risk of obesity (BMI > 30) causing disease in men and women
   *(National Audit Office, 2001)*

| | Relative increase in risk for: | |
|---|---|---|
| **Disease** | **women (BMI > 30)** | **men (BMI > 30)** |
| Type 2 diabetes | 12.7 | 5.2 |
| Hypertension | 4.2 | 2.6 |
| Myocardial infarction | 3.2 | 1.5 |
| Colon cancer | 2.7 | 3.0 |
| Angina | 1.8 | 1.8 |
| Cholecystitis | 1.8 | 1.8 |
| Ovarian cancer | 1.7 | *Not applicable* |
| Osteoarthritis | 1.4 | 1.9 |
| Stroke | 1.3 | 1.3 |

NB: Relative risk BMI < 25 = 1

## Individual national campaigns

These play their part in health promotion, e.g. **'No Smoking Day'** and **'Walk to School Day'**. The collective initiative of everyone trying to change lifestyle has a positive effect. However, the long-term effect may not be so beneficial. Evidence suggests that in the longer term, reinforcement of the message is needed in an acceptable form. The problem of 'it doesn't happen to me' prevails!

## Contraception and teenage pregnancy

Advice is available from the GP surgery on contraception generally.

There has also been a recent campaign by practice nurses and school nurses to alert teenagers to the decision to allow **'the morning after pill'** (e.g. levonorgestrel), to be available without prescription at pharmacies, as well as available on prescription, issued, (under the **Patient Group Directives** scheme). The preparation requires two doses, twelve hours apart. The first should be taken within 72 hours of unprotected intercourse but earlier

administration increases its efficacy. The risk of **STDs** must always be considered.

These measures demonstrate the attempts to reduce the (still rapidly rising) number of teenage, single mothers.

## Sexually transmitted diseases (STD)

These include:

- **HIV** and **AIDS**
- **Gonorrhoea**
- **Syphilis**
- **Chlamydia** (a common cause of infertility in the female)

Advice leaflets and campaigns on these areas are well covered. Despite this, infections are increasing at an alarming rate. The recent decision to enable drug addicts to have clean needles and syringes, is a step to prevent spread of the viruses of HIV and **hepatitis B, C, D** and **E**.

With recent research indicating that new medications have a significant effect on delaying the onset of AIDS, in HIV positive patients, it is hoped that individuals will come forward for screening at an early stage, which may help to slow the transmission of HIV.

## Communicable disease control

The recent impact of **SARS (Severe Respiratory Disease Syndrome)**, demonstrated the essential influence of the **World Health Organisation**, together with the various international disease surveillance centres, in controlling and preventing the world-wide spread of diseases (**pandemics**). Incidentally, publicity given to the importance of frequent hand-washing, was beneficial in an educational context.

## Conventional and complementary medicine

Individuals are looking at a wider concept of health and taking initiative for themselves about the choices available.

Complementary medicine includes:

- **Yoga**
- **Osteopathy**
- **Chiropractic**
- **Homeopathy**
- **Acu-puncture**
- **Acu-pressure**
- **Reflexology**
- **Medical herbalism**
- **Aromatherapy**
- **Indian head massage**
- **Chinese medicine.**

These, together with the vast amount of readily, available information on the Internet, empower people to a degree, never seen before. Indeed, doctors have been alerted to available, authentic treatments, of which they were not aware, by their patients. Whilst it is accepted that vulnerable people need some protection, wise doctors *listen* to their patients!

## Chronic disease management clinics within the GP surgery

### Coronary heart disease (ischaemic heart disease)

This is a condition in which fatty deposits (**atheroma**) are laid down in the lining of arteries as plaques, causing narrowing of arteries (**arteriostenosis**). If walls are also hardened it is known as **atherosclerosis**. Those particularly affected are the coronary arteries supplying the heart muscle, itself with blood. These plaques can become inflamed and break away, completely blocking an artery, causing an acute heart attack (**myocardial infarction**). The sudden formation of a blood clot (**thrombus**), which blocks the artery is known as a **thrombosis** (or **coronary thrombosis** when it affects the coronary arteries).

### Stroke

Similarly, these changes can occur in the brain where blockage of an artery (**occlusion**) is known as a **stroke** (sometimes also referred to by the outdated term of cerebrovascular accident). Strokes can also occur due to bleeding from a blood vessel in the brain due to a weakness in the wall (**aneurysm**) or as the result of high blood pressure.

### Risk factors for heart disease, stroke and other cardiovascular disorders

The number of risk factors for the patient must be assessed (*see Figure 81*) and drugs which lower cholesterol (**statins**) are considered if indicated as well as the obvious treatment to lower blood pressure where required.

Risk factors include:

- **Family history**
- **High cholesterol** and **lipid levels**

    - A high cholesterol level is known as **hypercholesterolaemia**

    - High levels of certain fats (lipids) is known as **hyperlipidaemia**

    - High levels of **triglycerides** (also a type of lipid) is another risk factor.

## Risk factors for coronary heart disease

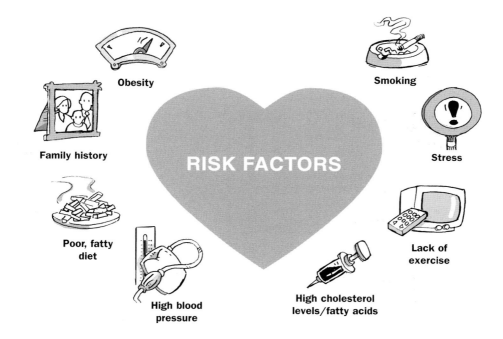

**Figure 81:** Risk factors for coronary heart disease

NB: **High density lipids (HDLs)** *are considered protective, whereas* **low density lipids (LDLs)** *are considered harmful. When measured together they are together known as* **total cholesterol (TC).**

- **High blood homocysteine** levels (a protein substance)

- **Smoking**

- **Obesity**

- **Lack of exercise**

- **High blood pressure (hypertension)**

- **Diabetes mellitus**

- **Asian origin**

- **Stress.**

*Cholesterol*

At present it is thought that the use of **'statins'** to lower cholesterol levels, considerably extends life expectancy for those with cardiovascular disease and especially for those who have already suffered a first, acute heart attack. As well as reducing cholesterol levels, it appears to reduce areas of inflammation in the fatty plaques of the artery linings, stopping them from breaking away and blocking the artery space (**lumen**).

Lifestyle changes are advised. Regular follow-up checks and blood tests are performed (as stated in the National Service Framework standards). Regular daily oral aspirin 75mg, is usually recommended, if appropriate for the patient, as a prevention of clot formation.

## The effects of asthma

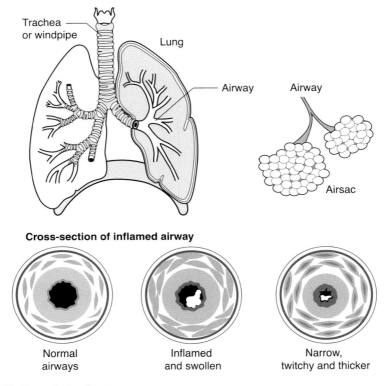

**Figure 82:** The effects of asthma

## Asthma

Asthma (*see Figure 82*) is a long-term, common condition in which:

- The lining of the **airways** in the lungs becomes inflamed and swollen with an increased **mucous secretion**

- Airways become narrower (**constriction**)

- Airway walls become thicker and 'twitchy'.

Triggers (including pollen, cold air, cigarette smoke and perfume), cause the asthma response.

### Signs and symptoms:

- Shortness of breath (**dyspnoea**)

- A feeling of **tightness** in the chest

- **Cough** usually episodic

- **Wheezing**

- **Being woken at night with increased shortness of breath**

- **Increased shortness of breath on waking** in the morning

- **Shortness of breath on exertion**

- **Inability to breathe out easily – decreased Peak Expiry Flow Rate (PEFR)**

Not all these may be present and a cough may be the only symptom presented. Some patients are encouraged to use an asthma symptom chart to monitor their condition (*see Figure 83*).

**Goals of treatment:**

- Be free from symptoms

- Normal or best Peak Flow reading to be restored and maintained (*see Figure 84*)

- Reduce the risk of severe attacks

- Minimise absence from school or work

- Restore normal living.

**Areas to be assessed:**

- The patient's understanding of the disease and the importance of prevention

- Compliance with drugs and recognition of effects of different inhaled medications
    - **Preventer** (brown) – e.g. beclometasone dipropionate (**corticosteroid**)

    - **Reliever** (blue) – e.g. salbutomol (**bronchodilator**)
    - **Protector** (green) – e.g . sodium cromoglycate

- Inhaler technique

- Measurement of Peak Flow reading and interpretation

- Recognition of worsening situation and response, e.g. need to increase inhaler use

- Number of days lost from school or work

- Asthma episodes disturbing sleep

- Any emergency situation requiring hospitalisation.

**ASTHMA IS A COMMON CAUSE OF SUDDEN DEATH and must never be treated as trivial!**

## Asthma symptom chart

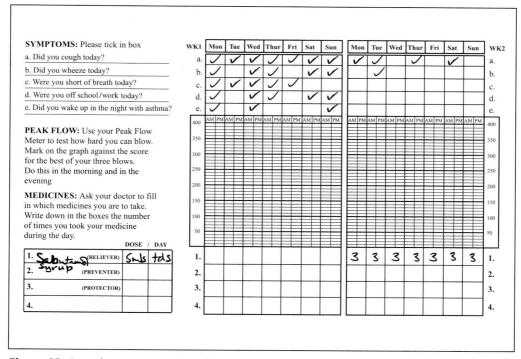

**Figure 83:** An asthma symptom chart for use by the patient

## Normal peak expiry flow (PEF)

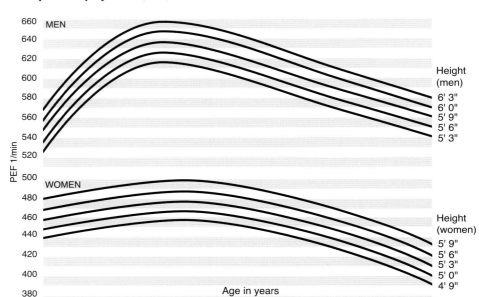

**Figure 84:** Normal peak expiry flow (PEF) values for men and women of different ages and heights

## Chronic obstructive pulmonary disease (COPD)

This chronic, slowly progressive disorder, is usually a result of **chronic smoking**, although chronic asthma may produce similar deformities.

The permanently **constricted airway** (caused by loss of elasticity in the tissues), does not completely respond to **bronchodilators** although symptoms are relieved on their administration.

Deformity of the chest and the so-called 'barrel chest' develop due to the inability to breathe out properly (**expiration**). These patients are usually in the >45 age range. They may eventually require **oxygen** administration. The conditions of air in the pleural cavity, (**emphysema**) and dilatation of the bronchioles, (**bronchiectasis**) are usually present, resulting in foul smelling **sputum** being coughed up from the lungs. **Spirometry** testing usually confirms the diagnosis.

## Diabetes mellitus

A condition in which the body is **unable to metabolise glucose** (i.e. convert it to energy or store it in the body). In people with diabetes, the pancreas (*see Figure 85*) does not produce enough of the hormone **insulin**, or the insulin it produces does not work properly. (In healthy people, insulin is produced by small organs in the pancreas which are called the **Islets of Langerhan.**) In people who have diabetes, sugar builds up in the tissues of the body and is excreted in the urine (**glycosuria**).

There are two types of diabetes:

**Type 1** previously known as **IDDM** (insulin dependent diabetes mellitus) or 'Early Onset' diabetes

**Type 2** previously known as **NIDDM** (non-insulin dependent diabetes mellitus) or 'Maturity Onset' diabetes.

## Type 1

Also known as **'Early Onset Diabetes'**. It affects children and young people. This disease is thought to be caused by the affects of a virus on the cells of the pancreas (**Islets of Langerhan**) which produce the hormone insulin or to the body's reaction to the secretion of insulin. There appears to be an hereditary factor.

As insulin is destroyed by the gastric secretions in the stomach it cannot be taken by mouth. Insulin replacement **injections** are required throughout life usually from two to four times a day. (The transplantation of pancreatic cells is being researched as a potential future treatment).

*Signs and symptoms:*

- **Loss of weight**

- **Thirst**

- Increased passing of urine (**polyuria**) especially at night (**nocturia**)

- **Tiredness**

- Itching/soreness of external genitalia (**pruritis vulva**), **thrush** infections

- **Recurring skin infections**

If not diagnosed, Type 1 diabetes can result in:

- **Ketones** building up in the blood as fats are unable to be burnt efficiently into carbon dioxide and water by the body, without the presence of glucose.

- **Unconsciousness, coma** and **death** due to high levels of sugar in the blood and tissues (**hyperglycaemia**).

## Type 2

Associated with obesity, lack of exercise and middle age, although there is great concern as young people are beginning to develop this disease through bad lifestyle.

Also, although not normally required, it has been necessary to treat some of these categories of patient with insulin injections in order to control blood sugar.

## The pancreas

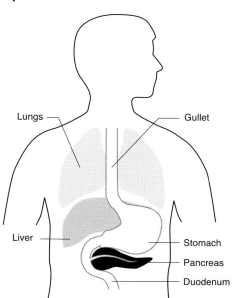

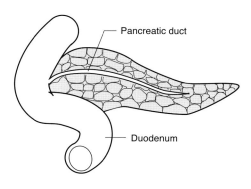

**Figure 85:** The pancreas

The main causes are that the body no longer responds normally to its own insulin and/or that the body does not produce enough insulin. There appears to be a family connection and also genetic: It tends to be more common in Asian and African-Caribbean communities.

*Signs and symptoms:*

Similar to Type 1 but Type 2 develops slowly and symptoms are generally less severe. Some people may not notice any symptoms and it is then only diagnosed at a routine medical check up. Many put their symptoms down to 'getting older' or 'overwork'.

In both types of diabetes early treatment reduces the chances of developing serious health problems such as **coronary heart disease, stroke, hypertension, circulation problems,** nerve damage (**neuropathy**), kidney (**nephropathy**) and eye damage (**retinopathy** and **cataract**) leading to blindness.

*Treatment*

- **Control of blood glucose levels,** if necessary by various types of medication for Type 2 and regular insulin injections for Type 1 (for life)

- **Control blood pressure** levels

- **Diet** – eating healthily

- **Control of weight**

- **Regular physical exercise**

- **No smoking**

- **Regular medical check ups** – to detect health problems early – at least annually

*Acute medical emergency – hypoglycaemia*

It is important to remember that any inbalance of insulin and glucose in the body resulting in too much insulin and too little glucose causing very low blood sugar (**hypoglycaemia**) can result in **unconsciousness** and **death**.

This is an acute medical emergency and should be treated with the immediate administration of **sugar by mouth** (orally) in any form, *before* the patient loses consciousness. (Unconscious patients must *never* be given anything by mouth as this could block their airway and cause death).

Patients on insulin are made aware of the symptoms and signs of a hypoglycaemic attack before they are discharged from hospital at their initial stabilisation treatment. They are also advised to carry sugar lumps in their pockets as well as wearing **'medic alert'** diabetic identity bracelet or necklace. It should be noted that antibiotics may temporally affect the level (**threshold**) at which sugar is found in the urine. Pregnancy can also cause similar effect, (**gestational glycosuria**).

# New GP Contracts 2003 and 2004

The **new GP Contract**, which was accepted by GPs in June 2003 (and renegotiated by GPs in 2004), is the most radical change to general practice since 1948, and applies to those GPs still working under the **General Medical Services scheme**.

**At the heart of the contract is:**

- A new categorisation of services will help GPs to manage their workload by enabling practices to transfer responsibility for providing some services e.g. out-of-hours care, contraceptive care and chronic disease management, to other practices or their PCO

- Individual GP patient lists will be replaced by a combined list for the whole practice

- Payment will be provided for an identified population, rather than for items of service

- Each practice will be given an allocation to cover their staffing and running costs, based on a formula reflecting the needs of local patients

- Greater and fairer remuneration for GPs, who will be rewarded according to the quality of care they provide rather than the number of patients they treat

- A new quality framework, setting standards of care based on evidence, with two thirds of the increased investment for practices linked to a new system of quality payments

- A guarantee that all patients will receive the full range of existing services, with greater choice for some services and faster access

- Set services provided will still include essential services for ill patients, but different levels of payment will be available for individual practices across the PCO that supply enhanced services or extend the range of services provided

- Enhanced services include; ENT, trauma and orthopaedics, dermatology, ophthalmology, chronic disorders, including diabetes or CHD, anticoagulant therapy, advanced minor surgery etc., where treatment in primary care can offer a more convenient service to patients and reduce demands on hospitals

- Supporting practices where extended evening, weekend or open access surgeries are offered in response to patient preferences, allowing fast and convenient patient access to PHC with GP appointments available within 48 hours

- A recruitment and retention package to tackle GP shortages

- The new contract will be accompanied by an unprecedented increase in investment to revitalise general practice and transform services for patients, and investment in GP premises and IT.

*(Sources NHS Confederation 2002 and 2003)*

Not all practices with GMS contracts will provide services other than those classified as **'essential'**.

## Essential services (ES)

These cover:

- Management of patients who are ill or believe themselves to be ill, with conditions from which recovery is generally expected, for the duration of that condition, including relevant health promotion advice and referral as appropriate, reflecting the patient choice wherever practicable

- General management of patients who are terminally ill

- Management of chronic disease in the manner determined by the practice in discussion with the patient.

**'Enhanced Services' include:**

- Ear, nose and throat (ENT)
- Trauma and orthopaedics
- Dermatology
- Ophthalmology
- Extended minor surgery
- Chronic disorders, including:
  - Diabetes mellitus
  - CHD (coronary heart disease)
  - Anticoagulant therapy.

## Directed Enhanced Services (DES)

Enhanced services which are under national direction with national specification and benchmarked pricing which all PCOs must commission to cover their relevant population. These cover:

- Support services to staff and the public in respect of care and treatment of patients who are violent

- Improved access

- Childhood vaccinations and immunisations

- Influenza immunisations

- Quality information preparation

- Advanced minor surgery.

## National Enhanced Services (NES)

These have national specifications and benchmark pricing, but are NOT directed. They include:

- Intrapartum care
- Anticoagulant monitoring
- Intra-uterine contraceptive device fitting, more specialised drug and alcohol misuse services
- More specialised sexual health services
- More specialised depression services
- Multiple sclerosis
- Enhanced care of terminally ill
- Enhanced care of the homeless
- Enhanced services for people with learning disabilities
- Immediate care and first response care and minor injury services.

## Local Enhanced Services (LES)

These are services developed locally according to the special needs of the area. Terms and conditions will be discussed and agreed locally between the PCO and the practice with, if wished, the involvement of the LMC.

There are other specialties, e.g. Holistic Services, Expert Patient Initiatives etc. which can be provide and attract extra income for the practice.

Practices will choose which services they wish to provide. PCOs will be responsible for ensuring all services are supplied in the area and SHAs will audit and monitor services.

PMS contracts allow GPs to transfer their contracts for patient care to PCOs and become employed instead of being self-employed (independent contractors).

Finally, the government, through its many agencies and the **Commission for Health Improvement**, monitors and audits services, establishing the cost-benefit analysis of all these treatments and methods of care.

However, the value to the individual and the family is incalculable, a loved one's life being irreplaceable, beyond any costing system produced by authorities or statisticians!

# Abbreviations
## (New GP Contracts 2003/2004)

| | |
|---|---|
| **AP** | Aspiration Payments |
| **CHI** | Commission for Health Improvement |
| **CPPIH** | Commission for Patient and Public Involvement in Health |
| **DES** | Directed Enhanced Services |
| **EPI** | Expert Patient Initiatives |
| **ES** | Essential Services |
| **HCP** | Holistic Care Payments |
| **HDA** | Health Development Agency |
| **HPE** | Health Promotion England |
| **LES** | Local Enhanced Services |
| **NCAA** | National Clinical Assessment Authority |
| **NES** | National Enhanced Services |
| **NICE** | National Institute for Clinical Excellence |
| **NSF** | National Service Framework |
| **OSC** | Overview and Scrutiny Committee |
| **PCO** | Primary Care Organisation |
| **PALS** | Patient Advisory and Liaison Service |
| **PCT** | Primary Care Trust |
| **PF** | Patient's Forum |
| **SHA** | Strategic Health Authority |
| **SSDP** | Strategic Service Development Plan |

(Other abbreviations and terms appear in the previous chapters).

Chapter **20**

# Screening tests

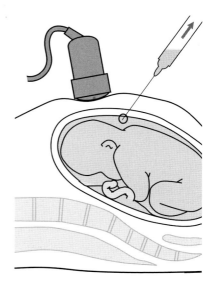

# Screening

Screening is the detection of disease before the presence of symptoms.

It is a form of secondary preventive medicine, aiming to detect the presence or absence of a disease or condition. It may be done on an individual (**opportunistic screening** at the practice) or through **mass screening** of the whole population.

The purpose of screening is to prevent early death, reduce disease, and improve the quality of life. The principle is based on the fact that certain diseases and conditions can be recognised by a simple test well before any serious disease has developed or symptoms occurred.

There are certain ethical requirements before screening is approved:

- The disease being searched for should always be a **serious** one

- The screening test itself should always be **simple** to perform and **not give false results**

- As far as possible the test should be an **objective rather than a subjective** test; i.e. the results must be clear and not left to individual opinion

- The test should be **safe** and **not induce undue fear** in people tested; counselling of participants is important, they must understand its nature

- **Effective treatment** must be available for the disease or condition for which the screening is being performed.

## Antenatal screening

Tests performed on pregnant women are important in detecting abnormalities of both mother and fetus at an early stage. One of the main aims is to ensure that a healthy baby is born to a healthy mother.

The following screening tests are performed:

- **Urine testing** to detect any abnormal content e.g. albumin may suggest a urine infection or kidney disease. Its occurrence later in pregnancy may indicate developing **toxaemia** of pregnancy. Sugar can indicate **diabetes mellitus**.

- **Blood pressure** to detect its state at the start of pregnancy and watch for any sign of **hypertension** developing – indicative of developing **toxaemia** of pregnancy (see terminology of the female reproductive system, Chapter 11). All measurements should be done with the pregnant patient either **sitting or lying on their left side** as lying on their back (**supine**) may produce a large drop in blood pressure.

## Blood tests

Antenatal blood tests are carried out to:

- determine **blood group** and **Rhesus factor**

- detect **anaemia**

- determine random **blood glucose**

- detect immunity to **rubella** (German measles)

- detect **syphilis** if present in order to treat and prevent fetal deformities

- detect **hepatitis B** antibodies

- detect **HIV** antibodies

- detect **sickle-cell anaemia** and **thalassaemia** (test offered to women of West Indian, African and Mediterranean origin).

An examination **per vaginam** may be performed at first visit to detect any abnormality of the reproductive system and the size of the uterus.

## Later visits

Urine, blood pressure, weight, height of fundus of uterus and any fluid retention (**oedema**) will be checked at each visit. The main aim of detecting the early onset of **toxaemia of pregnancy (PET)** in order to avoid **eclampsia** where fits occur and death of baby and mother can result, is paramount in antenatal care. Rapid weight gain, fluid retention, albumin in the urine and hypertension are all signs of the developing condition.

*Blood tests at 28 weeks*

- Full **blood count**

- **Antibody screening**

- Random **blood glucose**.

## Ultrasound scan

Ultrasound waves build up a picture of the fetus in the uterus (*see Figure 72, in Chapter 17, page 164*). This is used to:

- check fetus' **measurements**, size for dates, growth etc.

- check for **multiple pregnancy**

- detect **abnormalities**, particularly of head or spine (**spina bifida**)

- check position of placenta (**placenta praevia**).

*Procedure*

The woman is asked to drink plenty of fluid as a full bladder produces a better picture of the uterus by pushing it up into the abdominal cavity. Jelly is then placed on the abdomen with the patient lying on her back.

An instrument is passed backwards and forwards over the skin and high frequency sound is beamed through the abdomen. This is reflected back and creates a picture on the screen.

## Nuchal translucency scan:

This ultrasound scan measures the thickest tissue of the nape of the neck to detect **Down's syndrome** and **neural tube (brain and spinal chord) defects**. It is carried out at between 11 and 13 weeks.

# Amniocentesis

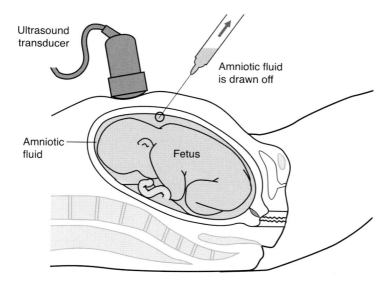

**Figure 86:** Amniocentesis

## Alpha-fetoprotein test

This is a blood test performed at about 16-18 weeks of pregnancy; used to determine the level of **alpha-fetoprotein (AF)** in the blood which, if raised, may indicate a **neural tube defect**, such as **spina bifida** or **ancencephaly** (undeveloped brain). low levels may suggest other abnormalities such as **Down's syndrome**.

## 'Triple screening' or 'triple plus' test

This is a blood test for **Down's syndrome**. It combines the levels of AFP with levels of two hormones present in the mother's blood and predicts the likelihood of Down's syndrome.

## Amniocentesis

The test (*see Figure 86*) may be offered at 12-18 weeks of pregnancy to older women (over 35 years) where the risk of Down's syndrome is higher, or where there is a family history of the condition. Positive testing for spina bifida or Down's syndrome with the AFP test will usually be followed by **amniocentesis**. It produces a very small increase in the risk of **spontaneous abortion** (miscarriage).

### Procedure

An ultrasound test will first determine the position of the fetus and placenta. After a local anaesthetic, a needle is passed through the wall of the abdomen to withdraw amniotic fluid which surrounds the fetus. This fluid is sent to the laboratory for testing for chemical content and also the genetic content of cells. In Down's syndrome the chromosomes are abnormal – a splitting of number 21 or the presence of an extra chromosome. Other abnormalities will also be investigated.

## Chorionic villus sampling

This test, available in some hospitals, can be carried out earlier than amniocentesis at eight to 11 weeks of pregnancy. It has a higher risk of abortion than amniocentesis. It is used to detect:

- **Down's syndrome**
- inherited diseases, such as **sickle-cell anaemia** or **thalassaemia**
- some sex-linked diseases, for example **haemophilia**.

It will not detect spina bifida. The full effects of this test upon the developing fetus are not yet known.

### Procedure

Using ultrasound as a guide, a fine tube is passed through the vagina and cervix, or sometimes through the abdomen, and a small piece of the developing placenta, called **chorionic tissue**, is withdrawn. This is sent to the laboratory for testing.

## Fetoscopy

This is a direct inspection of the fetus via a tube in the uterus or a camera attached to the needle piercing into the amniotic fluid. Performed at 15 – 18 weeks. It increases the risk of miscarriage and infection.

## Cordocentesis

This is the direct sampling of fetal blood through the **umbilical cord** or **intra-hepatic vein** of the fetus, to detect genetic abnormalities, infection or well-being of the fetus (performed from 12 weeks onwards).

# Tests on the newborn

A baby is completely examined soon after birth, to detect any **congenital abnormalities** so that measures can be introduced to minimise resulting problems. Conditions such as **club foot** or **cleft palate** are an obvious handicap. The screening for **undescended testicles** in males and other conditions is continued throughout infancy and childhood.

## Apgar rating (see also Chapter 11, page 108)

This is a test performed on all newborn and involves awarding of a rating for the following:

- **heart rate**
- **respiratory effort**
- **muscle tone**
- **reflex state**
- **colour.**

A baby in the perfect state at birth will score two points for each category giving a total score of 10.

This test is repeated at certain intervals following birth. It gives good indication of the probability of developmental problems and/or epilepsy, due to lack of oxygen at birth.

## Blood tests

These include blood tests for the detection of:

- **Phenylketonuria (Guthrie test)**

- **Hypothyroidism** or cretinism.

The Guthrie test, also known as **'the heel-prick test'** as the blood is taken from the newborn's heel, is performed after feeding has been established (usually at five days). It is used to detect a chemical known as **phenylketone** which is an abnormality present in babies unable to properly break down certain proteins. If not detected at birth and special diet implemented, it causes damage to mental development.

**Hypothyroidism**, if detected, can be treated by the administration of **thyroxine** and the abnormal mental development will be prevented.

## Otalani's test

Otalani's test for **congenital dislocation of hip** is done following birth. It is also known as the 'click test'. When the baby's hips are rotated a click is heard if a dislocation is present.

# Children

Screening tests for children are done routinely by the health visitor, medical officer or GP in **child health surveillance**.

These tests are done at different ages, the main concentration being in the infant and preschool periods.

Five main areas are involved for developmental screening:

- **locomotion** and **posture**

- **muscle control** and **function**

- **speech** and **language**

- **growth**

- **social development**.

**Hearing testing** is an important area of screening, and **routine testing** is an important tool for preventing loss of language development due to unidentified problems. **Squints** are usually minimised if early detection is made.

# Adult screening

Tests for recognising **precancerous conditions** are now recommended and include those for **carcinoma of the cervix, breast cancer, large bowel cancer** and **testicular and prostate cancer**.

Screening for coronary **heart disease, hypertension** and **obesity** are also very important. These are discussed in Chapter 19.

## Cervical smears

The **'Pap' test**, named after the man who introduced it – Papanicolaou – is one of the foremost screening tests at present. In England and Wales a programme of screening for women aged from 25 years to 64 years is available on the NHS (20 to 60 years in Scotland), although women may request the test after this age. Targets are at present set at 80% for the higher level and 50% for the lower. This will exclude those women who have had a hysterectomy with the removal of the cervix. An automatic three-year **recall scheme** is in operation, although some PCOs still only recall five-yearly. It is planned that the age ranges will be extended by 2004 to 70 years of age.

The smear must not be taken during **menstruation**. Cells are removed with a special spatula (**Aylesbury**) or **cytobrush** from the area of the cervical canal. It is important that they are removed from the correct area. These are then placed on a glass slide and immediately **'fixed'** with fixing solution. This prevents the cells from drying out so that the laboratory can read the smear. The 'fixed' smear should be placed in a cool area and allowed to dry for 20 minutes (*see page 176*).

The patient's details are written on the slide and the **cervical cytology form** must be completed. The slide is dispatched to the cytology section of the pathology department for examination and reporting.

It is of vital importance that the patient is informed how she will obtain the results of the test. Patients should be informed in writing of any abnormal result or request for repeat of the test if an inadequate smear has been sent. Deaths have occurred due to failure to follow this procedure.

The following are some factors predisposing to cervical cancer:

- **Early age at first intercourse**

- **Many sexual partners**

- **Genital warts** (including those on partners)

- **Genital herpes**

- **Smoking** – 20 cigarettes per day increases the risk by seven times.

**Promiscuity** is considered to be a factor as the more partners involved the more likely the causative factor (the wart virus is a strong suspect) may be encountered.

Positive results state findings such as:

- **dysplasia**      abnormal form

- **dyskaryosis**    abnormal nucleus

- **koilocytosis**   having a spoon-shaped appearance, warty changes.

Depending on the degree of abnormality of the cervical smear, the patient may be checked in six months or referred to the gynaecologist for a colposcopy and treatment.

## Liquid-based cytology (LBC)

**NICE** (National Institute for Clinical Excellence) has recently approved the use of this test for cervical cytology on the grounds of cost and efficiency. At present, many cervical smears (Pap test) are classed as 'inadequate', requiring further smear tests. Reading of these is often marred by mistakes.

In this new test (known about for several years but only recently available on the NHS), a brush-like device collects cells from the neck of the womb (**cervix**). This is then rinsed in a preservative, making the test reading by technicians, easier to analyse. It is estimated that more lives will be saved by this new method.

## Breast examination

Self-examination (*see Figure 87*) is still recommended for detection of this condition, but unfortunately if the lump can be felt the cancer is usually already well established. In the UK one in 12 women suffer from breast cancer at some time in their lives.

It is important that women are "breast aware", i.e. they should be familiar with the look and feel of their breasts and be able to recognise any changes.

Figure 87 shows the recommended procedure for self-examination of the breast. Women who find any changes in their breasts should immediately go to their GP, practice nurse of well-woman clinic. Most breast changes are **not** cancer – but it is important that any change is investigated quickly.

## Mammography

This X-ray examination is recommended for women of **50 years to 64 years** although patients are able to request their inclusion beyond this age. It is presently proposed to extend the recommended age from 64 years to 70 years by 2004. Breast tissue in women younger than 50 is not considered to provide an accurate reading due to its density, prior to the effects of the **menopause**.

It should be remembered that, although rare, men (as well as women) are susceptible to breast cancer. A high fat diet is thought to increase the risk of its development in both sexes.

The following are danger signs and should be reported immediately to the doctor:

- **Change in the shape or size of the breast**

- **An inversion, change in position or in colour, of the nipple**

- **Nipple discharge, dimpling, denting or discolouration of the skin**

- **A lump or swelling in the breast, in the armpit, or in the arm near the collar bone (clavicle)**

- **Pain in the breast or the armpit.**

# Examining your own breasts

During each of the following stages, you should turn from side to side whilst carefully looking at your breasts in a mirror:

**A** Place your hands by your sides

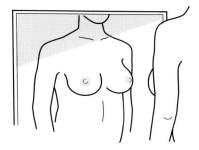

**B** Raise your arms above your head

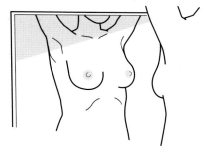

**C** Place your hands on your hips with your elbows pushed forward

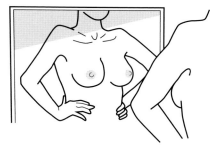

**How to feel for changes:**

**D** Feel each breast in turn. Keeping your fingers together and flat, firmly move over the whole breast, including the nipple and armpit

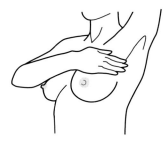

**E** You may prefer to do this lying down

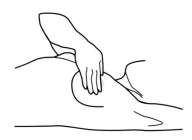

**Figure 87:** Self-examination of the breasts *(adapted from North West Thames Breast Programme leaflet)*

Health Care Trusts have introduced mass screening for women of the appropriate ages and a three-year **recall scheme** is in operation.

## Testicular screening

Testicular screening is recommended for men, and routine **manual examination** of the scrotum is advised for detecting any abnormal development. Advances have been made in the treatment of this rapidly growing cancer.

## Prostate cancer

For men with **prostatism** (enlargement of the prostate gland) a blood test for **PSA (prostatic-specific antigen)** will detect an increase in levels of this substance which may indicate the presence of carcinoma. There is growing pressure to increase the use of this test in men as is done in the USA.

## Cancer code

There is a 10-point European **cancer code** which aims to encourage people to live a healthy lifestyle to help avoid development of cancer. It includes:

- Stop smoking

- Go easy on the alcohol – 21 units for men and 14 for women are the recommended weekly maximums

- Avoid being overweight

- Take care in the sun

- Observe the Health and Safety at Work Regulations

- Cut down on fatty foods

- Eat plenty of fresh fruit and vegetables and other foods containing fibre

- See your doctor if there is an unexplained change in your normal health which lasts for more than two weeks.

## Cholesterol levels

A blood test for cholesterol levels is included in routine screening of at-risk adults. This is one of the fat components of the blood and is thought to be a factor in disease. A **cholesterol level** above 5.0 mmol/l is considered an unnecessary risk . The aim should be to reduce it by 20% - 25%. **LDL** levels should be <3.0 and, if greater, the aim should be to reduce them by 30%.

Levels should be checked in those with a family history of premature coronary disease and hypercholesterolaemia (high levels of cholesterol in the blood).

**Diet** is the first action to be taken in trying to reduce cholesterol/lipid levels. The **'statin'** group of drugs is now being widely prescribed for those with **CHD risk**. Research indicates that **high density lipids, (HDLs)** are beneficial. They also reduce inflammation found at the site of fatty plaque deposits in the lining of arteries. This reduces the risk of these detaching and causing blockage (**occlusion**) of coronary arteries. (The **low density lipids, LDLs** are considered harmful).

## Other tests

There are many other conditions where screening would benefit the patient, including:

- **glaucoma**

- **tuberculosis**

- **large bowel cancer**

- **diabetes mellitus**

- **hypertension.**

Many of relevant tests are covered in Chapter 21.

## HIV screening

The screening to detect antibodies to **human immunodeficiency virus (HIV)** is very carefully controlled. As there is no cure and the financial and social problems resulting are so devastating for the patient, counselling must be given before any test is undertaken. Anonymous testing is being performed on blood taken from patients for other reasons. This is never associated back to the source and is purely to gain some knowledge of the spread of the disease.

## New patient screening

This is a form of screening which is required under the 1990 Contract and continues with the **2003 GP Contract**. Routine testing of urine and taking of **blood pressure** will often identify undetected health problems. Information on **lifestyle** and **family history** should identify at-risk individuals.

## Screening of elderly people

Routine yearly screening of patients of **75 years and over** is also a requirement for GPs and various factors are assessed (*Figure 88*), including:

- **sensory function**
- **mobility**
- **mental condition**
- **physical condition including continence**
- **social environment**
- **use of medicines.**

Elderly people are often suffering from the **side-effects of medication**, as with a reduced liver and kidney function due to the ageing process, smaller dosages may be required.

## Screening of the elderly card

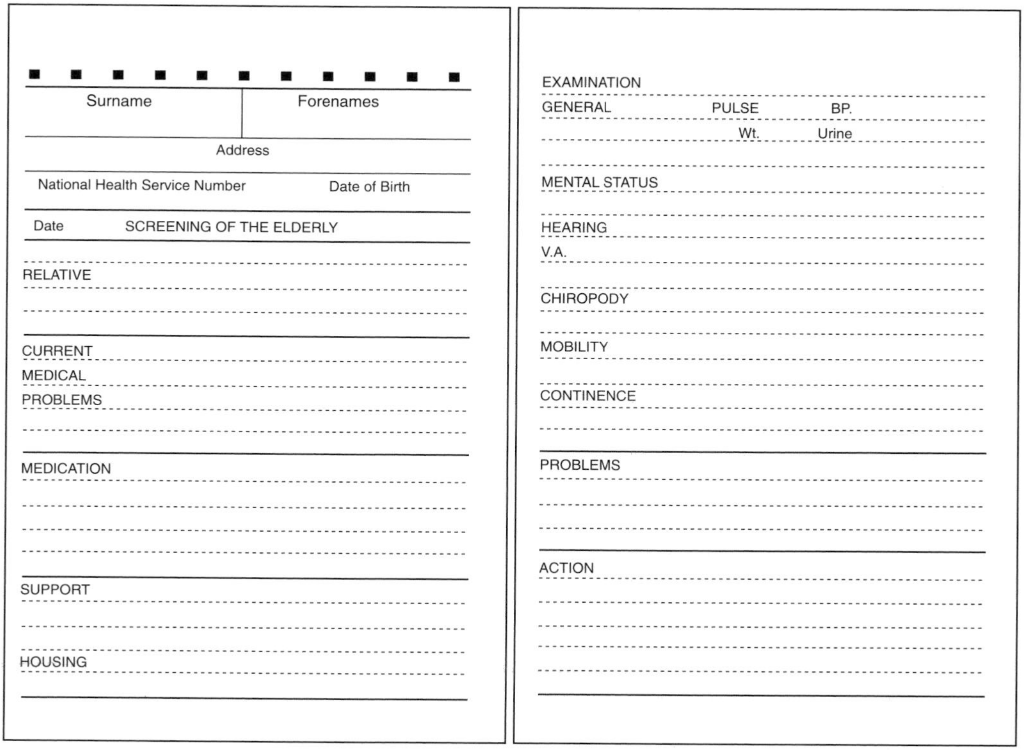

Surname | Forenames
Address
National Health Service Number | Date of Birth
Date | SCREENING OF THE ELDERLY
RELATIVE
CURRENT MEDICAL PROBLEMS
MEDICATION
SUPPORT
HOUSING

EXAMINATION
GENERAL | PULSE | BP.
Wt. | Urine
MENTAL STATUS
HEARING
V.A.
CHIROPODY
MOBILITY
CONTINENCE
PROBLEMS
ACTION

**Figure 88:** Screening of the elderly card

## Abbreviations

| | |
|---|---|
| **AFP** | Alpha-fetoprotein |
| **AIDS** | Acquired immuno-deficiency syndrome |
| **CHD** | Coronary heart disease |
| **CIN I-IV** | Cervical intra-epithelial neoplasia (classified according to the invasiveness of the neoplasm. CIN I denotes non-invasive) |
| **CVS** | Chorionic villus sampling |
| **HDL** | High density lipids |
| **HIV** | Human immunodeficiency virus |
| **LDL** | Low density lipids |
| **LBC** | Liquid-based cytology |
| **NICE** | National Institute for Clinical Excellence |
| **PET** | Pre-eclamptic toxaemia (of pregnancy) |
| **PSA** | Prostatic-specific antigen |
| **TC** | Total cholesterol |

## Terminology

| | |
|---|---|
| **Dyskaryosis** | Abnormal nucleus |
| **Dysplasia** | Abnormal form |
| **Koilocytosis** | Having a spoon-shaped appearance, warty changes |
| **Metaplasia** | Type of cells found to be growing outside their normal area, e.g. cells that are normally only found in the lining of the stomach are found to have spread to the oesophagus |

# Chapter 21 | Miscellaneous tests

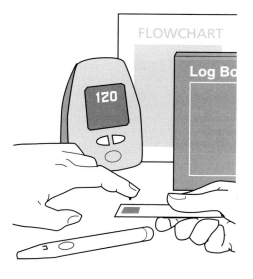

# Blood pressure measurement

This is a common test used in general practice to measure **arterial blood pressure**. Arterial blood pressure is the tension/pressure exerted in the walls of the arteries.

It is affected by the following factors (all of which can alter with age or illness (see Chapter 5):

- Beating of the heart (**cardiac output**)

- Amount (**volume**) and thickness (**viscosity**) of the **circulating blood**

- Resistance of the **peripheral arterioles** (diameter of the small arteries)

- The **elasticity** of the walls of the **main arteries**.

The blood pressure is measured in **millimeters of mercury - mmHg.**

The **systolic pressure** is the pressure exerted against the walls of the arteries when the ventricles are contracting. The **diastolic pressure** is the pressure exerted on the walls of the arteries when the heart is relaxed. The condition of **hypertension** is diagnosed when the readings are abnormally high on three separate occasions.

Blood pressure fluctuates throughout the day and night and is usually lower in the evening than in the morning.

## Procedure

Blood pressure can be measured using a **sphygmomanometer** (*see Figure 89*) a special cuff is applied to the arm of the patient, who should be lying or sitting and be relaxed. With patients who are on **antihypertensive** drugs, it should also be recorded with the patient standing.

The **pulse** should be felt (**palpated**) by hand, at the **brachial artery** (*see Figure 90*) after the cuff has been attached to the patient's arm and connected to the sphygmomanometer. The cuff should now be inflated until the brachial pulse can no longer be felt. The measurement should be noted. The cuff should be released and the patient allowed to rest for 1 to 2 minutes. The cuff is now reflated and pumped up to 30 mmHg **above** the reading where the pulse disappeared previously.

A **stethoscope** is applied to the pulse of the brachial artery at the inner aspect of the **elbow** flexure. The cuff is inflated to obliterate the pulse and then the air in the cuff is slowly released. The pulse will return as a tapping sound. This will be the reading of the systolic pressure. These sounds will continue but will then become fainter and rapidly diminish until they disappear. It will be at this point that the diastolic pressure will be interpreted. Readings should be measured to the nearest 2mmHg.

Sphygmomanometers containing mercury are being phased out (in favour of new electronic meters), although they have *not* been banned by the **Medical Devices Agency** at the present time. Most health professionals consider that sphygmomanometers give more accurate readings.

There are many causes for false readings, including:

- Temperature

- Smoking

- Recent consumption of caffeine or alcohol

- Taking of vigorous exercise, within the last 30 minutes

- Incorrect stance

- Incorrect application

- Incorrect size and height of the cuff

- Incorrect gauge at the incorrect level

- Recording on the relevant arm of those who have had a mastectomy.

In very low blood pressure (e.g. in severe shock) the systolic pressure may be obtained by palpation of the radial pulse. There will be no obtainable diastolic reading.

## Ambulatory monitoring of blood pressure (ABPM)

In some people the blood pressure is higher when measured by a health professional (so called **'white coat hypertension'**). Normal readings are likely to be lower when taken at home (by **ABPM**). A device to measure blood pressure is worn by the patient while they

---

### Korotkoff sounds

(the sounds heard when measuring blood pressure with a sphygmomanometer).

**Five Phases of Blood Pressure**

| Phase | Sounds |
|-------|--------|
| I | Faint tapping sounds heard as the cuff deflates (systolic reading) |
| II | Soft swishing sounds |
| III | Rhythmic, sharp, distinct tapping sounds |
| IV | Soft tapping sounds that become faint |
| V | No sound (diastolic reading) |

---

## Equipment used to measure blood pressure

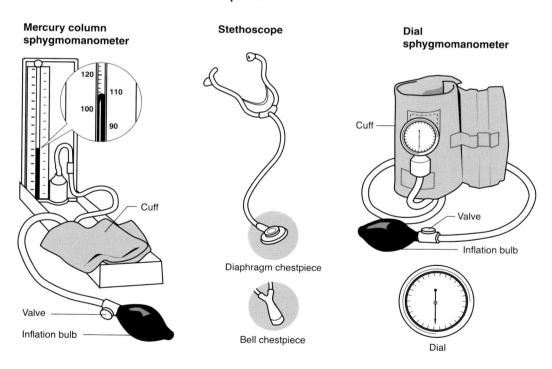

**Mercury column sphygmomanometer**

Cuff

Valve

Inflation bulb

**Stethoscope**

Diaphragm chestpiece

Bell chestpiece

**Dial sphygmomanometer**

Cuff

Valve

Inflation bulb

Dial

**Figure 89:** Equipment used to measure blood pressure

## Veins and arteries of the elbow

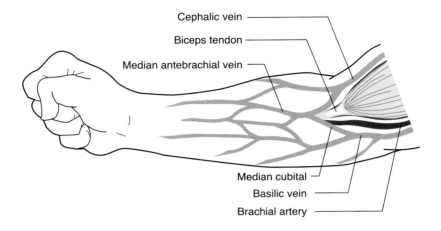

Cephalic vein

Biceps tendon

Median antebrachial vein

Median cubital

Basilic vein

Brachial artery

**Figure 90:** The veins and arteries of the elbow

continue with their normal activities. Blood pressure is usually recorded over a 24-hour period and normal activity should continue, excepting when the automatic recordings are being made. During these periods, the arm should be kept still and driving should not take place. A diary of activities of the patient, during the recording period can be most helpful. Recordings by day are usually taken every 20-30 minutes, whilst by night they are usually every 1 – 2 hours.

## Electrocardiography (ECG)

An electrocardiogram (ECG) is a recording of the electrical impulses of the heart muscle as it beats. The apparatus transfers the impulses into a graph tracing so that they can be read and interpreted (*see Figure 91*). It is used to detect possible irregular rhythm and damage caused by myocardial infarct (coronary thrombosis). Most general practices have their own portable apparatus.

### Tracings

The normal tracing of the heart is shown as the following:

| | |
|---|---|
| **The P-wave** | illustrates the **contraction of the atria** |
| **The QRS complex** | illustrates the conduction of the nerve impulse through the **bundle of His** in the **ventricular septum** of the heart into the ventricles |
| **The T-wave** | illustrates the recovery of the ventricles. |

### Procedure

The leads, which are labelled for arms, legs and chest are placed on the patient, who must be at rest and lying on his/her back (*see Figure 92*). Special conducting jelly is applied to the plates attached and any excessive hair is removed with the patient's permission, by shaving.

# Electrocardiography

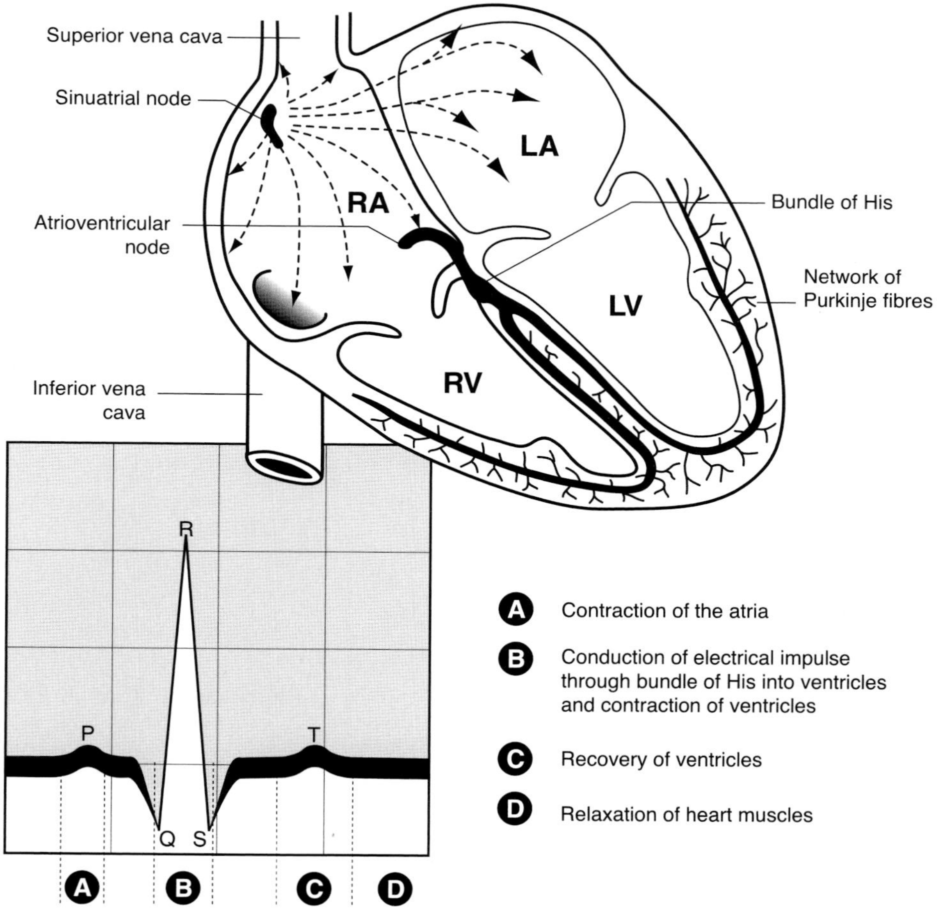

**Figure 91:** The conducting system in the heart

Any electrical interference must be eliminated; this may be from:

- wrist watch
- other electrical apparatus,
- shivering of the patient if cold or apprehensive
- main lead passing too close to the limb leads
- nearby electric radiator.

# Angiography

This shows the state of the blood vessels, when a **radio-opaque medium** (a dye that shows up under X-rays) is inserted intravenously into the patient's arm. Pictures are taken, which enable the physician to see any blockage or narrowing indicating lack of blood supply (**ischaemia**) to an area, especially to the heart

## Electrocardiography: position of the chest leads

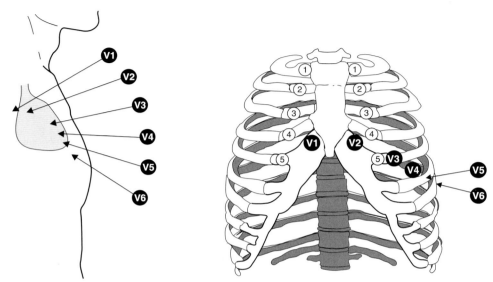

**Figure 92:** Electrocardiography: position of the chest leads

muscle itself. It is performed prior to making a decision to perform a **coronary bypass graft** operation or the insertion of a **'stent'**.

### Exercise stress test

The patient is wired up for an **ECG** and tracings recorded, as increasing **exercise** is performed. This may demonstrate a hidden problem with the functioning of the heart, which may only show under pressure.

### Thallium scanning (radionuclide)

This procedure is used to demonstrate the width of the blood vessels of the heart (**patency of the lumen**), which has not been demonstrated on other tests. Radioactive thallium is injected, intravenously and pictures of the heart taken. The thallium is shown in the vessels, which would otherwise be seen merely as shadows. It is used to demonstrate hidden deficiency in the blood supply to the heart

muscle itself (**ischaemic heart disease**), in some family members, where siblings have suffered sudden death from unsuspected heart disease at an early age. A special type of camera is used. It should be noted that women who are breast feeding must not do so, for at least 48 hours following this test, as the milk will remain radioactive.

### Insertion of stent

**Narrowing of a coronary artery**, due to fatty plaques and loss of its elasticity, can be temporarily treated with the insertion of a **'stent'** which hold open the artery **stricture**, so that a better blood supply is delivered to the heart muscle. This is a quicker measure provided, when a coronary bypass is unattainable but immediate treatment is required, as is shown by the prior performance of an angiogram. (See Chapter 16, page 51 for an angiograph of a stent).

242

## Electroencephalography (EEG)

An electroencephalogram (EEG) is used to detect **abnormal electrical activity of the brain** in the diagnosis of **epilepsy** and other **lesions** (abnormalities) such as **tumours** of the brain. The electrical activity is converted by the apparatus into a graph which can be read and interpreted.

Special **conducting jelly** is applied to the scalp and the leads attached. Differing areas are read and at one point lights are flashed to detect any abnormal response. Readings are taken with the patient's eyes closed and then open. The effect of **hyperventilation** (over-breathing) is also recorded.

### Types of waves

These include **alpha, beta** and **theta** waves, the names given to the various types of electrical discharge from the brain.

## Early morning urine specimen (EMU)

This is a test for **pregnancy**. It is usually performed in the laboratory and the specimen collected must be a concentrated one, i.e. the first urine passed in the morning before drinking, and it must be uncontaminated by blood (in cases of threatened abortion etc.). If necessary a tampon must be inserted before the urine is passed.

The chemical test is based on the presence of **HCG** (**human chorionic gonadotrophic hormone**) present in the urine in pregnancy and verifies the presence of this chemical which is produced by the developing chorionic layer of the embryo.

*A negative test does not necessarily signify that the patient is not pregnant.* The test should be repeated. It is necessary for sufficient of the HCG to be present to give a positive result.

## Midstream specimen of urine (MSU)

This test is performed to detect the presence of **protein** and **micro-organisms** in urine.

*It is essential that the specimen is free from contamination by body fluids* which may be present on the external genitalia and it is for this reason that it is the middle part, or 'mid-stream', is used. The patient is requested to wash the external genitalia before passing the specimen.

The first urine is passed in the normal way into the toilet, thus washing away any mucus present in the urethra. The next urine passed is received into the receptacle provided for the specimen, while the surplus urine is again passed into the toilet.

*It is important that all specimens are immediately and correctly labelled* to avoid any mistakes occurring. *Children or other vulnerable patients should never be left alone or given a glass receptacle for this test.* A suitable sterile jug or receiver should be used.

If the patient is to collect the specimen at home, a handout with full instructions on how to collect it is invaluable.

The specimen will usually be sent to the laboratory for culture and sensitivity (see Chapter 17).

## Routine urine testing

This consists of testing for a variety of abnormalities.

Normal fresh urine is a sterile aromatic amber liquid with a specific gravity of 1.005 to 1.030 and a pH of five to seven (slightly acid).

The specific gravity will depend on the concentration of the urine. It can indicate disease of the kidney and other conditions, e.g. diabetes insipidus.

Abnormal pH may indicate renal or other disease, but fever and diarrhoea will also affect this reading as well as the specific gravity.

Abnormal constituents tested for are:

| | |
|---|---|
| **Bile salts** | present in certain types of jaundice |
| **Bilirubin** | present in certain types of jaundice |
| **Blood** | present in tumours of the bladder, cystitis, urethritis and kidney stones |

| | |
|---|---|
| **Glucose** | present in diabetes mellitus and when taking certain drugs |
| **Ketones** also known as **acetone** | present when fats are inadequately burnt by body; present in diabetes mellitus imbalance acidosis and starvation states |
| **Nitrites** | present in bacterial infection of the urine |
| **Phenylketones** | present when the patient is unable to metabolise properly the nutrient phenylalanine. Accumulation of this in blood stream can cause mental retardation. |
| **Protein** | usually albumin and blood – present in infection, hypertension etc. |
| **Urobilinogen** | present in certain types of jaundice. |

There are numerous **reagent test strips** on the market and it is vital that the urine is fresh and that the 'in-date' reagent strips are read at the correct time limits. *Instructions must be carefully followed, both for testing and storage of the components.*

# Blood tests performed at practice premises

Many practices offer onsite blood testing as a fast service to patients, although these have decreased since concern of cross-infection from body fluids has been highlighted.

## Glucose estimation

This determines the current levels present in blood. It is used for assisting in diagnosis of diabetes mellitus, routine monitoring of glucose levels and screening of patients where appropriate. Further laboratory tests are used to ensure accuracy. Reagent strips are used as in urine testing. There are also meters which measure content. Capillary blood is used, gathered from finger/heel prick as appropriate.

## Cholesterol estimation

This is often offered as part of the 'well-person' check and can be used to back up dietary advice and assess patients' response to diet or medication (See also Chapter 20, page 234 for information on cholesterol testing).

## Other tests

Some surgeries offer the following tests:

| | |
|---|---|
| **Haemoglobin** | measure of the oxygen-carrying capacity of the blood |
| **Erythrocyte sedimentation rate (ESR)** | rate at which red blood cells separate from plasma. |

# Lumbar puncture (LP)

This is a common **neurological invasive test**, performed to detect abnormality of pressure of the **cerebrospinal fluid** (as in a **tumour**) or **infection** (**meningitis**).

Cerebrospinal fluid (**CSF**) is drawn off from the spinal canal space of the **meninges** at the level, of the **3rd and 4th lumbar vertebra** in an adult. (In adults, the spinal cord terminates above the 2nd lumbar vertebra, so there is no danger of hitting the cord itself).

The patient is usually curled into the fetal position and must remain very still. The fluid is placed into a sterile specimen pot for laboratory investigation, (chemical content, culture and sensitivity), after a meter has been attached to measure pressure within the meninges. It is observed whether the fluid is cloudy or clear or under pressure. A cloudy fluid would indicate infection is present.

This procedure is also used to insert drugs such as **antibiotics** in the treatment of infections or **cytotoxic drugs** (able to kill primitive dividing cells) to treat **leukaemia**.

It is important to ensure that the area does not leak any fluid, after the test has been completed and that the dressing remains dry. Lying flat, following the test, will help prevent the patient from having a severe headache.

## Monitoring blood glucose at home

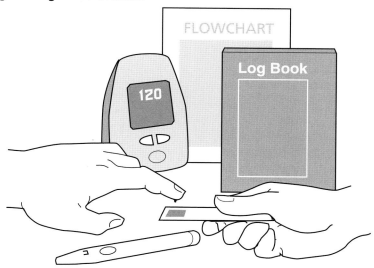

The patient pricks their finger (usually with a special "pen" designed for this purpose) and collects a drop of blood on a reagent strip. The strip is then put into an electronic monitoring device that provides an accurate reading of the blood glucose level. The patient records the reading in a log book.

**Figure 93:** Monitoring blood glucose at home

## Temperature, pulse and respirations (TPR)

The common tests performed to indicate whether there is any indication of abnormality such as fever, infection, bleeding etc. It is the vital centres in the brain stem which control these body functions.

### Temperature

There are many types of **thermometer** (*see Figures 94 and 95*). The thermometer used mostly at the GP's surgery is the **electronic ear thermometer**. New disposable covers must be used for each patient for all types of thermometers to prevent cross-infection.

| Normal temperature measurements | |
|---|---|
| **Oral** | 37°C |
| **Rectal** | 37.6°C |
| **Axillary** (armpit) | 36.4°C |
| **Tympanic** (ear) | 37°C |

**35°C** and below is called **hypothermia**

**40°C** and above is called **hyperpyrexia**

## Electronic thermometers

The **electronic ear thermometer** (*see Figure 95*) must be inserted far enough into the canal and left in place, until a bleep is heard. Mercury thermometers have generally been replaced by digital or electronic ones. They should never be placed in the mouth of anyone under 5 years or anyone who has fits or other similar conditions. Rectal measurement must only be used by professionals trained to understand the process and its dangers.

## Types of thermometer

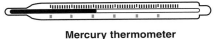

**Mercury thermometer**

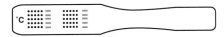

**Thermodot thermometer**

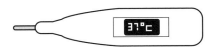

**LCD thermometer**

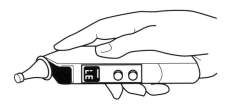

**Electronic ear thermometer**

**Figure 94:** Types of thermometers

### Hypothermia

Hypothermia in the very young, the elderly and those exposed to freezing conditions, is usually measured with a special low reading thermometer. This condition occurs when the core temperature drops to 35°C and below. Once the temperature falls to < 30°C, it is usually fatal as very little can be done to reverse the process.

### Hyperpyrexia

Hyperpyrexia is a condition in which the body temperature rises to 40°C and above. At this temperature, the body cells start to 'cook' and the 'thermostat' in the brain no longer works. Causes are fever from **infection**, prolonged **exposure to heat** and the use of drugs such as **'ecstasy'**. The pulse is full (strong) and bounding. **'Heat-stroke'** is the lay term for this condition.

With these two extremes, the temperature control centre in the brain is no longer capable of maintaining mechanisms for achieving correction of heat.

## Pulse

The pulse can be felt where an artery crosses a bone, near the surface of the body. It reflects the pumping of the heart and the rebound in the artery wall. It is felt using 2 or 3 fingers (not the thumb, which has its own pulse) placed upon the pulse area – usually at the wrist (radial) on the thumb side and gently pressed.

Measurement will indicate any deviation from the normal range. If the temperature is elevated, the pulse will normally increase accordingly. However, **emotion, fever** and **exercise** will all affect it.

The rate, **volume** (strength) and rhythm should be recorded over one minute. In **shock**, the volume will be very weak and the pulse easily compressed, but also very rapid (120 plus). Panic attacks will also produce a rapid pulse.

The act of breathing may cause an irregular pulse. Asking the patient to hold their breath for a few seconds will quickly result in return to a normal rhythm (**sinus rhythm**), if this is the cause of the irregularity.

## Using an electronic ear thermometer

**A** For children under one year, pull the ear straight back

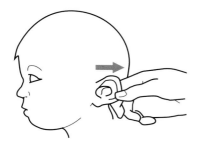

**B** For children over one year and for adults, pull the ear up and back

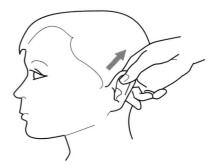

**C** Place the probe gently into the ear canal ensuring a snug fit

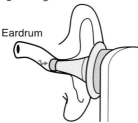

**D** Press the start button. Some models may 'beep' when the temperature has been recorded

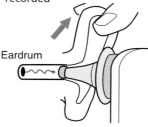

**Figure 95:** Using an electronic ear thermometer

### Normal pulse range (number of beats per minute)

| | |
|---|---|
| In the newborn | **140** |
| Infants | **120** |
| Children at 10 years | **80 - 90** |
| Adults | **60 - 80** |
| | (average 72) |

Emotion, exercise, age and health will all affect the pulse rate.

### Respirations

Respiration reflects the **metabolism** of the body and will vary according to the activity being performed. Measurement of this will indicate any increase or decrease from the normal range.

The number of times the chest rises and falls is counted per minute (**inspirations** and **expirations**). The breathing in and out, counts as one respiration.

There are many reasons for changes in respiration rates, and other factors will be taken into consideration when interpreting the results. If a person is aware that their respiration is being counted, the normal breathing pattern will alter. It is therefore often recorded at the same time as their pulse so that the patient is unaware that their respirations are being observed. In cases of **severe haemorrhage** (bleeding), the respirations will eventually become gasping, and are known as **'air-hunger'**. This indicates the lack of oxygen available to the tissues caused by insufficient red blood cells to transport it.

**Chest infections** and **heart failure** are also among conditions which will cause rapid breathing.

*Note: if a patient has recently had a hot or cold drink, been smoking or had any alcohol or other drug, e.g. caffeine, the TPRs will be affected.*

### Dual energy X-ray absorptometry (DEXA)

This **bone density screening test** may be performed to determine the loss of normal density of bone (**osteoporosis**) and those who may be at risk of this condition. The bone becomes spongy in this condition as the normal **calcium salts** and the **protein** and **collagen**, are unable to be deposited. This leads to an increase in the risk of breaking bones (**fractures**) in every normal day to day activity. Loss of **oestrogen** in the female after **menopause** is an important factor but men also develop this condition.

Those recommended for DEXA screening by the National Osteoporosis Foundation are:

- Postmenopausal women below 65 who have risk factors for osteoporosis

- Women aged 65 years and older

- Postmenopausal women with fractures

- Women whose decision to use medication to stop bone loss will depend on the result of the screening.

If bone density screening is done, it is recommended it should only be performed on those willing to be treated.

## Abbreviations

| | |
|---|---|
| **ABMP** | ambulatory blood pressure monitoring |
| **BP** | blood pressure |
| **BS** | blood sugar |
| **C°** | celsius |
| **DEXA** | dual energy x-ray absorptometry (for the diagnosis of osteoporosis) |
| **ECG** | electrocardiograph |
| **EEG** | electro-encephalograph |
| **EMU** | early morning urine |
| **ESR** | erythrocyte sedimentation rate |
| **FBS** | fasting blood sugar |
| **HCG** | human chorionic gonadotrophic hormone |
| **LP** | lumbar puncture |
| **mmHg** | millimetres of mercury |
| **MSU** | midstream urine/ specimen of urine |
| **TPR** | temperature, pulse and respirations |

## Terminology

| | |
|---|---|
| **Diastole** | phase when the heart is relaxing |
| **Systole** | phase when the heart is contracting |
| **Urinalysis** | testing of urine |

# Chapter 22

# Immunisation

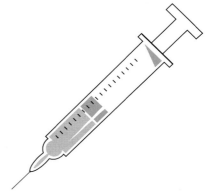

## Introduction

This is one of the most important areas of preventive medicine. It is concerned with the protection of the individual from specific diseases. The first instance of immunisation in the modern world, in the late 18th century, was carried out by **Jenner** who vaccinated people with the cowpox virus to produce immunity against the killer virus of **smallpox**.

## Immunity

Immunity is the ability of the body to fight disease. It may be **natural** or **artificial**.

### Natural immunity

Natural immunity is either an **inbuilt resistance** to a disease, (e.g. human beings do not suffer from distemper found in dogs), or one that is **'acquired'** by coming into contact with the actual disease and overcoming it.

### Active immunity

This is a state in which the body has produced antibodies to a disease. It may be **natural** (by suffering an attack of the disease) or **artificial**, i.e. by introducing the weakened disease, or its poisons, into the body to allow the body to produce antibodies to the disease without suffering the harmful effects of the disease itself. This is the principle of immunisation.

Live viruses, such as the measles virus, are **attenuated** (weakened) so that they do not cause damage to the body but are still able to stimulate the body's immune system to produce antibodies against the virus.

Dead viruses, or bacteria, are also used in some vaccines as well as **weakened toxins**, e.g. **diphtheria, tetanus** and **pertussis** (whooping cough) **vaccines**.

Several doses at differing intervals usually have to be given to produce a sufficiently high level of **antibodies** to achieve immunity. This immunity will be **long-lasting** as the body has learnt how to produce the specific antibodies to the disease. It will immediately recognise the foreign protein of the disease should the person subsequently come into contact with it.

### Passive immunity

This is achieved when **antibodies**, or **antitoxins**, produced by **another person or animal** are introduced into a person's body to fight disease. This immunity only lasts as long as the anti-bodies are present in the body, as the individual does *not* produce his/her own antibodies. Therefore this is only a **temporary immunity**, e.g. occurring naturally in **breast feeding** and artificially when **immunoglobulin**, containing **hepatitis A** antibodies, is given to travellers, or susceptible people are given immunoglobulin against an attack of chicken-pox.

## Reasons for immunisation

Immunisation is carried out to:

- **Protect** the individual

- **Limit the spread** of a disease

- Produce a **'herd' immunity**

- Assist in **eradication** of a disease.

## Recommended schedules

The Department of Health, through its Chief Medical Officer, recommends a schedule for children and travellers (see the **'Green Book'** – *Immunisation against infectious disease*, HMSO).

**Advice should always be sought from the Community Physician/Medical Officer when there is any query regarding suitablility and dosage for the individual patient.**

Table 9 shows the present recommendations for children and young persons:

- **Live vaccines** (BCG, oral poliomyelitis, measles, mumps, rubella) are either given together or separated by 3 weeks.

- **DTwP** contains whole cell pertussis vaccine

- **DTaP** contains acellular pertusis vaccine

- **DTwP** is more likely to cause reactions. The acellular version **DTaP** is less likely to cause a reaction and is now given instead

**Table 9:** Recommended schedules for immunisation

| ROUTINE CHILDHOOD IMMUNISATION PROGRAMME IN 2008 | | |
|---|---|---|
| Each vaccination is given as a single injection into the muscle of the thigh or upper arm | | |
| **When to immunise** | **Diseases protected against** | **Vaccine given** |
| Two months | Diphtheria, tetanus, pertussis (whooping cough), polio and Haemophilus influenza type b (Hib) Pneumococcal infection | **DtaP/IPV/HiB +Pneumococcal conjugate vaccine (PCV)** |
| Three months | Diphtheria, tetanus, pertussis (whooping cough), polio and Haemophilus influenza type b (Hib) Meningitis C | **DtaP/IPV/HiB +MenC** |
| Four months | Diphtheria, tetanus, pertussis (whooping cough), polio and Haemophilus influenza type b (Hib) Meningitis C Pneumococcal infection | **DtaP/IPV/HiB +MenC +PCV** |
| Around 12 months | Haemophilus influenza type b (HiB) Meningitis C | **HiB/MenC** |
| Around 13 months | Measles, mumps and rubella Pneumococcal infection | **MMR +PCV** |
| Three years 4 months or soon after | Diphtheria, tetanus, pertussis and polio Measles, mumps & rubella | **DtaP/IPV or dTaP/IPV +MMR** |
| Thirteen to eighteen years | Diphtheria, tetanus, polio | **Td/IPV** |
| **FROM SEPT 2008** Girls: twelve to thirteen years | Human Papilloma Virus (cervical cancer) A 2 year follow up programme from Autumn 2009 for girls up to 18 years | **HPV vaccine** |
| **Non-routine Immunisations** | | |
| Babies who are more likely to come into contact with TB than the general population: | | |
| At birth | Tuberculosis | **BCG** |
| Babies whose mothers are hepatitis B positive: | | |
| At birth | Hepatitis B | **Hep B** |

The DTwP vaccine has been replaced with an acellular Pertussis combined vaccine (**DTaP**: see above). It is thought that this will cause less side-effects although it is stated to be just as effective.

The Oral Poliomyelitis Vaccine (OPV), a live type of vaccine, is replaced by the less effective Inactivated Poliomyelitis (IPV), administered by injection. Global control of this disease is said to allow this change.

These new vaccines are thiomersal free (a mercury compound). This will meet the internationally agreed aim of reducing the exposure of children to mercury if it can be avoided. Further information can be found on the website: http:/www.immunisation.nhs.uk

Td is a tetanus and a low dose diphtheria vaccine.

- Requirements for children up to 4 years old to have a further booster injection for **HIB** is the result of the use in recent years of the acellular, vaccine for diphtheria, tetanus and pertussis, combined with **HIB**, being used routinely. Unfortunately, it has been found that levels of immunity to **HIB** have been lowered - hence the requirement.

## Relevant childhood diseases

### Diphtheria

This **acute upper respiratory disease**, caused by bacteria, is unfortunately increasing in its occurrence after having been relatively well-controlled through the routine immunisation of children. The toxins produced by the causative organism *Corynebacteria diphtheriae* can cause damage to the heart and nervous system. It can also cause an acute and rapid onset in difficulty in breathing as a result of the production of a greyish membrane in the airway, causing death in severe cases. It is an **airborne** disease usually spread by droplet infection and contact with **fomites** (objects contaminated by an infected person).

The vaccine is composed of **weakened toxins**.

### Tetanus

Tetanus is caused by **contact** with the bacteria *Tetanus bacillus* which is commonly found in soil. The organism is capable of producing **protective spores** which enable it to survive in **anaerobic** (without air) conditions. Entrance to the body may be through cuts, burns or scratches (e.g. from roses). In developing countries such as Africa and Asia, the newborn baby's umbilical stump sometimes becomes infected.

Tetanus is not transmitted from person to person. The toxins produced by the bacteria may cause spasms and paralysis, and the inability to breath can cause death if treatment is delayed; emergency **tracheostomy** (artificial opening into the windpipe) is used to treat this complication.

The vaccine is composed of **weakened toxins**.

### Pertussis (whooping cough)

Pertussis is a killer disease and in unimmunised children produces prolonged coughing spasms and a characteristic 'whoop' as air rushes into the airway as a spasm ceases. The toxins produced by the bacteria cause vomiting and periods of **apnoea** (absence of breathing), and death from choking (and other complications e.g. **bronchopneumonia**) is common in children under 6 months of age. This highly infectious **airborne disease**, caused by the bacteria *Bordetella pertussis*, is spread by droplet infection.

The vaccine is composed of **dead bacteria**.

### HIB (Haemophilus influenzae type B) and meningitis

HIB causes serious illnesses, such as **meningitis, pneumonia, epiglottitis** and other problems in young children. The vaccine is mainly given to prevent meningitis, but is only active against the specific infection caused by HIB and **does not prevent meningitis caused by other organisms,** e.g. meningococcal meningitis and viral meningitis.

The HIB bacteria are airborne, spread by droplet infection. Incidence of the disease, usually found in children under 1 year, has dropped dramatically since the introduction of the HIB vaccine schedule. The vaccine does not consist of live organisms.

The early signs and symptoms of meningitis are headache, fever, irritability, restlessness, vomiting and refusal of feeds (common with the symptoms of other illnesses such as colds and influenza). Babies can become seriously ill within hours; the presence of a high-pitched, moaning cry together with drowsiness are both signs. In older children, dislike of light and neck rigidity are warning signs. The presence of a red or purple skin rash, which does not fade under pressure, indicates **septicaemia**.

Advice can be obtained from the leaflet *A Guide to Childhood Immunisations* produced by the Health Education Authority, which also provides specific advice on what to look for in babies and children and how to act accordingly.

## Meningitis: what to look for

### in babies:

- A high-pitched, moaning cry
- The child being difficult to wake
- Refusing to feed
- Pale or blotchy skin
- Red or purple spots that do not fade under pressure – do the 'Glass Test' (see below)

### in older children:

- Red or purple spots that do not fade under pressure
- Stiffness in the neck – can the child kiss his/her knee, or touch his/her forehead to the knee?
- Drowsiness or confusion
- A severe headache
- A dislike of bright light

### The 'Glass Test':

Press the side of a glass firmly against the rash – you will be able to see it if it fades and loses colour under the pressure. If it doesn't change colour, contact your doctor immediately.

- If your child becomes ill with one or more of these symptoms and signs, contact your doctor urgently. You may be asked to go straight to the surgery.
- If your child has a rash of red or purple spots or bruises, get medical help immediately.

*Source: Health Education Authority (1997): A Guide to Childhood Immunisation.*

### Poliomyelitis

Polio is caused by a viral infection which, following invasion of the gastrointestinal tract, attacks the grey matter in the **central nervous system**. Spread via **water** and **faeces**, it can cause paralysis and death from the inability to breath.

*The faeces passed by the recently immunised child or person can cause the illness to develop in an unprotected person.* Baby carers who change the immunised child's nappies should ensure that they are properly protected and immunised (oral vaccine only). The recommended new programme removes the risk by using an inactivated polio vaccine by injection.

Poliomyelitis remains **endemic** in many developing countries. In industrialised countries, such as the UK, there are sporadic outbreaks, usually associated with unimmunised individuals.

The **oral vaccine** consists of a **live attenuated** (weakened) virus.

### Measles

Measles is highly infectious and can kill, so it is important that routine immunisation is given. General **malaise, coryza** (runny nose) and **headache** herald the beginning of the infection. On approximately the fourth day of the disease a distinctive skin rash appears consisting of **macules**. **Koplik spots** in the mouth may be apparent prior to the skin rash and will determine a differential diagnosis of this condition. Measles occurs due to an **airborne virus** which can cause high fever, **otitis media** (inflammation of the middle ear), **conjunctivitis, convulsions**, respiratory infection such as **bronchopneumonia**, and **brain damage**.

The vaccine given is a **live attenuated** preparation.

### Mumps

Mumps is an **airborne, viral** infection and causes inflammation and swelling of the **salivary glands**, especially the **parotid glands**. Complications can cause **deafness, pancreatitis** (inflammation of the pancreas) and swelling of the **testicles** and **ovaries**, which may result in sterility. Spread by **droplet infection**, mumps may also inflame the brain, causing **meningitis** and **encephalitis**.

The vaccine contains a **live attenuated** virus.

### Rubella

Rubella (commonly known as German measles) is caused by an **airborne virus** spread by **droplet infection**. It usually produces a mild illness characterised by a fleeting rash similar to measles and a fever. **Serological** investigation, where indicated, is required for proof of the infection as many diseases produce a similar skin rash. However, if a woman catches the disease in **early pregnancy**, **deformity** of the developing fetus is common. Damage may also be done if the woman is not aware that she is pregnant. The routine immunisation of girls in their early teens has now been replaced with the routine **MMR immunisation** of all children at an earlier age.

The vaccine is a **live attenuated** one.

### Tuberculosis
Tuberculosis is caused by an infection with bacteria (e.g. *Myobacterium tuberculosis*). It is an **airborne** infection which is easily spread by **droplet infection**. Infection of the lungs is the most common form of the disease, but other organs can become infected as a result of drinking milk from infected animals, particularly in developing countries. Unfortunately, drug-resistant strains have emerged and are increasing worldwide. Despite the increase in reported cases, the disease is relatively rare in the UK.

### BCG *(Bacillus Calmette-Guérin)* vaccine
BCG is a **live attenuated** vaccine given to protect against tuberculosis. A routine skin test (**Heaf** or **Mantoux** test) is performed on the arm by introducing dead tuberculin bacilli intradermally in order to determine the person's antibody levels to tuberculosis. If the person has been exposed to the disease, the results of the skin test will show a **positive** reaction. The vaccine will not be given if the skin test is positive. Cases of positive reaction will be screened for active tuberculosis.

### Varicella (chickenpox)
Varicella is a highly infectious disease caused by a virus. **Papules, vesicles** and subsequently **pustules** appear on the face and scalp, spreading to the trunk, abdomen and limbs. The major distribution is towards the centre of the body surface, and lesions also occur on the **mucous membranes** of the respiratory tract.

The three stages of skin eruption will be present as successive crops of papules arise throughout the course of the disease. Eventually all lesions will dry up and the scabs will be shed. The disease is spread by **droplet infection, personal contact** and **fomites**.

**Shingles** *(herpes zoster)* is a condition in which the varicella virus is reactivated in the body of an individual who has previously recovered from a case of chickenpox.

At present there is **no active vaccine** available in this country, but a **live attenuated** one is licenced in other countries such as the USA.

## Some other childhood diseases
### Slapped cheek syndrome *(Erythema infectosum)*
Caused by a virus, this causes a 'slapped cheek' appearance with a measles-type rash appearing on the face but spreading to give a 'lacy' appearance over the trunk and limbs. A mild fever is usually present. No treatment is required.

### Hand, foot and mouth disease *(Coxsackie virus)*
A relatively mild infection causing blistering of the hands, feet and mouth. Fever and a feeling of being unwell (malaise) are usually present. No treatment is necessary but parents require reassurance.

### Roseola *(Roseola infantum)*
A viral disease which produces a pink measles type rash on the third or fourth day after infection. Commonly affects children at around the age of 2 years.

### Impetigo
Caused by a bacteria (*staphylococcus*) and is extremely contagious, spread through direct contact. The commonest site is the face but can occur anywhere on the body. It produces yellow crusty areas (**lesions**), which spread rapidly. Treatment is by antibiotics either topical or by mouth (oral). Strict hygiene is required and children should be isolated from school or play areas until scabs fall off.

## Adult immunisation

It is recommended that adults receive **booster immunisations** for **tetanus** and **poliomyelitis**. It is advisable to check the immunisation status of all new patients. The continued coverage of protection against **diphtheria** is also vital to stop the disease recurring in this country.

### Tetanus

At present a booster dose is recommended **every 10** years (previously five years). Checking of current status is important for all new patients.

### Poliomyelitis

Adults under the age of 40 years should receive boosters every 10 years if travelling outside the UK, and parents should receive boosters at the same time as their baby commences immunisation (oral vaccine only).

### Diphtheria

A low-dose vaccine is available for those individuals over the age of 10 years. Primary immunisation is indicated for all adults not previously protected. (The old **Schick test** for susceptibility to the disease is now no longer used.)

## Contraindications to immunisation

Each case must be looked at individually by the physician responsible for administering the vaccine.

The following should be considered as **contraindications** (reasons not to proceed) to immunisation in children:

- If the child is **unwell** or has a **fever**

- If the child has had a **reaction** to previous immunisations

- If the child has had previous **severe allergic** reaction to eating **eggs**.

- If the child is **taking medicines** for other conditions (especially **steroids**), is **immunodeficient**, or has recently received **passive immunisation** of immunoglobulin

- If the child suffers from **fits** or there is a close family history, the doctor will discuss and review any likely problem with the parent. Stable neurological conditions may not indicate contraindication.

Contraindications for **adults** are similar, but **pregnancy** is also included as any immunisation may damage the fetus.

When **live vaccines** are to be given, special consideration of risks must be made in order to ensure the patient's immune response is not impaired because of any already existing condition or disease. Certain live vaccines must not be given within a fixed period of each other.

## Consent

Consent from the parent for **children under 16 years** is normally essential and there should be a protocol to be followed for children accompanied by someone other than the parent. *This is extremely important from a legal aspect.* Written consent is not essential but provides permanent **proof** of agreement should future problems arise. Consent is required for each immunisation given.

Any likely side-effect etc., must be discussed by the doctor with the parent before consent is given. **It should be noted** that **a young person under 16 years of age** may give or refuse consent for immunisation or treatment provided that he/she understands fully the benefits and risks involved. Whether giving or refusing consent, the child should always be encouraged to involve the parent or guardian in the decision. **Immunisation should not be given against the young person's wishes.**

## Vaccine damage payments

Unfortunately, a few children suffer damage as a result of immunisation. There is now a single tax-free payment for people who have suffered **severe mental and/or physical disablement** of 80% or more as a result of immunisation against one or more of the following diseases:

- Diphtheria
- Tetanus
- Pertussis
- Poliomyelitis
- Rubella
- Measles
- Tuberculosis
- Mumps
- Smallpox
- *Haemophilus influenzae* type B (HIB)

There is a time and age limitation to this compensation award.

## Reporting of adverse reactions

Any adverse reaction to immunisation should be reported on the 'yellow card' system and sent to the Medicines and Health Care Products Regulatory Agency (MHRA). Information should include vaccine and batch numbers, which will alert the authority to any general problems arising and so prevent further damage (as seen in the 'thalidomide' disaster when a drug was prescribed to women in the first trimester of pregnancy which resulted in children being born with varying degrees of deformity, especially the presence of only rudimentary limbs).

Evidence is considered by the Joint Committee on Vaccination and Immunisation (JCVI), an independent body providing expert advice on policy, safety and efficacy of vaccines.

Reporting is voluntary for doctors, but is a statutory requirement for drug companies and vaccine manufacturers.

## Targets

Prior to the introduction of new requirements, the Primary Care Trusts are expected to immunise 90% of children under five years against diphtheria, tetanus, pertussis, poliomyelitis and HIB to achieve the higher target payment and 70% to receive the lower payment.

## Role of the receptionist

The receptionist will be involved in recall of children for immunisation and in keeping records. It is important that all data are properly recorded and notes are properly filed (*see Figure 96*).

The immediate reporting to the doctor or nurse, of any information that may have been told to the receptionist by the parent, concerning a baby's reaction to a previous immunisation or fears concerning a particular injection, such as pertussis, is most important. This can avoid problems as often these fears are not repeated to the person administering the vaccine.

The provision of current health education leaflets and posters is also an important requirement.

It is also important that the receptionist is aware of the need to be alert to patients who visit the doctor following recent return from abroad. If illness occurs within three weeks, it is necessary to isolate the patient from other patients in the waiting room in order to avoid cross-infection. *Until the patient has been diagnosed s/he must be considered a health risk to others.*

## Batch numbers and expiry dates

These are recorded on the special forms by the person giving the injection and records must be kept in case of any reaction.

## Storage

Vaccines must be kept at the correct temperature as stated on the bottle and in the literature. *A refrigerator, other than the one used for food and milk etc., must be kept for this purpose and temperature levels must be carefully checked;* a temperature of between 2 and 8°C is the usual requirement, although some polio vaccines require storage at 0 – 4°C. The contents and strength of the vaccine will be adversely affected if it is incorrectly stored.

The temperature should never be allowed to sink below 0°C, as freezing can damage the efficacy of the vaccine and also break the container.

## Immunisation record card

**1. YOUR TRAVEL VACCINE RECORD**

✓ Visit your surgery well in advance as some vaccines need to be given a month or more before you go.

✓ Remember that for some vaccines, to ensure long-term protection, you will need to come back for a booster vaccination.

| Vaccine | | Date received | Booster due date |
|---|---|---|---|
| Hepatitis A | Primary | | |
| | First Booster | | |
| Typhoid | | | |
| Meningococcal A+C | | | |
| Yellow Fever | | | |
| Diphtheria/Tetanus | | | |
| Tetanus | | | |
| Polio | | | |

*Continued on inside back cover*

**1. YOUR TRAVEL VACCINE RECORD (cont.)**

| Vaccine | | Date received | Booster due date |
|---|---|---|---|
| Japanese Enc | Dose 1 | | |
| | Dose 2 | | |
| | (Dose 3) | | |
| Tick-borne encephalitis | | | |
| Rabies | Dose 1 | | |
| | Dose 2 | | |
| | Dose 3 | | |
| Hepatitis B | Dose 1 | | |
| | Dose 2 | | |
| | Dose 3 | | |
| | (Dose 4) | | |
| Other | | | |
| Malaria | Remember to ask your doctor/nurse/pharmacist for advice where appropriate | | |

**Figure 96:** Immunisation record card *(Reproduced with kind permission from Pasteur Mérieux MSD Ltd.)*

**Position** in the refrigerator is also important; shelves or compartments in the **door must never be used**. Specialist refrigerators designed for medicine and vaccines are obtainable.

Maximum and minimum temperatures should be recorded regularly, preferably daily. Written procedures should be provided and, if the temperature requirements are breached, necessary reporting to the appropriate person. There should be clear designated responsibility for both monitoring and reporting.

Arrangements for cold storage must be made to allow regular defrosting of refrigerators if an alternative one is not available.

## Transportation of vaccines

Transportation of vaccines must be carefully monitored to ensure damage to their content does not occur. **Temperature control** must be maintained and monitored throughout the period of transportation.

If vaccines have been sent by post, they **should not be accepted if more than 48 hours have elapsed** since the time of dispatch.

First-class post must be used and all necessary instructions regarding the materials and hazards should be followed.

## Disposal

Great care must be taken to ensure **safe disposal** of empty or unused, expired vials by **incineration** or **heat inactivation**. The requirements of the **Environmental Protection Act 1990** and regulations governing the disposal of clinical waste must be strictly followed and written procedures should be provided. Disposal in the **'sharps' bin** followed by incineration is usually the required procedure in general practice. Information and advice may be obtained from the local consultant in Communicable Disease Control.

## Travellers

Travellers require special protection according to the area in which they are to be travelling. Information and advice is available to doctors from the **Communicable Disease Surveillance Centre**. The newspaper **Pulse** issues **monthly bulletins** on these requirements. This is based on recommendations issued from the **World Health Organisation**.

### Recommended schedule for travellers

As well as the following schedule for travellers, a recent special health education card produced by the Health Education Authority with advice on preventing HIV risk is shown in Figure 97.

Travellers to remote areas or developing countries are also advised to carry a **sterile set of basic dental and surgical requirements**, including an intravenous 'giving set'. The reuse of injection needles is a common occurrence in these areas, and travellers have been **cross-infected** with **Hepatitis B** and **HIV**. **Hepatitis C** is also a hazard and at present there is no vaccine available. Hepatitis B is far more virulent than HIV; it is not killed by boiling the equipment and requires strict **autoclaving procedures** for its elimination.

All travellers are recommended for immunisation against **diphtheria**, **poliomyelitis** and **tetanus** if not previously immunised.

The current immunisation schedules are:

| | |
|---|---|
| All areas except North and West Europe, North America, Australia and New Zealand | **poliomyelitis** |
| All areas with poor standards of hygiene and sanitation | **typhoid and hepatitis A** |
| Infected areas as advised | **anti-malaria tablets, precautions against mosquitoes, yellow fever, tuberculosis** |
| In some circumstances | **diphtheria, hepatitis B, rabies, Japanese encephalitis, tick encephalitis, meningococcal meningitis** |

## International certificates

These are internationally recognised certificates verifying that the named person has received immunisation against a particular disease. They are available for **yellow fever**, but **not for cholera** as people do not require immunisation against it. **At present, a signed medical statement to this effect can be issued to those travelling to an epidemic area.**

International certificates are signed by the doctor responsible for administering the vaccine. It is compulsory to have an international certificate for entry to some countries.

**Figure 97:** The "TravelSafe" Code card
*(Source: Health Education Authority).*

The special vaccines available for travellers are:

### Yellow fever

This is a **live vaccine** and is only available from **special centres**. Special storage is required. An initial immunisation is followed by booster injection every 10 years.

### Cholera

Currently, there is **no vaccine** available in this country. However, an oral vaccine is being developed which will hopefully prove more efficient than previous ones.

### Typhoid

There are **three vaccines** available at present; two for **injection** and one **live attenuated oral** preparation. Requirements of dosage and boosters vary according to the preparation used. The current recommended final boosters are required at **3-year intervals**, however manufacturer's suggestions should be followed. **Immunity to paratyphoid infection is not provided.**

### Smallpox

This is now no longer required as the disease has been eradicated.

### Hepatitis A

This is advised for visitors to developing countries or areas where sanitation is poor. **Until recently** this has been a **passive form** of immunisation provided by the administration of human immunoglobulin containing antibodies to the disease. However, there is now an **active immunisation** available, which has replaced the need for passive immunisation.

The single protection vaccines for hepatitis A active immunity advise booster doses **every 10 years** following the initial schedule. Manufacturer's recommendations vary according to the product.

### Hepatitis A and B

There is now a **combined vaccine** available for both hepatitis A and B which, following the administration of the initial recommended schedule, gives protection for 5 years. Antibody levels must be measured to ensure protection.

Three injections are required; two within a month and a third injection 6 months later. Antibody levels must be checked to ensure successful immunisation. Booster doses are required at **3- to 5-yearly intervals** according to levels of **antibody titre**.

### Poliomyelitis

This immunisation should be given to travellers to developing countries where **hygiene** is primitive. A booster dose is required **every 10 years**.

### Tetanus

This is recommended for **all travellers** if their present immunisation against tetanus is not up to date. A **10-yearly booster** is recommended.

### Diphtheria

Those previously covered by routine immunisations should be offered **low-dose** immunisation **every 10–20 years**. Travellers to **Russia** and certain **eastern European countries** where the disease is **endemic** should be offered boosters. (**Primary** immunisation is indicated for individuals who have never received immunisation for this disease.)

## Meningococcal meningitis

This is a vaccine available to protect travellers against certain strains of this bacterial infection. Travellers to **sub-Saharan** areas of **Africa** are advised to be immunised with this vaccine.

## Meningococcal ACWY

A certificate is required for pilgrims to the **Hajj** in **Saudi Arabia**.

## Malaria

Travellers to declared areas of **known malarial risk** should be advised to take precautions to avoid this disease. The **mosquito** is the carrier for this disease and it is prevalent in tropical and subtropical areas over a wide area, e.g. **India** and **Africa**.

Unfortunately, due to mosquitoes entering **aeroplanes**, it is also possible to contract malaria from airports en route, where the disease of malaria would not be expected. There have even been cases thought to have been contracted in this way close to **Gatwick Airport** in England.

The sharing of **infected needles** is also a means of infection.

Advice concerning prevention of mosquito bites must be given. **Special tablets must be started at least a week before departure and continued for a period of one month following return.** However, manufacturers' recommendations should always be followed and those using **'mefloquine'** are advised to commence the treatment at least two to three weeks prior to departure.

Unfortunately, **resistance** is increasing to many forms of treatments and the drug given will depend upon the area to be visited.

## Japanese B encephalitis

This vaccine may be offered to those travellers residing in **south-east Asia** for 1 month or more. It is a viral infection and the vaccine is composed of a **killed virus**.

## White Nile Fever

This is related to Japanese Encephalitis and is prevalent in the **USA** as well as present in **Canada, Central America** and the **Caribbean**. There is **no licenced vaccine** available and prevention is by vector control. The USA has a comprehensive spraying policy. **Bite prevention** measures are vital during outbreaks. It is spread by the **Culex mosquito** and is caused by a virus.

## Other immunisations available

Other immunisations available include those against **influenza, pneumococcal disease** and **hepatitis B**. Vaccines are also available against **anthrax** for those workers at risk and **rabies** (hydrophobia) for those persons who may have been bitten by a rabid animal.

### Influenza

This is commonly given to patients 'at risk', i.e. **elderly people**, patients with **asthma** and those with other **chronic respiratory** or **cardio-vascular disease**. It is usual to have campaigns alerting patients to protect themselves against the yearly epidemics which occur. Booster doses are given **yearly** and the vaccine is developed wherever possible to combat the particular strain of the virus. Special fees are payable at present.

### Pneumococcal infections

This vaccine is offered routinely to those at risk from **bacterial respiratory infections**. Patients recommended for this vaccine include those with **immunodeficiency, diabetes mellitus, chronic liver, lung** and **heart disease**, and individuals who have had their **spleen removed**. One dose is given and booster doses are not normally administered.

### Hepatitis B

This **active immunisation** is available for those at risk, whether due to their **lifestyle** or **occupation**.

**Practice staff who are likely to come into contact with body fluids from infected persons need to be protected (a requirement under regulations of the Health and Safety at Work).**

It is not always known who is infected with this virus as the incubation period can be up to 6 months and carriers have no symptoms.

**Three injections are required;** two within a month and a third injection 6 months later. Antibody levels must be checked to ensure successful immunisation. Booster doses are required at **3- to 5-yearly intervals**, according to levels of antibody titre. There are different varieties of vaccine and the manufacturer's recommendations must be followed.

A **passive immunisation** of a specific immunoglobulin (**Hepatitis B immune globulin**) is also available for immediate temporary protection in cases of **accidental inoculation**, **'needle-stick'** injuries, or contamination with **antigen-positive blood**. This specific passive immunity does not affect the development of active immunity, so combined passive/active immunisation is recommended in certain cases of post-exposure treatment.

NB: *It should be noted that immunisation schedules are subject to change and immunisation information should be checked regularly.*

## Anaphylactic shock

There is always the risk of a patient being administered a vaccine and developing **anaphylactic shock**. This potentially fatal condition, occurring in response to the administration of a foreign protein, can happen rapidly without any warning, producing a variety of clinical features, ranging from **respiratory difficulties** to immediate **cardiovascular collapse** and **death**.

Signs may include **skin rash**, noisy breathing due to **bronchospasm** and **oedema**, and **loss of consciousness**. Immediate resuscitation techniques must be available and life-support drugs such as adrenaline must always be available whenever immunisation is being performed. Guidelines are available from the Department of Health and the local community physician/medical officer.

## Abbreviations

**DTaP**          Diphtheria, Tetanus,
                  acellular Pertussis

**IPV**           Inactivated Poliomyelitis
                  vaccine

## Instructions to parents/carers following immunisation of a child

If your child has a fever there are several things you can do to control it. You should consult your GP if your child appears unusually ill or if the fever persists. The following measures will help to lower your child's temperature:

### Skin exposure

A child loses heat through his skin. If your child feels hot, take off most of his clothes. *Do not* wrap up the child because this will raise his/her temperature.

### Fluids

Give plenty of fluids. Frequently a child with a temperature does not feel hungry – plenty of fluids will prevent dehydration, may reduce the temperature and will make the child more comfortable.

### Medication

A slight temperature is not dangerous and does not always require paracetamol.

Paracetamol is only given to babies under 12 weeks for fever following vaccination.

- **For babies age 8 weeks** the dose is 60mg (2.5ml paediatric paracetamol solution e.g. Calpol)

- **For children 3 months -1 year** the dose is 60-120 mg (2.5ml - 5ml)

- **For children 1 - 5 years** the dose is 120-250mg (5ml - 10ml).

This dose may be repeated every 6 hours, but for no longer than 24 hours.

**Always follow the instructions on the bottle. Paracetamol taken in excess can be dangerous so return the bottle to a safe place after every dose.**

### Tepid Sponging

If you are unable to control the temperature with the above measures, sponge the child with *lukewarm* water. Do not use cold water as this will take the blood away from the skin and therefore delay cooling. Rub the skin briskly so that the blood will come to the skin surface where it can be cooled. Sponge no more frequently than every 2 hours and no longer than half an hour at a time. If an electric fan is available, this will help with the cooling.

### Convulsions

Convulsions are fits - which commonly occur in children up to the age of about 4 years if their temperature rises unduly highly and rapidly. If a child has a fit, lie them on their side so that any moisture in the throat will drain out. *Do not attempt to put anything between the teeth and gums* and contact your GP immediately.

### Polio

If you or anyone who will be changing the baby's nappies has not been immunised against polio, there is a risk of infection. Please discuss this with the nurse or doctor. **NB:** The new inactivated polio injection does *not* carry this risk as it is not a live vaccine.

Chapter **23**

# Miscellaneous terminology

R<sub>x</sub>

+ve

−ve

↑/↓

## Terminology of medical specialties

**Anaesthesia (anaesthetist)**
concerning the administration of anaesthetics

**Cardiology (cardiologist)**
concerning the heart and blood vessels

**Dermatology (dermatologist)**
concerning skin

**Endocrinology (endocrinologist)**
concerning the endocrine system

**Gastroenterology (gastroenterologist)**
concerning the digestive system

**Genitourinary (genitourinary physician)**
concerning the urinary system and male
reproductive system

**Geriatrics (geriatrician)**
concerning disorders of elderly people

**Gynaecology (gynaecologist)**
concerning the female reproductive system

**Haematology (haematologist)**
concerning the blood

**Immunology (immunologist)**
concerning immunity (defence of the body)

**Nephrology (nephrologist)**
concerning the urinary system
(particularly the kidneys)

**Neurology (neurologist)**
concerning the nervous system

**Obstetrics (obstetrician)**
concerning pregnancy and childbirth

**Ophthalmology (ophthalmologist)**
concerning eye disease

**Orthopaedics (orthopaedic surgeon)**
concerning disorders of the locomotor system

**Otorhinolaryngology (ENT physician/surgeon)**
concerning ear, nose and throat disorders

**Paediatrics (paediatrician)**
concerning children's diseases

**Pathology (pathologist)**
concerning diagnosis of disease and examination of patient samples and dead bodies by
post-mortem

  *Forensic pathology:* criminal investigation

**Physician**
concerning medical conditions
(as opposed to surgical)

**Psychiatry (psychiatrist)**
concerning mental illness

**Radiology (radiologist)**
concerning use of X-rays in diagnosis
and treatment

**Rheumatology (rheumatologist)**
concerning disease and conditions
of connective tissue

**Surgery (surgeon)**
concerning surgery
(as opposed to medical treatment)

**Urology (urologist)**
concerning the urinary system

**Venereology (venereologist)**
concerning sexually transmitted diseases.

## Non-medical specialties

**Audiometry (audiometrist)**
concerned with the measurement of hearing

**Gerontology (geriatrician)**
the study of old age

**Optometry (optician)**
concerning the measurement of refraction
(ability to focus) of the eye and dispensing
spectacles

**Orthodontistry (orthodontist)**
concerning correction of teeth (dentition)

**Orthoptics (orthoptist)**
treatment and diagnosis of squints etc.

**Physiotherapy (physiotherapist)**
concerning treatment by physical exercise etc.

**Psychology (psychologist)**
concerning behaviour including the normal

**Radiography (radiographer)**
concerning the taking of X-rays
and delivery of treatment.

## Classification of diseases and associated terms

| | |
|---|---|
| **Acquired** | occurring after birth |
| **Acute** | of sudden onset |
| **Aetiology** | the scientific study of the cause of disease |
| **Allergic** | hypersensitivity to foreign protein |
| **Atrophy** | wastage or shrinking of an organ |

| | |
|---|---|
| **Benign** | not malignant – has a good prognosis |
| **Chronic** | of long, slow duration |
| **Congenital** | present at birth |
| **Diagnosis** | deciding what is wrong with the patient by considering signs and symptoms |
| **Differential diagnosis** | One of a list of possible diagnoses, given the signs and symptoms presented, e.g. differential diagnoses of chest pains include indigestion, myocardial infarction etc. |
| **Dystrophy** | abnormal nourishment or function of an organ |
| **Empirical** | treatment that is given because it works although there is no known scientific reason why it does |
| **Epidemiology** | study of the cause of disease including social factors |
| **Exacerbate** | make worse |
| **Functional** | effects the body function |
| **Hypertrophy** | excessive growth or development of an organ with its own tissue |
| **Iatrogenic** | condition caused by the doctor, usually by side-effects of medication |
| **Idiopathic** | of unknown origin |
| **Infective(ious)** | a disease capable of being spread from one person to others |
| **Malignant** | harmful, damaging, e.g. cancer |
| **Metabolic** | concerning the basic working or metabolism of the body |
| **Morbid** | abnormal |
| **Neoplastic** | producing new growths, i.e. cancerous |
| **Organic** | effects the structure of the body |
| **Prognosis** | the forecast of the probable course and outcome of a disease |

| | |
|---|---|
| **Sub-clinical** | not producing any obvious signs or symptoms |
| **Syndrome** | a collection of three or more signs and symptoms which together form a disease, e.g. Down's syndrome |
| **Systemic** | widespread/throughout the body |
| **Toxic** | caused by poisons – poisonous |
| **Traumatic** | caused by injury/damage. |

## Miscellaneous abbreviations

| | |
|---|---|
| **A&E** | accident and emergency |
| **AET** or **aet** | aged |
| **ARC** | AIDS-related complex |
| **BID** | brought in dead |
| **BP** | blood pressure |
| **BS** | breath sounds |
| **Ca** | carcinoma (or calcium) |
| **C/O** or **CO** | complains of (or carbon monoxide) |
| **Cx** | cervix |
| **Dec** | deceased |
| **DNA** | did not attend (or deoxyribonucleic acid) |
| **DNR** | do not resuscitate |
| **DOA** | dead on arrival |
| **DOB/dob** | date of birth |
| **Dxr** | deep X-ray |
| **ENT** | ear, nose and throat |
| **ESN** | educationally sub-normal |
| **FH** | family history (or fetal heart) |
| **FNA** | fine needle aspiration (for cytology investigation) |
| **GOK** | god only knows |
| **HAI** | hospital acquired infection |
| **HDU** | high dependency unit |
| **HI** or **hi** | hyperdermic injection |
| **H/O** | history of |
| **Hx** | history |

| | |
|---|---|
| IA, i.a. | intra-articular |
| ICU | intensive care unit |
| IgA | immunoglobulin (gamma) A |
| IgBF | immunoglobulin (gamma) binding factor |
| IgD | immunoglobulin (gamma) D |
| IgE | immunoglobulin (gamma) E |
| IgG | immunoglobulin (gamma) G |
| IgM | immunoglobulin (gamma) M |
| IM, i.m. | intramuscular |
| IP | inpatient |
| IQ | intelligence quotient |
| ISQ | in status quo (no change) |
| IT | intrathecal |
| ITU | intensive therapy unit |
| IV, i.v. | intravenous |
| K | potassium |
| NAD | no abnormality detected/demonstrated |
| NG | new growth (neoplasm) |
| NOAD | no other abnormality detected |
| NOS | no other symptoms/signs |
| OA | on arrival/osteoarthritis |
| OE | on examination |
| OP | outpatient |
| OPD | outpatient department |
| PCO | patient complains of |
| PH | past history |
| PMH | past medical history |
| POP | plaster of Paris |
| PP | private patient |
| PR | per rectum (rectal examination) |
| PUO | pyrexia of unknown origin |
| PV | per vaginam |
| RSI | repetitive strain injury |
| RTA | road traffic accident |
| SMI | school medical inspection |
| SOB | shortness of breath |
| Sx | surgery (or suction, or symptoms and signs) |
| TATT | tired all the time |

| | |
|---|---|
| TCA | to come again |
| TCI | to come in |
| TLC | tender loving care |
| TPR | temperature, pulse and respirations |
| TTA | to take away |
| UPLD | upper limb disorder |
| WRULD | work related upper limb disorder |
| YOB | year of birth |

## Signs and symbols

| | |
|---|---|
| $\Delta$ | diagnosis |
| $\Delta\Delta$ | differential diagnoses |
| > | greater than |
| < | less than |
| +ve | positive |
| –ve | negative |
| ↑/↓ | increase/decrease |
| $R_x$ | recipe/take (prescription) |
| c. | with |
| s. | without |
| 3/7 | three days |
| 1/52 | one week |
| 1/12 | one month |
| °jaundice | no jaundice |
| °oedema | no oedema |
| # | fracture |
| $\mu g$ | microgram |
| ↔ or N | normal |
| Ψ | psychiatric |
| ♀ | female |
| ♂ | male |
| † | deceased |
| ⋆ | birth |
| ♀♀ | female homosexual |
| ♂♂ | male homosexual |

Chapter **24**

# Notifiable and infectious diseases

Acute encephalitis ✓

Cholera ☐

Diphtheria ☐

Erysipelas ☐

Food poisoning ☐

# Infectious diseases

An infectious disease is one that is easily transmitted. It may be passed from person to person or from animals or insects to humans.

**Transmission may be:**

- **Airborne** (**droplet** infection) – from sneezing, coughing, talking and dust

- **Waterborne** (contaminated water, food etc)

- Through **contact** – **direct transmission** including from touching an infected person, body fluids etc or **indirect contact** by transfer from inanimate objects (fomites) such as door handles, pens etc

- By **vectors** – from animals (known as **'zoonosis'**) or insects.

**Entry to the body may be by:**

- **Ingestion** (via the mouth)

- **Inhalation** (via the lungs)

- **Inoculation** (via the skin or mucous membranes; or through animal/insect bites or 'needle-stick' injury).

**Carriers of disease** may include persons incubating or suffering from the disease.

**Silent carriers** are those persons who display no signs or symptoms of disease but remain able to transmit organisms to infect others. They may have recovered from the disease itself (e.g. hepatitis B) but also, may not actually know that they have been infected.

Certain infectious illnesses and food poisoning are reportable (*see Table 10*).

In England and Wales this is governed by:

- **The Public Health (Control of Diseases) Act 1984**

- **The Public Health (Infectious Diseases) Regulations 1968 and 1985 (concerning AIDS) and various other regulations.**

In Scotland the following legislation applies:

- **Infectious Diseases (Notification Act 1889)**

- **Public Health (Scotland) Act 1897**

- **Food and Drugs (Scotland) Act 1957.**

If the medical practitioner considers or suspects that a patient is suffering from a notifiable disease, it is a legal requirement to immediately inform the **'proper officer'**. The proper officer is usually, but not always, the Medical Officer of the Environmental Health Department of the Local Authority. Similarly, in Scotland it may be the Chief Administrative Medical Officer to the Health Board.

Doctors are **paid a nominal fee** for the notification, and special forms are provided by the Public Health Department for this purpose. The certificate (completed by the attending physician) is normally the means of notification and requires information on the patient's:

- **Name**
- **Address**
- **Sex and age**
- **Name of the disease**
- **Date of the onset of the illness.**

If the patient is in hospital, then further details are required, including:

- The **address** from which the patient was admitted

- **Date** of admission

- An opinion as to whether the disease or poisoning from which the patient is, or is suspected to be, suffering from **was contracted in hospital.**

The purpose of this requirement is to:

- Identify the responsible **organism**

- Identify the **source** and **mode** of spread of the infection

- Identify **carriers**

- Identify **contacts**

- **Control** the spread of the disease by appropriate means.

According to the seriousness of the threat to the community, certain diseases are required to be notified immediately by telephone to the 'proper officer', e.g. suspicion of typhoid fever. Further powers under the regulations provide compulsory examination of those suspected of suffering from, or being 'carriers' of, the notifiable disease. The Health Protection

**Table 10:** Notifiable Diseases *(Source: The Medical Protection Society, 1988)*

## Notifiable diseases

| England and Wales | Northern Ireland | Scotland |
|---|---|---|
| Acute encephalitis | Acute encephalitis/ | Anthrax |
| Acute poliomyelitis | meningitis: bacterial | Chickenpox |
| Anthrax | Acute encephalitis/ | Cholera |
| Cholera | meningitis: viral | Diphtheria |
| Diphtheria | Anthrax | Dysentery (bacillary) |
| Dysentery (amoebic | Chickenpox | Erysipelas |
| or bacillary) | Cholera | Food poisoning |
| Food poisoning (all sources) | Diphtheria | Legionellosis |
| Leprosy | Dysentery | Lyme disease |
| Leptospirosis | Food poisoning | Measles |
| Malaria | Gastroenteritis (persons | Membranous croup |
| Measles | under two years of age only) | Meningococcal infectiom |
| Meningitis | Hepatitis | Mumps |
| Meningococcal septicaemia | A Hepatitis | Paratyphoid fever |
| (without meningitis) | B Hepatitis | Plague |
| Mumps | unspecified: viral | Poliomyelitis |
| Opthalmia neonatorum | Legionnaire's disease | Puerperal fever |
| Paratyphoid fever | Leptospirosis | Rabies |
| Plague | Malaria | Relapsing fever |
| Rabies | Measles | Rubella |
| Relapsing fever | Meningococcal septicaemia | Scarlet fever |
| Rubella | Mumps | Smallpox |
| Scarlet fever | Paratyphoid fever | Tetanus |
| Smallpox | Plague | Toxoplasmosis |
| Tetanus | Poliomyelitis: acute | Tuberculosis |
| Tuberculosis | Rabies | Typhoid fever |
| Typhoid fever | Relapsing fever | Typhus |
| Typhus | Rubella | Viral haemorrhagic fevers |
| Viral haemorrhagic fevers | Scarlet fever | Viral hepatitis |
| Viral hepatitis | Smallpox | Whooping cough |
| Whooping cough | Tetanus | |
| Yellow fever | Tuberculosis: pulmonary | |
| | and non-pulmonary | |
| | Typhoid fever | |
| | Typhus | |
| | Viral haemorrhagic fevers | |
| | Whooping cough | |
| | Yellow fever | |

**NB:** Although smallpox disease has been eliminated, it remains a notifiable disease.

Agency is also involved in the reporting process and certain diseases are reported directly to their staff.

It is an offence in Scotland to send a child to school with a notifiable infectious disease.

Environmental Health Officers are widely involved with disease prevention and control. The Medical Officer is responsible for ensuring necessary procedures are carried out and that all authorities liaise with and take advice from the Chief Medical Officer of Health at the Department of Health together with liaison with the Health Protection Agency. There are Health Protection Units set up locally who work closely with each Primary Care Trust and Local Authority. Further liaison with the various International Centres for Communicable Disease Control and the World Health Organisation helps to ensure the pattern of disease is monitored and pandemics (world-wide epidemics) are anticipated, prevented, controlled and monitored.

## Communicable Disease Surveillance Centre (CDSC)

The CDSC in Colindale, London, coordinates information and response acting on behalf of the Health Protection Agency for those **national** duties concerning control, surveillance and provision of expert advice on control of infectious diseases.

### The tasks of the CDSC include:

- Leading at a national level on the surveillance, alerting and response functions for infectious disease

- Responding to, and coordinating control measures in an infectious disease outbreak, incident or issue that is national (or of national significance) or involves a number of regions

- Providing a comprehensive authoritative public health information and news service for infectious diseases, including publishing the Communicable Disease Report and the relevant portions of the HPA web-site

- Providing authoritative, expert public health advice for those responsible for controlling infectious disease

- Participating in training programmes for those involved in the surveillance and control of infectious diseases

- Supporting national policy development by the Department of Health and other Government bodies, for example on vaccines and vaccine preventable diseases

- Undertaking research and development to support the above public health responsibilities

- Working with other national bodies to deliver UK wide protection against infectious diseases and provides the public health point of contact in the UK for those working to control infection across Europe (the European Commission and WHO-Europe) and the rest of the World (WHO-CSR)

All this is undertaken in collaboration with laboratory, clinical, and public health colleagues within the Agency and elsewhere.

## Health Protection Agency (HPA)

Following publication of the White paper *Getting Ahead of the Curve* in 2002, the Chief Medical Officer for Health, announced the need for an agency (the Health Protection Agency) which would ensure that skills and expertise in a number of organisations would work in a more coordinated way. This was intended to reduce the burden and consequences of various health protection threats or disease. The examples of the problems of BSE and newer terrorist threats, of anthrax contamination etc had highlighted a need for fast tracking and response by government.

### Specialists in the HPA*

- **Specialists in communicable disease control** – who tackle outbreaks of infectious diseases and prevent the spread of disease through vaccination and other measures

- **Public health specialists**

- **Infection control nurses**

- **Emergency planning advisers**

- **Microbiologists** – who study the organisms that cause infectious diseases

- **Epidemiologists** – who monitor the spread of disease

- **Toxicologists** – who study the effects of chemicals and poisons on the body

- **Laboratory scientists and technicians**

- **Information specialists**

- **Scientists**

- **Information technologists.**

Many of these staff have national and international reputations for their work.

(*Source: The HPA website:* www.hpa.org.uk)

*The role of the HPA**

- **Advising government** on public health protection policies and programmes

- **Delivering services** and supporting the NHS and other agencies to protect people from infectious diseases, poisons, chemical and radiological hazards

- Providing an impartial and authoritative source of **information and advice** to professionals and the public

- **Responding to new threats** to public health

- Providing a **rapid response** to health protection emergencies, including the deliberate release of biological, chemical, poison or radioactive substances

- **Improving knowledge** of health protection, through research, development, education and training.

(*Source: The HPA website:* www.hpa.org.uk)

Recently the HPA has been directly involved in the drawing up of contingency plans for reaction to the incidence of possible cases of **Sudden Acute Respiratory Syndrome (SARS)** and **White Nile Fever** (a viral disease similar to Japanese Encephalitis carried by the mosquito), arising in the country. At present these are *not* notifiable diseases. Whilst risks are low, there is a need to prepare for the possibility of a UK acquired case. Plans include the definition of roles and responsibilities of parties involved in tackling the diseases should the need arise and presents a strategy for limiting the impact of the viruses.

## Sexually transmitted diseases (STD)

**It should be noted that sexually-transmitted diseases, e.g. HIV, AIDS and gonorrhoea, are not normally reportable. This is because it is feared that people would be inhibited from seeking treatment.** However, there are various measures which can be taken if there is **imminent danger** to the public.

It is essential that necessary **reporting** is carried out; practice staff may be involved in ensuring that certificates are dispatched to the appropriate person in the area. There is also a special 'spotter' scheme of reporting, via the Royal College of General Practitioners. Those persons attending surgery who have **recently returned from abroad** and are complaining of illness should be **isolated** in order to ensure other patients are not **exposed** to infectious illness. Similarly, patients who appear to have skin rashes due to infectious disease should be **separated** from others in the waiting room until they are seen by the doctor and a **diagnosis** is made.

## Abbreviations

| | |
|---|---|
| **BCG** | bacillus Camille-Guérin – vaccine against tuberculosis |
| **DT** | diphtheria, tetanus – vaccine |
| **DtaP** | vaccine of diphtheria, tetanus and acellular pertussis (whooping cough) – not so effective as DTwP but causes less reaction (better tolerated) |
| **DTP** | diphtheria, tetanus, pertussis (whooping cough) – vaccine against the three diseases |
| **DTwP** | vaccine of diphtheria, tetanus and whole cell pertussis (whooping cough) |
| **Hep A** | hepatitis A viral infection (water-borne) |
| **Hep B** | hepatitis B viral infection (body fluids), also known as serum hepatitis |
| **Hep C** | hepatitis C viral infection |

**Hep non A**
**Hep non B**
**Hep non C** } hepatitis caused by virus other than A, B or C. These are now recognised as D and E

**HIB***     Haemophilus influenzae bacillus – immunisation for babies against meningitis caused by bacteria

**IPV**     inactivated polio vaccine

**MMR**     measles, mumps, rubella – vaccine against the three diseases

**SARS**     sudden acute respiratory syndrome

**STD**     sexually transmitted diseases

**Td**     low-dose diphtheria vaccine

*N.B. Hib vaccine is now usually combined with DTP vaccine or DT.*

# Appendices
# I - VII

## Appendix I: Prefixes

| Prefix | Meaning |
|---|---|
| *a-* | absence of |
| *ab-* | away from |
| *acou-* | hearing |
| *acro-* | extremities |
| *ad-* | towards |
| *aero-* | air |
| *af-* | towards/near |
| *agora-* | open space |
| *ambi-* | both |
| *amblyo-* | dim/dull |
| *an-* | absence of |
| *ana-* | up/excessive |
| *aniso-* | unequal |
| *ankylo-* | crooked/bent |
| *ante-* | before |
| *anti-* | against |
| *apo-* | away from |
| *audio-* | hearing |
| *auto-* | self |
| *baso-* | basic |
| *bi-* | two |
| *bin-* | double/two |
| *bio-* | life |
| *blasto-* | immature/germ cell |
| *brady-* | slow |
| *cata-* | down |
| *centi-* | a hundredth |
| *chemo-* | chemical |
| *chromo-/ chromato-* | colour |
| *circum-* | around |
| *co-/con-* | together/joined |
| *contra-* | against |
| *cryo-* | cold |
| *crypto-* | hidden |
| *cyano* | blue |
| *de-* | away, from/removing |
| *deca-* | ten |
| *deci-* | tenth |

| Prefix | Meaning |
|---|---|
| *demi-* | half |
| *dextra-* | to the right |
| *di-* | two |
| *dia-* | through |
| *diplo-* | double |
| *dis-* | against/separation |
| *disto-* | far |
| *dorso-* | dorsal (back) |
| *dys-* | difficult/abnormal/painful |
| *ec-* | out of/away from |
| *ecto-* | external/outside/without |
| *em-* | in |
| *en-/endo-* | within/in/into |
| *ent-* | within |
| *epi-* | upon/above/on |
| *ery-/erythro* | red |
| *eu-* | well/good/normal |
| *ex-/exo-* | out of/away from |
| *extra-* | outside |
| *flav-* | yellow |
| *fore-* | before/in front of |
| *gen-* | birth or producing |
| *hecta-* | one hundred |
| *hemi-* | half |
| *hetero-* | unlike/dissimilar |
| *hexa-* | six |
| *homeo-/homo* | like, similar, same |
| *hyper-* | above/high/in excess of normal |
| *hypo-* | low/below/under/less than normal |
| *ichthyo-* | dry/scaly |
| *idio-* | peculiar to individual/own |
| *in-* | not/into/within |
| *infra-* | below |
| *inter-* | between |
| *intra-* | within/inside |
| *intro-* | inward |
| *iso-* | equal |
| *juxta-* | next to |
| *kilo-* | one thousand |

| Prefix | Meaning |
|---|---|
| koilo- | spoon |
| kypho- | crooked/humped/rounded |
| latero- | side |
| leavo- | left |
| lepto- | thin/soft |
| leuco-/leuko- | white |
| lordo- | bent forward |
| macro- | large |
| mal- | poor/abnormal |
| mano- | pressure |
| medi- | middle |
| mega-/megalo- | big/enlarged |
| melano- | black/dark/pigment |
| meso- | middle |
| meta- | after/beyond |
| micro- | small/one-millionth |
| milli- | thousandth |
| mio- | smaller |
| mono- | one/single |
| multi- | many |
| narco- | stupor |
| neo- | new |
| nocto-/nycto- | night |
| nulli- | none |
| oct- | eight |
| oligo- | scanty/deficiency |
| opistho- | backwards |
| ortho- | straight |
| os- | opening or bone |
| pachy- | thick |
| pan- | all |
| para- | alongside |
| ped- | foot or child |
| penta- | five |
| per- | through/by |
| peri- | around |
| photo- | light |
| pluri- | many |
| polio- | grey |
| poly- | many |

| Prefix | Meaning |
|---|---|
| post- | after |
| pre-/pro- | before |
| presbyo- | old age |
| proto- | first |
| proximo- | near |
| pseudo- | false |
| quadri- | four |
| quinqu- | five |
| re- | again/back |
| retro- | backwards/behind |
| sapro- | dead/decayed |
| sarco- | flesh |
| sclero- | hard |
| scolio- | crooked |
| scota- | darkness |
| semi- | half |
| sex- | six |
| sono- | sound |
| squamo- | scaly |
| staphylo- | grapes/cluster |
| steno- | narrow |
| strepto- | chain |
| sub- | below |
| super-/supra- | above |
| syn- | with/together/union |
| tachy- | rapid/fast |
| tact- | touching |
| ter- | three |
| tetra- | four |
| trans- | across/through |
| tri- | three |
| ultra- | beyond |
| uni- | one |
| ventro- | front/anterior |
| xantho- | yellow |
| xero- | dry |

## Appendix II: Word roots

| Word root | Meaning |
|---|---|
| abdomino- | abdomen |
| acetabulo- | acetabulum (part of the hip) |
| actino- | ray/sun |
| adeno- | gland (any) |
| adipo- | fat |
| adreno- | adrenal gland |
| albumen-/ albumin- | albumin |
| alveolo- | air sac |
| amylo- | starch |
| ano- | anus |
| andro- | man |
| angio- | vessel |
| antro- | antrum |
| aorto- | aorta |
| appendico- | appendix |
| aqua- | water |
| arterio- | artery |
| athero- | plaque lining blood vessels/porridge |
| arthro- | joint |
| articulo- | joint |
| atrio- | atrium (upper chamber of heart) |
| auri | ear |
| axillo- | axilla (armpit) |
| balano- | penis |
| bili- | bile |
| blenno- | mucus |
| blepharo- | eyelid |
| brachio- | arm |
| broncho- | bronchus |
| bronchiolo- | bronchiole |
| bucco- | cheek |
| caeco- | caecum |
| cardio- | heart |
| carpo- | wrist, part of hand |
| cephalo- | head |

| Word root | Meaning |
|---|---|
| cerebello- | part of brain (cerebellum) |
| cerebro- | brain |
| cervico- | cervix/neck |
| cheil- | lip |
| cheiro- | hand |
| cholangio- | bile/biliary vessels |
| chole- | bile |
| choroido- | choroid (layer of eye) |
| cholecysto- | gallbladder |
| choledocho- | common bile duct |
| chondro- | cartilage |
| claviculo- | clavicle (collar bone) |
| colo-/colono- | colon (large intestine) |
| cor-/coreo- | pupil |
| coro- | pupil/dermis |
| corono- | heart |
| corporo- | body |
| costo- | rib |
| coxygo- | coccyx |
| cranio- | part of skull containing brain |
| culdo- | recto-uterine sac (Pouch of Douglas) |
| cyclo- | ciliary body (of eye) |
| cysto- | bladder |
| cyto- | cell |
| dacryo- | tear/tear duct |
| dactyl- | finger |
| dento- | tooth |
| derm-/dermato- | skin |
| digit- | finger/toe |
| disc- | disc between vertebrae |
| duodeno- | duodenum (part of intestine) |
| electro- | electricity |
| embolo- | plug |
| encephalo- | brain |
| endocardio- | lining of heart |
| endometrio- | endometrium (lining of uterus) |
| entero- | intestine |
| epiglotto- | epiglottis |

| Word root | Meaning |
|---|---|
| ery-/erythro- | red |
| ethmoid- | part of the cranium |
| faci- | face/surface |
| femoro- | femur (thigh bone) |
| ferri-/ferro- | iron |
| feto-/foeto- | fetus |
| fibulo- | fibula (lower leg bone) |
| fronto- | front part of cranium |
| galacto- | milk |
| gastro- | stomach |
| genito- | genital |
| gingivo- | gums |
| glomerulo- | glomerulus (part of nephron) |
| glosso- | tongue |
| glyco- | sugar |
| gnatho- | jaw |
| gyno-/gynaeco- | woman |
| haemo-/haemato- | blood |
| hallux- | great toe |
| hep-/hepato- | liver |
| hernio- | hernia, rupture, protrusion |
| hidro- | perspiration |
| histo- | tissue |
| humero- | humerus (upper arm) |
| hydro- | water |
| hygro- | moisture |
| hystero- | womb |
| iatro- | physician |
| ileo- | ileum (part of intestine) |
| ilio- | ilium (bone of the pelvis) |
| immuno- | immunity |
| irido- | iris (of eye) |
| ischio- | ischium (part of hip bone) |
| jejuno- | jejunum (part of intestine) |
| kalo- | potassium |
| karyo- | nucleus |
| kerato- | cornea/skin |
| labyrintho- | labyrinth (part of ear) |

| Word root | Meaning |
|---|---|
| lacrimo-/lachrymo-/lacrymo- | tear |
| lacto- | milk |
| lamino- | lamina (part of vertebra) |
| laparo- | abdomen/abdominal wall |
| laryngo- | larynx |
| leuco- | white |
| linguo- | tongue |
| lipo- | fat |
| lobo- | lobe |
| lympho- | lymphatic, lymph |
| lymphadeno- | lymph gland |
| lymphangio- | lymph vessel |
| malo-/malar | cheek bone |
| mammo-/masto- | breast |
| mandibulo- | lower jaw |
| mastoido- | mastoid (part of ear) |
| maxillo- | upper jaw |
| meningo- | meninges |
| menisco- | meniscus (knee cartilage) |
| metacarpo- | hand bones |
| metatarso- | foot bones |
| metro- | womb |
| morpho- | form/dream |
| myc-/myco-/myceto- | fungus |
| myelo- | marrow/spinal cord |
| myo-/myos- | muscle |
| myocardio- | myocardium (heart muscle) |
| myometrio- | myometrium (muscle of uterus) |
| myringo- | ear drum |
| myxo- | mucous membrane |
| narco- | deep sleep/stupor |
| natro- | sodium |
| naso- | nose |
| necro- | death |
| nephro- | kidney |
| neuro- | nerve |
| nocto- | night |

| Word root | Meaning |
|---|---|
| **nucleo-** | nucleus |
| **nycto-** | night |
| **occipito-** | part of the cranium (occipital bone) |
| **oculo-** | eye |
| **odonto-** | tooth |
| **olecrano-** | part of the elbow |
| **onycho-** | nail |
| **oesophago-** | oesophagus (gullet) |
| **oestro-** | oestrogen |
| **onco-** | tumour |
| **oo-** | egg/ovum |
| **oophoro-** | ovary |
| **ophthalmo-** | eye |
| **opto-** | sight |
| **orbito-** | part of the eye socket |
| **orchio-/orchido-** | testis |
| **oro-** | mouth |
| **os-** | bone/mouth |
| **ossic-/ossiculo-** | ossicles (ear bones) |
| **osteo-** | bone |
| **oto-** | ear |
| **ovari-** | ovary |
| **paedo-** | child |
| **palato-** | roof of the mouth |
| **pancreato-** | pancreas |
| **parieto-** | part of the cranium (parietal bone) |
| **paroto-** | parotid gland |
| **patello-** | knee cap |
| **patho-** | disease |
| **ped-** | foot |
| **pericardio-** | outer layer of heart (covering of heart) |
| **perineo-** | perineum |
| **peritoneo-** | peritoneum |
| **phago-** | swallow, eat |
| **phako-** | lens |
| **phalangio-** | fingers, toes |
| **phallo-** | penis |
| **pharmaco-** | drug |

| Word root | Meaning |
|---|---|
| **pharyngo-** | pharynx (throat) |
| **phlebo-** | vein |
| **phono-** | voice |
| **phreno-** | diaphragm/mind |
| **pilo-** | hair |
| **pleuro-** | covering of lung |
| **pneumo-/ pneumono-** | air/gas/lung |
| **podo-** | foot |
| **pollex-** | thumb |
| **procto-** | anus/rectum |
| **psycho-** | mind |
| **ptyalo-** | saliva |
| **pubo-** | pubis |
| **pyelo-** | pelvis of the kidney |
| **pyloro-** | pylorus of the stomach |
| **pyo-** | pus |
| **pyro-** | fever |
| **prostato-** | prostate gland |
| **rachio-** | spine |
| **radiculo-** | nerve root |
| **radio-** | radiation/main bone of lower arm |
| **recto-** | rectum |
| **ren-** | kidney |
| **retino-** | retina |
| **rhabdomyo-** | striated muscle |
| **rhino-** | nose |
| **saccharo-** | sugar |
| **sacro-** | sacrum |
| **salpingo-** | fallopian/uterine/ eustachian tube |
| **sanguino-** | blood |
| **sarco-** | flesh |
| **scapulo-** | shoulder blade |
| **sero-** | serum |
| **sialo-** | salivary gland |
| **sigmoido-** | sigmoid colon |
| **sino-** | space/sinus |
| **socio-** | sociology |
| **somato-** | body |

| Word root | Meaning |
|---|---|
| **splancho-** | viscera/organs |
| **spermato-** | spermatazoa/semen |
| **sphenoido-** | part of the cranium |
| **sphygmo-** | pulse |
| **spiro-** | breath |
| **spleno-** | spleen |
| **spondylo-** | vertebra |
| **steato-** | fat |
| **sterno-** | breast bone (sternum) |
| **stetho-** | chest |
| **stoma-/stomato-** | mouth |
| **synovo-** | synovial |
| **syringo-** | cavity/tube |
| **tabo-** | tabes |
| **tarso-** | foot/eyelid |
| **temporo-** | part of the cranium (temporal bone) |
| **tendino-/teno-** | tendon |
| **thelo-** | nipples |
| **thermo-** | heat |
| **thoraco-/ thoracico-** | chest/thorax |
| **thrombo-** | blood clot |
| **thymo-** | thymus gland |
| **thyro-** | thyroid |
| **tibio-** | tibia (main lower leg bone) |
| **tilo-** | breast |
| **tonsillo-** | tonsils |
| **tox-/toxico-** | poison |
| **tracheo-** | windpipe/trachea |
| **tricho-** | hair |
| **tropho-** | nourishment |
| **turbino-** | bone in the nose (turbinate) |
| **tympano-** | ear drum |
| **ulno-** | lower arm bone (ulna) |
| **uretero-** | ureter |
| **urethro-** | urethra |
| **urino-** | urine |
| **uro-** | urine/urinary organs |
| **utero-** | womb |

| Word root | Meaning |
|---|---|
| **uveo-** | uveal tract (part of eye) |
| **uvulo-** | uvula |
| **valvo-/valvulo-** | valve |
| **varico-** | varicose veins |
| **vasculo-** | blood vessel |
| **vaso-** | vessel |
| **veno-** | vein |
| **ventrico-/ ventriculo** | ventricle (lower chamber of heart) |
| **vertibro-** | vertibra |
| **vesico-** | vesicle/bladder/ fluid-filled blister |
| **vestibulo-** | vestibule of inner ear |
| **volo-** | palm |
| **zoo-** | animal |
| **zygo-/zygomato-** | cheek bone (zygomatic) |

# Appendix III: Suffixes

| Suffix | Meaning |
|---|---|
| **-a** | condition of |
| **-aemia** | blood |
| **-ac** | concerning/pertaining |
| **-aesthesia** | feeling/sensibility |
| **-al** | concerning/pertaining to |
| **-algia** | pain |
| **-an** | concerning/pertaining to |
| **-ase** | enzyme |
| **-ate** | a salt |
| **-blast** | immature cell |
| **-cele** | swelling/protrusion |
| **-centesis** | to puncture/tapping |
| **-cide** | kill/destroy |
| **-cision** | cutting |
| **-clasis** | destruction of/breaking |
| **-clysis** | injection/infusion |
| **-coccus** | round cell, type of bacteria |
| **-crine** | secrete |
| **-cyte** | cell |
| **-derm** | skin |
| **-desis** | binding together |
| **-dipsia** | thirst |
| **-drome** | running together |
| **-dynia** | pain |
| **-ectasis** | dilatation |
| **-ectomy** | surgical removal of |
| **-form** | having the formation or shape of |
| **-fuge** | expelling |
| **-gen** | |
| **-genesis** | producing/forming/origin |
| **-genic** | |
| **-gogue** | increasing flow |
| **-gram** | picture/tracing |
| **-graph** | machine that records/tracing |
| **-graphy** | procedure of recording/tracing |
| **-gravid/-gravida** | pregnancy |

| Suffix | Meaning |
|---|---|
| **-ia/-iasis** | condition of/state of |
| **-iac** | pertaining to |
| **-iatric** | pertaining to medicine/physician |
| **-ic** | concerning/pertaining to |
| **-iosis/-ism** | condition of/state of |
| **-itis** | inflammation of |
| **-kinesis** | movement/activity |
| **-lalia** | speech |
| **-lith** | stone |
| **-lithesis** | slipping |
| **-lithiasis** | condition/presence of stones |
| **-lysis** | destruction/splitting/breaking down |
| **-malacia** | softening |
| **-megaly** | enlargement of |
| **-meter** | measure |
| **-oedema** | swelling caused by excess fluid |
| **-oid** | likeness/resemblance |
| **-ology** | study of/science of |
| **-oma** | tumour |
| **-opia** | condition of the eye/vision |
| **-opsia** | vision |
| **-opsy** | looking at |
| **-orrhaphy** | sewing or repair |
| **-oscopy** | examination with a lighted instrument |
| **-ose** | sugar |
| **-osis** | condition of |
| **-ostomy** | artificial opening into |
| **-otomy** | cutting into/dividing/incision |
| **-ous** | like/similar to |
| **-para** | given birth |
| **-paresis** | weakness |
| **-pathy** | disease |
| **-penia** | lack of/decreased |
| **-pexy** | fixation of |
| **-phage/-phagia** | eating/ingesting/swallowing |

| Suffix | Meaning |
|---|---|
| **-phakia** | lens (of the eye) |
| **-phasia** | speech |
| **-philia** | liking/loving/affinity for |
| **-phobia** | irrational fear |
| **-phylaxis** | protection/prevention |
| **-plasia** | formation |
| **-plasty** | form/mould/reconstruct |
| **-plegia** | paralysis |
| **-pnoea** | breathing |
| **-poiesis** | making/production |
| **-ptosis** | drooping/falling |
| **-ptysis** | cough |
| **-rrhage** | burst forth/bleeding |
| **-rrhagia** | condition of heavy bleeding |
| **-rrhaphy** | sew/repair/suture |
| **-rrhexis** | rupture/break |
| **-rrhoea** | flow/discharge |
| **-rrhythmia** | rhythm |
| **-sclerosis** | hardening |
| **-scope** | lighted instrument used to examine |
| **-scopy** | examination with a lighted instrument |
| **-scotoma** | blind spot |
| **-somatic** | pertaining to the body |
| **-sonic** | sound |
| **-spadia** | to draw out |
| **-stasis** | cessation of movement/flow |
| **-stat** | an agent to prevent moving or change |
| **-staxis** | dripping (blood)/ continuous slight loss |
| **-stenosis** | narrowing |
| **-sthenia/ -stheania** | strength |
| **-taxia** | co-ordination/order |
| **-tocia** | labour/birth |
| **-tome** | cutting instrument |
| **-tripsy** | crushing |

| Suffix | Meaning |
|---|---|
| **-triptor** | instrument used to crush |
| **-trophy** | nourishment/food |
| **-tropic/-trophic** | affinity/turning toward |
| **-tussis** | cough |
| **-uria** | condition of urine |

# Appendix IV:
## Abbreviations of degrees, qualifications, titles and awards

| Abbreviation | Meaning |
|---|---|
| BA | Bachelor of Arts |
| BAO | Bachelor of the Art of Obstetrics |
| BC or BCh or BChir | Bachelor of Surgery |
| BM | Bachelor of Medicine |
| BS | Bachelor of Surgery |
| BSc | Bachelor of Science |
| CCDC | Consultant in Communicable Disease Control |
| ChB or CChir | Bachelor of Surgery |
| CM or ChM | Master of Surgery |
| CPH | Certificate in Public Health |
| CPN | Community Psychiatric Nurse |
| DA | Diploma in Anaesthetics |
| DCH | Diploma in Child Health |
| DCh | Doctor of Surgery |
| DCP | Diploma in Clinical Pathology |
| DDS | Doctor of Dental Surgery |
| DHyg | Doctor of Hygiene |
| DIH | Diploma in Industrial Health |
| DLO | Diploma in Laryngology and Otology |
| DN | District Nurse |
| Dip Med Rehab | Diploma in Medical Rehabilitation |
| DM | Doctor of Medicine |
| DMR | Diploma in Medical Radiology |
| DO | Diploma in Ophthalmology |
| DObstRCOG | Diploma in Obstetrics of the Royal College of Obstetricians and Gynaecologists |
| DOMS | Diploma in Ophthalmological Medicine and Surgery |

| Abbreviation | Meaning |
|---|---|
| DPH | Diploma in Public Health |
| DPM | Diploma in Psychological Medicine |
| DR | Diploma in Radiology |
| DSc | Doctor of Science |
| DTH | Diploma in Tropical Hygiene |
| DTM | Diploma in Tropical Medicine |
| FAMS | Fellow of the Association of Managers, Medical Secretaries, Practice Administrators and Receptionists |
| FDS | Fellow of Dental Surgery |
| FFARCS | Fellow of Faculty of Anaesthetists, Royal College of Surgeons |
| FFHom | Fellow of Faculty of Homeopathy |
| FFR | Fellow of the Faculty of Radiologists |
| FRCGP | Fellow of the Royal College of General Practitioners |
| FRCOG | Fellow of the Royal College of Obstetricians and Gynaecologists |
| FRCP | Fellow of the Royal College of Physicians (London) |
| FRCPE or FRCPEd* or FRCPEdin* | Fellow of the Royal College of Physicians of Edinburgh |
| FRCPS | Fellow of the Royal College of Physicians and Surgeons |
| FRCPath | Fellow of the Royal College of Pathologists |
| FRCPsych | Fellow of the Royal College of Psychiatrists |
| FRCS | Fellow of the Royal College of Surgeons (England) |
| FRCSE* | Fellow of the Royal College of Surgeons of Edinburgh |
| FRIPHH | Fellow of the Royal Institute of Public Health and Hygiene |

| Abbreviation | Meaning |
|---|---|
| FRS | Fellow of the Royal Society |
| HVCert | Health Visitors Certificate |
| LAH | Licentiate of Apothecaries Hall (Dublin) |
| LDS | Licentiate in Dental Surgery |
| LM | Licentiate in Midwifery |
| LRCP | Licentiate of Royal College of Physicians |
| LSA | Licentiate of Society of Apothecaries |
| MA | Master of Arts |
| MAO | Master of the Art of Obstetrics |
| MAMS | Member of the Association of Medical Secretaries, Managers, Practice Administrators and Receptionists |
| MB | Bachelor of Medicine |
| MCh | Master of Surgery |
| MChD | Master of Dental Surgery |
| MChir | Master of Surgery |
| MChOrth | Master of Orthopaedic Surgery |
| MCPath | Member of College of Pathology |
| MCPS | Member of College of Physicians and Surgeons |
| MD | Doctor of Medicine |
| MDS | Master of Dental Surgery |
| MFCP | Member of the Faculty of Community Physicians |
| MFHom | Member of the Faculty of Homeopathy |
| MHyg | Master of Hygiene |
| MMSA | Master of Midwifery of Society of Apothecaries |
| MPH | Master of Public Health |
| MRCGP | Member of the Royal College of General Practitioners |
| MRCOG | Member of the Royal College of Obstetricians and Gynaecologists |

| Abbreviation | Meaning |
|---|---|
| MRCP | Member of the Royal College of Physicians (London) |
| MRCPath | Member of the Royal College of Pathologists |
| MRCPsych | Member of the Royal College of Psychiatrists |
| MRCS | Member of the Royal College of Surgeons (England) |
| MS | Master of Surgery |
| MSc | Master of Science |
| MSW | Medical Social Worker |
| OT | Occupational Therapist |
| PhD | Doctor of Philosophy |
| RGN | Registered General Nurse |
| RN | Registered Nurse |
| SEN | State Enrolled Nurse (old title) |
| SCM | State Certified Midwife |
| SRN | State Registered Nurse (old title) |
| SRP | State Registered Physiotherapist |

* It is correct to put the initial of the appropriate college after MRCS or FRCS, or LRCP and FRCP for the Royal Colleges of Scotland

## Appendix IV continued: Abbreviations of organisations and institutions associated with medical practice

| Abbreviation | Meaning |
|---|---|
| AMSPAR | Association of Medical Secretaries, Practice Managers, Administrators and Receptionists |
| AP | Aspiration Payemts |
| BMA | British Medical Association |
| BMJ | British Medical Journal |
| BRCS | British Red Cross Society |
| CDSC | Communicable Disease Surveillance Centre |

| Abbreviation | Meaning |
|---|---|
| CHI | Commision for Health Improvement |
| CPPIH | Commision for Patient and Public Involvement in Health |
| DES | Directed Enhanced Services |
| DoH | Department of Health |
| DSS | Department of Social Security |
| EHO | Environmental Health Officer |
| EPI | Expert Patient Initiatives |
| ES | Essential Services |
| FPA | Family Planning Association |
| GMC | General Medical Council |
| GMSC | General Medical Services Committee |
| HA | Health Authority |
| HCHS | Hospital and Community Health Services |
| HCP | Holistic Care Payments |
| HDA | Health Development Agency |
| HPA | Health Protection Agency |
| HPE | Health Promotion England |
| HPU | Health Protection Unit |
| IHSM | Institute of Health Service Managers |
| LES | Local Enhanced Services |
| LMC | Local Medical Committee |
| LMG | Local Medical Group |
| MAAG | Medical Audit Advisory Group |
| MASTA | Medical Advisory Service for Travellers Abroad |
| MDU | Medical Defence Union |
| MHRA | Medicines and Health Care Products Regulatory Agency |
| MPS | Medical Protection Society |
| MRC | Medical Research Council |
| NAHAT | National Association of Health Authorities and Trusts |

| Abbreviation | Meaning |
|---|---|
| NBTS | National Blood Transfusion Service |
| NCAA | National Clinical Assessment Authority |
| NES | National Enhanced Services |
| NHS | National Health Service |
| NICE | National Institute for (Health and) Clinical Excellence |
| NMC | Nursing and Midwifery Council |
| NPSA | National Patient Safety Agency |
| NSF | National Service Framework |
| OSC | Overview and Scrutiny Committee |
| PALS | Patient Advisory and Liaison Service |
| PCG | Primary Care Groups |
| PCO | Primary Care Organisation |
| PCT | Primary Care Trust |
| PF | Patient's Forum |
| RCGP | Royal College of General Practitioners |
| RCN | Royal College of Nursing |
| RHE | Regional Health Executive |
| SSDP | Strategic Service Development Plan |
| SHA | Strategic Health Authority |
| WHO | World Health Organisation |

## Appendix IV continued: General medical abbreviations

| Abbreviation | Meaning |
|---|---|
| µmol | micromole |
| A&E | accident and emergency |
| A&W | alive and well |
| ab | abortion |
| ABC | aspiration, biopsy, cytology |
| abd | abdomen/abdominal |
| abdo | abdomen/abdominal |

| Abbreviation | Meaning |
|---|---|
| **ABMP** | ambulatory blood pressure monitoring |
| **ABR** | auditory brain stem response |
| **Acc** | accommodation |
| **ACTH** | adrenocorticotropic hormone |
| **AD** | right ear (auris dextra) |
| **ad** | auris dextra (right ear) |
| **ADD** | attention deficit disorder |
| **ADH** | antidiuretic hormone |
| **ADHD** | attention deficit hyperactivity disorder |
| **AET/aet** | aged |
| **AFP** | alpha-fetoprotein |
| **AGN** | acute glomerulonephritis |
| **AHF** | antihaemophiliac factor |
| **AI** | artificial insemination |
| **AIA** | allergy induced autism |
| **AID** | artificial insemination by donor |
| **AIDS** | acquired immunodeficiency syndrome |
| **AIH** | artificial insemination by husband |
| **ALL** | acute lymphocytic leukaemia |
| **ALS** | amyotrophic lateral sclerosis |
| **AMD** | age-related macular degeneration |
| **AML** | acute myeloid leukaemia |
| **AN** | antenatal |
| **ANS** | autonomic nervous system |
| **AP** | artificial pneumothorax |
| **AP&L** | anterior, posterior and lateral |
| **APH** | antepartum haemorrhage |
| **APT** | activated prothrombin time |
| **APTT** | activated partial thromboplastin time |
| **ARC** | AIDS-related complex |
| **ARM** | artificial rupture of membranes |

| Abbreviation | Meaning |
|---|---|
| **ART** | assisted reproductive technology |
| **AS** | autistic spectrum disorder or left ear (auris sinister) or aortic stenosis |
| **ASD** | Asperger's syndrome disorder |
| **asD** | atrial septal defect |
| **ASHD** | arteriosclerotic heart disease |
| **Ast** | astigmatism |
| **AST** | aspartate transaminase (cardiac enzyme) |
| **AU** | both ears (aures unitas) or each ear |
| **au** | aures unitas (both ears) or auris uterque (each ear) |
| **BaE** | barium enema |
| **BaM** | barium meal |
| **BBA** | born before arrival |
| **BCG** | bacillus Camille-Guérin – vaccine against tuberculosis |
| **BI** | bone injury |
| **BID** | brought in dead |
| **BM** | bowel movement |
| **BNO** | bladder neck obstruction |
| **BO** | bowels open |
| **BP** | bipolar disorder or blood pressure |
| **BS** | breath sounds |
| **BS** | blood sugar |
| **BSE** | bovine spongiform encephalopathy ('mad cow' disease) |
| **BSO** | bilateral salpingo-oophorectomy (surgical removal fallopian tubes and ovaries) |
| **BUN** | blood urea nitrogen |
| **BW** | birth weight |
| **Bx** | biopsy |
| **C&S** | culture and sensitivity |
| **C/O** | complains of |
| **C1, C2,** etc | cervical vertebrae |

| Abbreviation | Meaning |
|---|---|
| Ca | carcinoma/calcium |
| CA | chronological age |
| CABG | coronary artery bypass graft |
| CABS | coronary artery bypass surgery |
| CAD | coronary artery disease |
| CAPD | continuous ambulatory peritoneal dialysis |
| CAT (CT) | scan – computerised X-ray of layers of tissues (computerised axial tomography) |
| CCF | congestive cardiac failure |
| CCU | coronary care unit |
| CD, cd or CD | controlled drugs |
| CDH | congenital dislocation of the hip |
| CHD | coronary heart disease |
| CHF | congestive heart failure |
| CIN I-IV | cervical intra-epithelial neoplasia |
| CIN | cervical intra-epithelial neoplasia |
| CJD | Creutzfeldt-Jacob disease |
| CLL | chronic lymphocytic leukaemia |
| CML | chronic myeloid leukaemia |
| CNS | central nervous system |
| CO | carbon monoxide |
| C˚ | Celsius |
| CO, C/O | complains of (or carbon monoxide) |
| $CO_2$ | carbon dioxide |
| COAD | chronic obstructive airway disease |
| COC | combined oral contraceptive pill |
| COHS | controlled ovarian hormone stimulation |
| COLD | chronic obstructive lung disease |

| Abbreviation | Meaning |
|---|---|
| COPD | chronic obstructive pulmonary disease |
| CPK | creatine phosphokinase (cardiac enzyme) |
| CPR | cardiopulmonary resuscitation |
| CPT | carpal tunnel syndrome |
| CRP | C-reactive protein indicates the presence of inflammation within the body |
| CSF | cerebrospinal fluid |
| CSU | catheter specimen of urine |
| CVA | cerebrovascular accident (stroke) |
| CVP | central venous pressure |
| CVS | chorionic villus sampling (to detect fetal abnormalities) or cardiovascular system |
| Cx | cervix (neck of womb) |
| D | diopter (lens strength) |
| D&C | dilatation and curettage (scraping out of womb) |
| D&V | diarrhoea and vomiting |
| db | decibel (measurement of hearing) |
| DCIS | ductal carcinoma in situ (a type of breast cancer) |
| Dec | deceased |
| DEXA | dual energy x-ray absorptometry (for the diagnosis of osteoporosis) |
| DLE | disseminated lupus erythematosus |
| DNA | did not attend or deoxyribonucleic acid |
| DNR | do not resuscitate |
| DOA | dead on arrival |
| DOB/dob | date of birth |
| DS | disseminated sclerosis (old term for MS) |
| DT | delirium tremens or diphtheria, tetanus – vaccine |

| Abbreviation | Meaning |
|---|---|
| DtaP | vaccine of diphtheria, tetanus and acellular pertussis |
| DTP | diphtheria, tetanus, pertussis (whooping cough) – vaccine |
| DTs | delirium tremens |
| DTaP | vaccine of diphtheria, tetanus and acellular pertussis |
| DTwP | vaccine of diphtheria, tetanus and whole cell pertussis |
| DU | duodenal ulcer |
| DUB | dysfunctional uterine bleeding |
| DVT | deep vein thrombosis |
| Dx | diagnosis |
| Dxr | deep X-ray |
| EBT | electron beam tomography |
| ECG | electrocardiogram |
| ECT | electroconvulsive therapy |
| EDC | expected date of confinement |
| EDD | expected date of delivery |
| EEG | electroencephalogram |
| EMG | electromyogram |
| EMU | early morning urine |
| ENT | ear, nose and throat |
| EOF | end organ failure |
| EOM | extraocular movement |
| ERCP | endoscopic retrograde cholangiopancreatography |
| ERPC | evacuation of retained products of conception |
| ESL | extracorporeal shock-wave lithotripsy |
| ESN | educationally subnormal |
| ESR | erythrocyte sedimentation rate |
| EUA | examination under anaesthetic |
| FAS | fetal abnormality syndrome |
| FB | foreign body |

| Abbreviation | Meaning |
|---|---|
| FBC | full blood count |
| FBS | fasting blood sugar to determine diabetes mellitus or low blood sugars |
| Fe | iron |
| $FEV_1$ | forced expiration volume (subscript shows timed interval in seconds) |
| FH | family history or fetal heart |
| FHH | fetal heart heard |
| FHNH | fetal heart not heard |
| FMF | fetal movement felt |
| FMRI | functional magnetic resonance imaging |
| FNA | fine needle aspiration |
| FSH | follicle-stimulating hormone |
| G&A | gas and air |
| GA | general anaesthetic |
| GAD | general anxiety disorder |
| GH | growth hormone |
| GI | gastrointestinal |
| GIFT | gamete intra-fallopian transplantation |
| GOK | God only knows |
| GORD | gastro-oesophageal reflux disease |
| GOT | glutamicoxalo-acetic transaminase (cardiac enzyme) |
| GPI | general paralysis of the insane |
| GTT | glucose tolerance test (to diagnose diabetes mellitus) |
| GU | genitourinary or gastric ulcer |
| GVHD | graft versus host disease (in transplants) |
| H/O | history of |
| $H_2O$ | water |
| HAI | hospital acquired infection |
| Hb | haemoglobin (pigmented protein which carries oxygen) |
| $HbA_1$ or $HBA_1$ | blood test for diabetes |

| Abbreviation | Meaning |
|---|---|
| HbA1c | blood test for diabetes |
| HCG | human chorionic gonadotrophic hormone |
| HCl | hydrochloric acid |
| HCM | see HoCM |
| HCT | Haematocrit |
| HDL | high-density lipoprotein |
| HDU | high dependency unit |
| Hep A | hepatitis A viral infection (water-borne) |
| Hep B | hepatitis B viral infection (body fluids), also known as serum hepatitis |
| Hep C | hepatitis C viral infection |
| Hg | mercury |
| HI | hypodermic injection |
| HIB | Haemophilus influenzae bacillus – immunisation for babies |
| HIV | human immunodeficiency virus |
| HM | hand movement |
| HNPU | has not passed urine |
| HoCM | hypertrophic (obstructive) cardiomyopathy |
| Hp | helicobacter pylori |
| HPL | human placental lactogen |
| HPU | has passed urine |
| HPV | human papilloma virus |
| HRT | hormone replacement therapy |
| HS | heart sounds |
| HSV | herpes simplex virus |
| HUS | haemolytic uraemic syndrome |
| HVGD | host versus graft disease |
| HVS | high vaginal swab |
| Hx | history |
| i.a. | intra-articular (into a joint) |
| IBS | irritable bowel syndrome/disease |
| ICU | intensive care unit |

| Abbreviation | Meaning |
|---|---|
| IDDM | insulin-dependent diabetes mellitus |
| Ig | immunoglobulin |
| IgA | immunoglogulin (gamma) A |
| IgBF | immunoglobulin (gamma) binding factor |
| IgD | immunoglobulin (gamma) D |
| IgE | immunoglobulin (gamma) E |
| IgG | immunoglobulin (gamma) G |
| IgM | immunoglobulin (gamma) M |
| IM or im | intramuscular |
| INR | international normalised ratio (prothrombin time) |
| IOFB | intraocular foreign body |
| IOP | intraocular pressure |
| IP | inpatient |
| IPPB | intermittent positive pressure breathing |
| IPV | inactivated polio virus/vaccine |
| IQ | intelligence quotient |
| ISQ | in status quo (no change) |
| IT | intrathecal |
| ITU | intensive therapy unit |
| IU or U | international unit |
| IUC | idiopathic ulcerative colitis |
| IUCD | intra-uterine contraceptive device |
| IUD | intra-uterine device or intra-uterine death |
| IUFB | intra-uterine foreign body |
| IV, i.v. | intravenous |
| IVC | intravenous cholangiography |
| IVF | in vitro fertilisation |
| IVP | intravenous pyelogram |
| IVU | intravenous urogram |
| K | potassium |
| KUB | kidney, ureter, and bladder (X-ray) |
| L&D | light and dark (perceived) |
| L1, L2, etc | lumbar vertebrae |

| Abbreviation | Meaning |
|---|---|
| **LA** | local anaesthetic/ left atrium |
| **LASIK** | laser *in situ* keratomileusia |
| **LBC** | liquid-based cytology |
| **LCS** | left convergent squint (eye turns inwards) |
| **LD** | learning disability or lactate dehydrogenase (cardiac enzyme) |
| **LDL** | low-density lipoprotein |
| **LDS** | left divergent squint (eye turns outwards) |
| **LFT** | liver function test (to diagnose liver disease) |
| **LH** | luteinising hormone |
| **LIF** | left iliac fossa |
| **LIH** | left inguinal hernia |
| **LLQ** | left lower quadrant |
| **LMP** | last menstrual period |
| **LOA** | left occipitoanterior |
| **LOL** | left occipitolateral |
| **LOP** | left occipitoposterior |
| **LOT** | left occipitotransverse – same as LOL (position of fetus in uterus) |
| **LP** | lumbar puncture |
| **LRTI** | lower respiratory tract infection |
| **LSCS** | lower segment caesarean section |
| **LTH** | luteotropic hormone (prolactin) |
| **LUQ** | left upper quadrant |
| **LV** | left ventricle |
| **MA** | mental age |
| **MAOI** | monoamine oxidase inhibitor (antidepressant) |
| **MC&S** | microscopy, culture and sensitivity |
| **MCH** | mean corpuscular haemoglobin |
| **MCHC** | mean corpuscular haemoglobin concentration |

| Abbreviation | Meaning |
|---|---|
| **MCV** | mean corpuscular volume (size of cell) |
| **Mg** | Magnesium |
| **mg** | milligram |
| **ml** | millilitre |
| **mmHg** | millimetres of mercury |
| **mmol** | millimole |
| **MMR** | measles, mumps, rubella – vaccine against the three diseases |
| **MND** | motor neurone disease |
| **MOF** | multiple organ failure |
| **MRI** | magnetic resonance imaging |
| **MRSA** | multiple-/methicillin-resistant Staphylococcus aureus |
| **MS** | multiple sclerosis |
| **MSH** | melanocyte-stimulating hormone |
| **MSU** | midstream specimen of urine |
| **N&V** | nausea and vomiting |
| **Na** | sodium |
| **NAD** | no abnormality detected/demonstrated |
| **NAI** | non-accidental injury |
| **NBI** | no bone injury |
| **ND** | normal delivery |
| **NFR** | not for resuscitation |
| **NG** | new growth or nasogastric (tube) |
| **NIDDM** | non-insulin-dependent diabetes mellitus |
| **nmol** | nanomole |
| **NMR** | nuclear magnetic resonance (scan – see MRI) |
| **NOAD** | no other abnormality detected |
| **NSAID** | non-steroidal anti-inflammatory drug |
| **NSCLC** | non-small cell lung carcinoma |

| Abbreviation | Meaning |
|---|---|
| NTDs | neural tube defects (of the brain, spinal cord or meninges ) e.g. spina bifida |
| NT-proBNB | blood test for heart failure |
| $O_2$ | oxygen |
| OA | on arrival or osteoarthritis |
| OCD | obsessive compulsive disorder |
| OD | oculus dexter (right eye) |
| OE | on examination |
| OGD | oesophagogastroduodenoscopy |
| OP | outpatient or original pack (manufacturer's own pack) |
| OPD | outpatient department |
| ORD | oesophageal reflux disease |
| OS/os | oculus sinister (left eye) |
| OU/ou | oculus uterque (each eye) |
| P or P | pharmacy only medicine |
| PAP | Papanicolaou smear (cervical smear test) |
| PAT | paroxysmal atrial tachycardia |
| PBI | protein-bound iodine |
| PCB | post-coital bleeding |
| PCO | patient complains of |
| PCO | see PCOS |
| PCOS | polycystic ovarian syndrome |
| PCP | Pneumocystis carinii pneumonia |
| PCV | packed cell volume |
| PDT | photodynamic therapy |
| PE | pulmonary embolism |
| PEFR | peak expiratory flow rate |
| PERLA/PERRLA | pupils equal (round), react to light and accommodation |
| PET | pre-eclamptic toxaemia or positron emission tomography |
| PGD | patient group direction |
| PH | past history |

| Abbreviation | Meaning |
|---|---|
| pH | acid/alkaline balance |
| PID | pelvic inflammatory disease or prolapsed intervertebral disc |
| PMB | postmenopausal bleeding |
| PMH | past medical history |
| PMS | premenstrual syndrome |
| PN | postnatal |
| PNC | postnatal clinic |
| PND | paroxysmal nocturnal dyspnoea or post-nasal drip |
| POD | pouch of Douglas (retro-uterine fold of peritoneum lying behind the womb) |
| POM or POM | prescription only medicine |
| POP | plaster of Paris or progestogen only pill (contraceptive) |
| PP | placenta praevia or private patient |
| PPH | postpartum haemorrhage |
| PPI | proton pump Inhibitor |
| PR | per rectum (rectal examination) |
| PRK | photo-refractive keratotomy |
| PSA | prostatic-specific antigen (test for cancer of prostate) |
| PTCA | percutaneous transluminal coronary angioplasty |
| PTH | parathyroid hormone |
| PTSD | post traumatic stress disorder |
| PU | peptic ulcer |
| PUO | pyrexia of unknown origin |
| PV | per vaginam |
| PVC | premature ventricular contraction |
| PVS | persistant vegetative state |
| RA | rheumatoid arthritis/right atrium |
| RAI | radioactive iodine |

| Abbreviation | Meaning |
|---|---|
| **RAIU** | radioactive iodine uptake |
| **RBC** | red blood cell |
| **RCS** | right convergent squint (eye turns outwards) |
| **RCS** | right convergent squint (eye turns inwards) |
| **RD** | respiratory disease |
| **RDS** | respiratory distress syndrome or right divergent squint (eye turns outwards) |
| **REM** | rapid eye movement |
| **RGP/RP** | retrograde pyelogram |
| **RIF** | right iliac fossa |
| **RIH** | right inguinal hernia |
| **RLQ** | right lower quadrant |
| **ROA** | right occipitoanterior |
| **ROL** | right occipitolateral (position of fetus in uterus) |
| **ROP** | right occipitoposterior (position of fetus in uterus) |
| **ROT** | right occipitotransverse – same as ROL (position of fetus in uterus) |
| **RP** | retrograde pyelogram |
| **RSI** | repetitive strain injury |
| **RT** | radiation therapy |
| **RTA** | road traffic accident |
| **RUQ** | right upper quadrant |
| **RV** | right ventricle |
| **RVS** | respiratory virus syndrome |
| **SA** | sarcoma |
| **SAD** | seasonal affective disorder |
| **SADS** | sudden adult death syndrome |
| **SAH** | subarachnoid haemorrhage |
| **SARS** | sudden acute respiratory syndrome |
| **SB** | still birth |
| **SC** | *sine correctione* (without correction-spectacles) |
| **SCAN** | suspected child abuse or neglect |

| Abbreviation | Meaning |
|---|---|
| **SCBU** | special care baby unit |
| **SCLC** | small cell lung cancer |
| **SGOT** | serum glutamic oxaloacetic transaminase (liver enzyme) |
| **SGPT** | serum glutamic pyruvic transaminase (liver enzyme) |
| **SI** | sexual intercourse or international system of units |
| **SIDS** | sudden infant death syndrome |
| **SLE** | systemic lupus erythematosus |
| **SMI** | school medical inspection |
| **SMR** | submucous resection |
| **SOB** | shortness of breath |
| **SOL** | space-occupying lesion |
| **SSRI** | selective serotonin reuptake inhibitor |
| **STD** | sexually transmitted disease |
| **STYCAR** | standard visual tests for young children and retards |
| **Sx** | surgery (or suction, or symptoms and signs) |
| **T−** | decreased intra-ocular pressure |
| **T** | tumour |
| **T&A** | tonsillectomy and adenoidectomy |
| **T+** | increased intra-ocular pressure |
| **T1, T2,** etc | thoracic vertebrae or tumour sizes |
| **T$_3$** | triiodothyronine (thyroid hormone) |
| **T$_4$** | serum thyroxine test for thyroid disease |
| **TAH** | total abdominal hysterectomy |
| **TATT** | tired all the time |
| **TB** | tuberculosis |
| **TC** | total cholesterol |

| Abbreviation | Meaning |
|---|---|
| TCA | to come again or tricyclic antidepressant (old type of antidepressant) |
| TCI | to come in |
| TCRE | transcervical resection of the endometrium |
| Td | low-dose diphtheria vaccine |
| TENS | transcutaneous electrical nerve stimulation |
| THR | total hip replacement |
| TIA | transient ischaemic attack (in the brain) |
| TIBC | total iron-binding capacity |
| TKR | total knee replacement |
| TLC | tender loving care |
| TLE | temporal lobe epilepsy |
| TMR | transmyocardial revascularisation |
| TNM | tumour nodes metastases |
| TOE | trans-oesophageal echocardiography |
| tomo | tomogram |
| TOP | termination of pregnancy |
| TPHA | Treponema pallidum haemagglutination assay (blood test for syphilis) |
| TPR | temperature, pulse and respiration |
| TS | Tourette's syndrome |
| TSH | thyroid-stimulating hormone |
| TSS | toxic shock syndrome |
| TTA | to take away |
| TUP | tubal uterine pregnancy |
| TUR | transurethral resection (of prostate gland) |
| TURB | transurethral resection of bladder |
| TURBT | transurethral resection of bladder tumour |
| TURP | transurethral resection of prostate gland |

| Abbreviation | Meaning |
|---|---|
| TV | *Trichomonas vaginalis* (infection of vagina causing frothy yellow discharge) |
| TVH | total vaginal hysterectomy |
| U&E | urea and electrolytes |
| UA | urinalysis |
| UC | ulcerative colitis |
| UGI | upper gastrointestinal |
| UPLD | upper limb disorder |
| URI | upper respiratory infection |
| URTI | upper respiratory tract infection |
| USS | ultrasound scan |
| UTI | urinary tract infection |
| VA | visual acuity (clarity or accuracy of vision) |
| VC | vital capacity of lungs |
| vCJD | variant Creutzfeldt-Jacob disease |
| VCU, VCUG | voiding cystourethrogram |
| VDRL | veneral disease research laboratory (for syphilis) |
| VF | visual field |
| VI | *virgo intacto* (virgin) |
| VSD | ventricular septal defect |
| Vx | vertex (the crown of the head of the fetus) |
| WBC | white blood count |
| WBC&diff. | white blood count and different percentages present |
| WRULD | work-related upper limb disorder |
| XX | female sex chromosomes |
| XY | male sex chromosomes |
| YOB | year of birth |
| ZIFT | zygote intra-fallopian transfer |

# Appendix V: Eponyms

The following are a list of eponyms: diseases, syndromes, procedures and tests named after the person or area associated with it.

**Addisonian anaemia**
pernicious anaemia

**Addison's disease**
destruction of the adrenal cortex causing deficiency of hormone production

**Albee's bone graft**
operation of spinal fixation

**Albee's operation**
producing fixation of hip

**Albers-Schonberg**
a type of osteoporosis disease ('marble bones')

**Allen-Master's sign**
pelvic pain resulting from old laceration of broad ligament during childbirth

**Alzheimer's disease**
early dementia

**Argyll Robertson pupils**
reacting to accommodation but not to light

**Aschoff's nodules**
nodules in heart muscle (myocardium) in rheumatism

**Asperger's syndrome**
a type of autism

**Babinski's reflex**
stroking of the sole of foot causing downward flexion (dorsiflexion)

**Bacillus Calmette–Guérin**
vaccine for immunisation against tuberculosis

**Bankart's operation**
treatment of recurrent dislocation of shoulder joint

**Banti's syndrome**
enlarged spleen in children due to backpressure of veins, anaemia, jaundice, etc.

**Bannwarth's syndrome**
neurological manifestation of Lyme disease

**Barbados leg**
elephant leg

**Barlow's disease**
infantile scurvy (vitamin C deficiency)

**Barrett's oesophagus**
chronic ulceration of lower oesophagus due to chronic inflammation and epithelial changes

**Bartholin's abscess**
an abscess of the glands of the vulva

**Bell's palsy**
one-sided facial paralysis due to pressure on VIIth cranial (facial) nerve

**Billroth's operation**
partial gastrectomy

**Binet's test**
IQ intelligence test

**Blalock's operation**
for correction of Fallot's tetralogy (congenital deformity of the heart)

**Boeck's disease**
sarcoidosis

**Bornholm disease**
pain in pleura

**Brandt–Andrew's technique**
method of delivering the placenta

**Braxton Hicks contractions**
irregular contractions of uterus occurring after third month of pregnancy

**Bright's disease**
nephritis

**Brodie's abscess**
chronic inflammation of the bone marrow (osteomyelitis)

**Brudzinski's sign**
knee and hip flexion when raising head from pillow

**Burkitt's tumour**
a form of malignant lymphoma found in African children caused by a virus

**Burow's operation**
technique for repairing defect of lip

**Caldwell-Luc operation**
technique for drainage of maxillary antrum (facial sinus)

**Charcot's joints**
effects of third stages of syphilis or other neurological defect

**Charcot's triad**
staccato speech, nystagmus (oscillation of eyeballs) and intention tremor in multiple sclerosis

**Christmas disease**
congenital bleeding disorder due to lack of clotting factor

**Chvostek's sign**
excessive facial twitching on stimulating facial nerve found in cases of tetanus

**Colles' fracture**
dinner fork deformity of wrist caused by fracture of lower end of radius

**Coombs' test**
blood test for antibodies

**Creutzfeldt–Jacob disease**
degenerative brain disease associated with BSE

**Cushing's syndrome**
effects of excessive corticosteroid hormones

**Da Costa's syndrome**
cardiac neurosis (psychological origin of heart symptoms)

**Delhi boil**
tropical sore

**Dengue fever**
a viral disease transmitted by mosquitos, occurring in epidemics in tropical and subtropical areas

**Derbyshire neck**
goitre (enlargement of thyroid gland caused by insufficient iodine in diet)

**Dick test**
for susceptibility to scarlet fever

**Down's syndrome**
deformity of chromosome 21 causing mental impairment, enlarged tongue, oval tilted eyes, squint, etc. (formerly known as mongolism)

**Duchenne's syndrome**
spinal paralysis with polyneuritis

**Dupuytren's contraction**
painless deformity causing contraction of fingers towards palm

**Ebola fever**
a haemorrhagic disease

**Erb's palsy**
deformity of hand causing finger flexion, known as 'waiter's tip paralysis'

**Ewing's tumour**
sarcoma of shaft of long bone in under 20-year-olds

**Fallot's tetralogy**
comprising of four congenital heart defects

**Felty's syndrome**
chronic arthritis associated with leukopenia (deficient number of white blood cells) and enlarged spleen (splenomegaly)

**Fothergill's operation**
surgical repair of uterine prolapse

**Freidreich's ataxia**
progressive disease of nervous system resulting in weakness of muscles and staggering

**Frölich's syndrome**
deficiency of pituitary hormones

**Graves' disease**
oversecretion of thyroid hormones

**Guillain–Barré syndrome**
a type of polyneuritis characterised by an ascending paralysis

**Gulf War syndrome**
a condition associated with participants in the Gulf War

**Hanta virus**
a virus causing haemorrhagic disease transmitted by rodents; first identified in USA

**Hashimoto's disease**
chronic auto-immune disease of the thyroid gland

**Haygarth's nodules**
swelling of finger joints in arthritis

**Henoch's purpura**
purple patches caused by bleeding into and from the tissues of the intestinal wall

**Hirschsprung's disease**
enlarged colon present at birth

**Hodgkin's disease**
tumour of the lymph glands caused by a virus

**Hunter's syndrome**
similar to Hurler's syndrome, but less severe

**Hurler's syndrome**
mental retardation, abnormal development of skeleton, dwarfism, and gargoyle-like facial development due to a metabolic disorder

**Huntington's chorea**
degenerative genetic disease of the nervous system

**Hutchinson's teeth**
abnormally notched teeth; part of the signs of congenital syphilis

**Jacksonian epilepsy**
epilepsy caused by injury or tumour of brain

**Kaposi's tumour**
pigmented tumour of the skin (common in AIDS)

**Kernig's sign**
inability to straighten leg at knee joint when thigh is bent at right angles; indicates irritation of meninges

**Klinefelter's syndrome**
abnormal chromosome content (47) with XXY chromosomes, causing aggression and sterility

**Koch's disease**
tuberculosis

**Koplik's spots**
white spots found in mouth in measles prior to the skin rash occurring; only present in measles

**Küntscher nail**
used for fixation of fractures of long bones

**Kveim test**
test for sarcoidosis; intradermal injection followed by later biopsy

**Lassa fever**
a haemorrhagic disease transmitted by rodents

**Legionnaires' disease**
acute infection; pneumonia/influenza-type illness caused by legionella pneumophilia

**Little's disease**
spastic paralysis; form of palsy

**Ludwig's angina**
inflammation of subcutaneous layer of skin of the neck (cellulitis)

**Lyme disease**
infectious disease caused by ticks, causing widespread neurological and arthritic symptoms

**McBurney's point**
area on abdomen where pain is felt when testing for appendicitis

**Malta fever**
undulant fever caused by drinking infected milk (also called brucellosis and Mediterranean fever)

**Mantoux test**
intradermal test for tuberculosis reaction

**Mendel's law**
a theory of hereditary

**Ménière's disease**
disease of inner ear affecting hearing and balance; causes ringing in ears (tinnitus)

**Osler's nodules**
small painful areas on fingertips in cases of bacterial inflammation of the lining of the heart (endocarditis)

**Paget's disease**
disease causing brittle bones and cancer of the nipple

**Parkinson's disease**
progressive disease of the brain producing 'shaking palsy'; treated with L-dopa

**Paul–Bunnell test**
blood test for glandular fever

**Pel–Ebstein fever**
recurring fever in Hodgkin's disease

**Pott's disease**
spinal lesions

**Pott's fracture**
fracture/dislocation of the ankle

**Queckenstedt's test**
test performed during lumbar puncture to determine obstruction to flow of cerebrospinal fluid

**Ramstedt's operation**
surgery to release tight constriction of pyloric sphincter muscle between stomach and duodenum in babies; the condition is congenital

**Raynaud's disease**
intermittent spasms of arteries supplying extremities

**Reiter's syndrome**
recurrent urethritis, arthritis, inflammation of the iris, lesions of the mucous membranes, diarrhoea

**Rett's syndrome**
progressive autism, dementia, etc. associated with metabolic abnormality, principally found in girls

**Reye's syndrome**
acute disease of brain in young children following a febrile illness (avoid aspirin medication)

**Richter's syndrome**
a type of lymphoma occurring in the course of chronic leukaemia

**Rinne's test**
test for deafness

**Romberg's sign**
inability to stand without swaying when eyes are closed and feet placed together

**Rose's test/Rose Waaler**
blood test for rheumatoid arthritis

**Rovsing's sign**
pressure applied to left iliac fossa which causes pain in right iliac fossa (aspirin advised)

**Sabin vaccine**
live, attenuated (weakened) oral vaccine for poliomyelitis

**Salk vaccine**
first vaccine developed using dead organisms (given by injection)

**Schick test**
determines susceptibility to diphtheria

**Schilling test**
special test using radioactive isotopes to determine the levels of vitamin B12 in urine (pernicious anaemia)

**Shirodkar's operation**
purse string suture applied to incompetent cervix during pregnancy to prevent miscarriage

**Simmonds' disease**
anterior pituitary hormone deficiency, usually developed following childbirth when low blood pressure (hypotension) due to haemorrhage has deprived the pituitary gland of its blood supply

**Smith-Peterson nail**
used to fix fractures of neck of femur (hip)

**Spitz-Holter valve**
inserted in the brain in hydrocephalus (CNS unable to circulate, causing pressure on brain)

**Still's disease**
a type of arthritis in children

**Stoke–Adam's syndrome**
attacks where the heart stops momentarily and loss of consciousness occurs

**Tay–Sach's disease**
progressive metabolic disease, occurring especially in the Jewish population, causing weakness in muscles and blindness in infancy

**Tourette's syndrome**
obsessive–compulsive disorder involving motor and vocal tics

**Turner's syndrome**
a congenital disorder in which there are only 45 chromosomes; the missing X chromosome causes dwarfism, etc.

**Wasserman test**
blood test for syphylis

**Weil's disease**
infection caught from the urine of rats; this is the most serious form of leptospirosis

**Widal's test**
blood test for typhoid

**Wilms' tumour**
malignant tumour of kidney found in young children

**Wilson's syndrome**
disorder causing cirrhosis of liver and widespread jaundice, abnormal metabolism of copper, brain disease, green deposits of pigment in cornea, etc.

**Zollinger–Ellison tumour**
tumour of the non-insulin-producing cells of the pancreas

## Appendix VI: Infection control and universal precautions

Infection Control Policy and Universal Precautions should address the following issues:

- Basic hygiene, for example **handwashing** which is the most important single action to prevent cross-infection (*see Figures 98 and 99*)

- **Pre-cleaning of instruments**

- Chemical **disinfectants** including advice on handling and storing

- When **protective clothing** should be worn, e.g. gloves, aprons, eye shields and protective footware. Recommended use of single use non-sterile latex or PVC gloves should be used to handle body fluids.

- **Body fluids**\* should be handled with the same precautions as blood.

- **Gloves changed** between patients – not washed.

- How to dispose of or clean **contaminated articles**

- **Prohibition of eating, drinking and smoking**, except in designated areas

- The use and maintenance of **decontamination equipment**, e.g. how to load and unload operate autoclaves, including guidance on changing water, switching on machines and frequency of servicing as well as recording of temperature and pressure readings on a regular basis.

- **Handling toxic materials**

- What constitutes **clinical waste**, its safe disposal, where to store it prior to collection (with particular reference to 'sharps')

- **Sharps** procedure to prevent 'needle-stick' injuries

- **Procedure for accidents**, in particular follow up required in the event of a 'sharps' or 'needle-stick' injury' and to whom it should be reported.

*\*As well as blood, body fluids include:*

- **Amniotic fluid**
- **Cerebrospinal fluid**
- **Peritoneal fluid**
- **Pleural fluid**
- **Pericardial fluid**
- **Synovial fluid**
- **Semen**
- **Vaginal secretions**
- **Saliva**
- **Urine and faeces.**

# REMEMBER, assess the risk of the task – NOT the patient!!!!!

**The Infection Control Nurse of your PCO should provide all guidance on this area**

## Hand washing

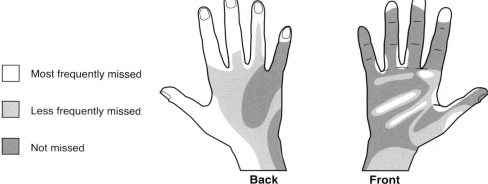

Most frequently missed

Less frequently missed

Not missed

**Back**  **Front**

**Figure 98:** The areas of the hands that are frequently missed in hand washing

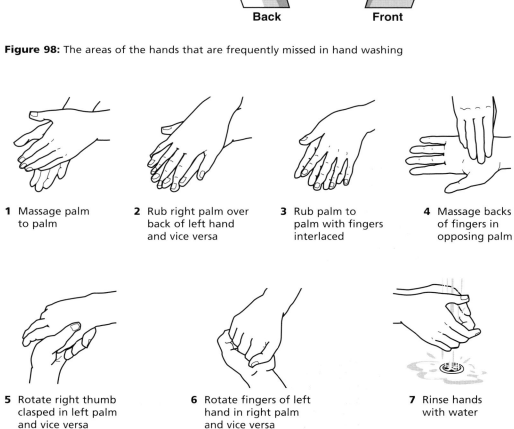

1 Massage palm to palm

2 Rub right palm over back of left hand and vice versa

3 Rub palm to palm with fingers interlaced

4 Massage backs of fingers in opposing palm

5 Rotate right thumb clasped in left palm and vice versa

6 Rotate fingers of left hand in right palm and vice versa

7 Rinse hands with water

**Figure 99:** The correct procedure for effective hand washing

# Appendix VII: The Caldicott Principles

## Data Protection Act 1998

The Data Protection Act 1998 came into force in 2000. It legislates for the control and protection personal data generally. The more stringent requirements of the Act do not apply to some kinds of healthcare research (e.g. research using anonymised unlinked data and some epidemiological research) because of an 'exemption' clause research in the Act. Adherence to this law and advice on compliance in the UK is monitored by the Information Commissioner.

> NB: The Act covers all identifiable, manual and computerised personal data and replaces the Access to Health Records Act 1990 for **living** persons. The Access to Health Records Act 1990 remains in force **only** for deceased patients' personal data.

## Main provisions of the Data Protection Act 1998

Personal data, in written or electronic form must be:

- Fairly and lawfully processed
- Processed for limited purposes
- Adequate, relevant and not excessive for the purpose
- Accurate
- Kept no longer than necessary
- Processed in accordance with the data subject's rights
- Secure
- Only transferred to countries with adequate data protection systems.

## The Caldicott Committee and the Caldicott Guardian

The Caldicott Principles go further than the 1998 Data Protection Act and were the result of the "Report on the Review of Patient-Identifiable Information' by the Caldicott Committee, Department of Health 1997 (http://www.doh.gov.uk/ipu/confiden/report/caldrep.pdf). The Caldicott Guardian in each Healthcare Trust is the person who is responsible for ensuring that these principles are respected and acted upon.

## The Caldicott Principles

The Caldicott Principles apply in addition to the requirements of the Data Protection Act 1998. They are:

### Principle 1 – Justify the purpose(s)

Every proposed use or transfer of patient-identifiable information within or from an organisation should be clearly defined and scrutinised, with continuing uses regularly reviewed by an appropriate guardian.

### Principle 2 – Don't use patient-identifiable information unless it is absolutely necessary

Patient-identifiable information items should not be used unless there is no alternative

### Principle 3 – Use the minimum necessary patient-identifiable information

Where use of patient-identifiable information is considered to he essential, each individual item of information should be justified with the aim of reducing identifiability.

### Principle 4 – Access to patient-identifiable information should be on a strict need to know basis

Only those individuals who need access to patient-identifiable information should have access to it, and they should only have access to the information items that they need to see.

### Principle 5 – Everyone should be aware of their responsibilities

Action should be taken to ensure that those handling patient-identifiable information – both clinical and non-clinical staff – are aware of their responsibilities and obligations to respect patient confidentiality.

### Principle 6 – Understand and comply with the law

Every use of patient-identifiable information must be lawful. Someone in each organisation should be responsible for ensuring that the organisation complies with legal requirements.

## Informed consent

Informed consent for the use of personal data should be sought wherever this is practically possible and will not cause more harm in terms of distress to the patient or their family. This should be balanced against the possibility of contributing to the advancement of medical knowledge. People are usually happy to allow access to their data: it is often the omission to ask which causes offence. There is a need for more research and public debate about the levels of access to personal data the public will allow without consent. Where consent is not sought this should be justified to the Research Ethics Committee.

## Practical tips

- Where informed consent is not possible, justify this in detail to the Research Ethics Committee.

- Identify the local Data Protection Officer for the Directorate in which you work.

- Store all non-electronic research data in locked filing cabinets (including cassette tapes, CD and video recordings).

- Make sure that sponsors (who have access to the data) do not remove it to a country outside the EU without adequate data protection systems.

- Remember that the Funders have no right to check patient records on which research is based unless they have taken on formal responsibility as 'sponsors' of research.

- Any researcher from outside the NHS must have an honorary contract with the Trust before they are allowed access to data, samples or patients.

- The principal or lead investigator is responsible for ensuring the appropriate archiving of data when the research has finished.

- Ensure data is stored securely for a minimum of 15 years.

# Index

# Index

# Index

# Index

# Index

Notes

Notes